Electronic
Health Records

Electronic Health Records

Understanding and Using Computerized Medical Records

RICHARD GARTEE

Upper Saddle River, New Jersey 07458

Library of Congress Cataloging-in-Publication Data

Gartee, Richard.
  Electronic health records : understanding and using computerized medical records / Richard Gartee.
    p. cm.
  ISBN 0-13-196079-2
  1. Medical records—Data processing.
  [DNLM: 1. Medical Records Systems, Computerized.   2. Forms and Records Control—methods.
    WX 173 G244e 2006]   I. Title.
  R864.G37 2006
  651.5—dc22

                                                                                        2006001606

Publisher: Julie Levin Alexander
Publisher's Assistant: Regina Bruno
Executive Editor: Joan Gill
Assistant Editor: Bronwen Glowacki
Director of Marketing: Karen Allman
Senior Marketing Manager: Harper Coles
Marketing Coordinator: Michael Sirinides
Marketing Assistant: Wayne Celia, Jr.
Director of Production and Manufacturing: Bruce Johnson
Managing Production Editor: Patrick Walsh
Production Liaison: Julie Li
Production Editor: Caterina Melara/Prepare, Inc.
Media Product Manager: John Jordan
Manager of Media Production: Amy Peltier
New Media Project Manager: Tina Rudowski
Manufacturing Manager: Ilene Sanford
Manufacturing Buyer: Pat Brown
Senior Design Coordinator: Mary Siener
Interior Designer: Solid State Graphics
Cover Designer: Solid State Graphics
Cover Photos: James Schnepf; Photo Researchers Inc./Frieder Michler, Astrid & Hanns; Index Stock Imagery, Inc.
Director, Image Resource Center: Melinda Reo
Manager, Rights and Permissions: Zina Arabia
Manager, Visual Research: Beth Brenzel
Manager, Cover Visual Research & Permissions: Karen Sanatar
Image Permission Coordinator: Carolyn Gauntt
Composition: Prepare, Inc.
Printing and Binding: Courier
Cover Printer: Phoenix Color Corporation

Cover photo 1: Depicting Touchworks on a laptop computer, courtesy of Allscripts, LLC.
Cover photo 2: Depicting Centricity® Physician Office EMR, courtesy of GE Healthcare. Centricity is a registered trademark of General Electric Company.
Cover photo 3: Depicts a clinician learning the Medcin Student Edition.

Pearson Education Ltd.
Pearson Education Singapore Pte. Ltd.
Pearson Education Canada, Ltd.
Pearson Education—Japan

Pearson Education Australia Pty. Limited
Pearson Education North Asia Ltd.
Pearson Educación de Mexico, S.A. de C.V.
Pearson Education Malaysia Pte. Ltd.

10 9 8 7
ISBN 0-13-196079-2

for Hayley

and R.J.

Contents

Chapter 1

Electronic Health Records—An Overview 1

Chapter 8

Privacy and Security of Health Records   371

Chapter 9

EHR and Technology   410

Preface

Introduction

Electronic Health Records are the "next big thing" in health care. There are many forces at work that will cause a change in health care from paper to electronic health records. Health care organizations, medical schools, employers, and even the government have recognized the importance of computerizing the various components of the medical record.

Major consultants such as the Gartner Group and CAPGemini report that Electronic Health Record systems are becoming a priority for medical practices.

National health care associations such as AHIMA, HIMSS, MGMA,* and the Medical Records Institute are focusing their members toward the implementation of Electronic Health Records.

President Bush has set a goal of 10 years for the complete transition of health care to an EHR. To that end, Congress has provided significant funding and the Department of Health and Human Services has set up a special office and appointed a National Coordinator for Health Information Technology.

With such a widespread push to adopt Electronic Health Records (EHR), a very large portion of the health care workforce is going to need to make a transition from the way medical records have been kept for the last 300 years to the way they are going to be kept in the future. For most doctors, nurses, medical assistants, and clinical staff, the thought of that transition is scary. The purpose of this book is to build, through practical experience, an understanding and a level of comfort with computerized medical records that can be applied directly to the clinical setting.

This book may be the first of its kind. EHR books previously available were oriented toward medical groups wishing to purchase and implement an EHR system. In most cases, they contained theoretical discussions of what to look for in a vendor or how to implement an EHR.

Instead, this book focuses on the users of an EHR—doctors, nurses, medical assistants, physician assistants, and other clinical staff. The text not only provides the learner with a thorough understanding of the terminology of Electronic Health Records (EHR) systems but also, more important, on the practical use of such systems in actual medical settings.

It is my hope that the widespread adoption of this text will alleviate the anxiety and fear that medical staff experience when changing from paper

*AHIMA—American Health Information Management Association; HIMSS—Healthcare Information and Management Systems Society; MGMA—Medical Group Management Association.

to electronic records by allowing them to understand the history and use of EHR before they are exposed to it in the workplace. Using the combination of textbook and software, we can create an educated clinical workforce that understands and is comfortable with computerized health records.

Learning Made Easy

This book makes learning about electronic health records easy because it reinforces theoretical material with hands-on experience.

Over 50 hands-on exercises facilitate the transfer of classroom concepts to actual applications in the medical office. This not only familiarizes learners with concepts of computerized Electronic Health Records but also helps them develop the confidence and skills necessary to become successful in a clinical setting.

Current EHR systems consist of components such as prescriptions, exam notes, lab orders and results, and even scanned images. The text covers each component of the EHR in a separate discussion, enabling the student to prepare for real-world situations in which a medical office has implemented only some components of the EHR.

Working in conjunction with physician experts and the developers of the leading EHR systems, the author draws on his extensive experience in the field of medical systems implementation and design to create the text. In areas where government regulations are explained, the text draws directly from the rules and guidance documents published by the U.S. government.

Complicated security regulations and mandated evaluation and management formulas are visually presented in easy to grasp tables.

Organization of the Text

The book organization provides learners with a comprehensive understanding of the history, theory, and potential benefits of Electronic Health Records. Each chapter builds on the knowledge acquired in previous chapters.

Chapter 1 Electronic Health Records—An Overview provides a foundation for student learning, introducing concepts and topics that are explained in depth in subsequent chapters. The chapter begins with a definition of Electronic Health Records, discusses why they are important, and the forces in our society driving their adoption. Workflow scenarios compare the flow of information into paper versus electronic charts, the workflow of physician orders, and the differences between inpatient and outpatient settings. Additional topics include the potential uses of EHR data for patient health management, decision support, and the electronic interchange of data between systems.

Chapter 2 Coding Standards explains that for the interchange of EHR data to occur, different computer systems must identify medical procedures and concepts in the same way. However, there exist today multiple coding standards. Chapter 2 describes the various forms of storing EHR data and the value of using standardized codes for that data. The chapter covers each of the prominent standards, their history, purpose, and relationship to each other.

The student not only achieves a knowledge of EHR coding systems and their history but also, in subsequent chapters, will acquire practical skills in the use of an EHR system through firsthand experience with medical record software.

Chapter 3 Learning Medical Record Software introduces the Medcin Student Edition software, which will be used for the remainder of the book. In a series of brief hands-on exercises, the student becomes familiar with EHR concepts, learns to navigate the software, and creates an actual exam note.

Chapter 4 Data Entry at the Point of Care continues to build the student's computer skills with additional methods to speed data entry. Additionally, students are introduced to computerized order entry and electronic prescriptions. Hands-on exercises are used for each feature.

One very practical fact of health care is that providers need to be paid for their work. The vast majority of those payments are the result of filing insurance claims that require standardized codes. **Chapter 5 Electronic Coding from Medical Records** expands on several of the standardized code sets introduced in Chapter 2. Hands-on exercises with the software simplify complicated billing rules and explain the relationship of the exam note to the billing codes in a very visual way. Chapter 5 also explores the relationship of the diagnosis to patient care plans and orders as well as tests to rule out a diagnosis.

Chapter 6 Advanced Techniques Speed Data Entry enlarges on concepts introduced in Chapters 1–4. Hands-on exercises allow the student to experiment with other methods of documenting the exam and introducing the concepts of patient management, problem lists, and graphing lab trends. Standards for electronic interchange of data discussed in Chapter 1 are given further meaning by explanations of medical devices and electronic lab interfaces in this chapter. The workflow of electronic lab order and result systems and the incorporation of patient entered data also are discussed.

Disease Management and Prevention are the focus of **Chapter 7 Using the EHR to Improve Patient Care**, in which students learn about flow sheets, pediatric wellness visits, immunizations, growth charts, and preventative care screening, all using hands-on exercises. Students extend their ability to analyze trends in the patient's health by learning to graph additional types of data. Chapter 7 also discusses generating medical alerts from EHR data and the drug interaction checking feature of electronic prescription writing software.

Chapter 8 Privacy and Security of Health Records provides a thorough presentation of HIPAA privacy and security regulations that are of paramount concern in any medical setting. Because both rules apply to patient data stored and transmitted electronically, understanding the rules is a prerequisite to portions of Chapter 9 concerning the Internet. Chapter 8 also explains data encryption, electronic signatures, and how records are signed electronically.

Chapter 9 EHR and Technology explores and compares an array of methods and devices used for EHR entry as well as alternative solutions that may improve the patient experience. How the style of a medical practice is reflected in the selection and placement of input devices as well as the recommended configurations is illustrated with numerous photos of medical personnel using the devices. An exercise teaches students how to annotate medical illustrations electronically for patient education or for documenting observations in the EHR.

Chapter 9 also includes a thorough discussion of medicine on the Internet, research tools, what is necessary for secure patient–provider communications, and the newest innovation, E-visits.

The Transfer of Acquired Skills to Actual EHR Systems

The combination of this text and the Student Edition software provides a complete learning system. Exercises using the Student Edition software are not aimed at teaching a particular brand of medical records software but, rather, at providing the student with practical experiences using an EHR that will be transferable to many prominent EHR systems.

The benefits of using an EHR include creating accessible, searchable, codified, patient charts. To make this possible, national standards of coding have been established. The software used with this book is based on one of the nationally accepted nomenclature standards, Medcin, which is further described in Chapter 2.

Although there is a large number of EHR vendors in the health care market, 10 of the top 15 EHR systems for medical offices use the Medcin nomenclature. Even EHR systems that may use proprietary or user defined nomenclatures still behave conceptually similar to the student software. These facts increase the likelihood that the student's knowledge will transfer easily to a commercial medical record system in use at a clinic.

Medcin is not the brand name of a commercial EHR but, rather, the licensed core technology in many prominent EHR systems. Medicomp Systems, the organization responsible for Medcin, has graciously provided the use of the server and software they license to these companies for the student to use for the exercises in this book.

The Student Edition software contains the entire Medcin nomenclature used in professional EHR systems.

A Few Words of Advice

When you finish an exercise, consider the amount of class time remaining before beginning the next exercise.

The two comprehensive exam exercises may require the full class time for the exercise. Consider the amount of class time remaining after the written exam before beginning the comprehensive exercise.

Exercises in the textbook have been designed to produce medically accurate exam notes; however, the notes do not necessarily represent a thorough medical exam. Exercises may omit certain routine elements of the exam that normally would be documented by a clinician. This is not a limitation of the Medcin knowledge base or of the physicians who reviewed the exercises. This is done solely to facilitate completion of exercises in the allotted class time.

Students of this course who are already medical professionals may recognize that the exams are not complete. Do not become distracted by this; the purpose of each exercise is to explore some new aspect of the EHR within the normal class time. Eliminating some elements of a full exam was unavoidable to achieve the goals of the exercise.

A Unique Approach to Learning the Electronic Health Record (EHR)

This textbook-software package introduces learners to the EHR through practical applications and Hands-On exercises. The text focuses on learners who will eventually become the end-user of the EHR, nurses, medical assistants, physician assistants, doctors, and other clinical staff. This text and software combination provides a complete learning system. Chapters integrate the history, theory, and benefits of EHR with the opportunity to experience the EHR environment first-hand by completing Hands-On exercises using the Student Edition Software. Each Chapter builds upon the knowledge acquired in previous chapters.

Applying Theory to Practice

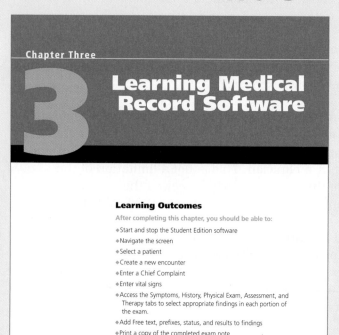

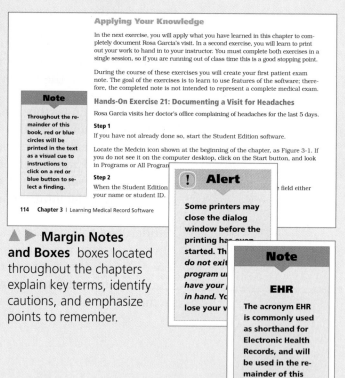

Applying Your Knowledge

In the next exercise, you will apply what you have learned in this chapter to completely document Rosa Garcia's visit. In a second exercise, you will learn to print out your work to hand in to your instructor. You must complete both exercises in a single session, so if you are running out of class time this is a good stopping point.

During the course of these exercises you will create your first patient exam note. The goal of the exercises is to learn to use features of the software; therefore, the completed note is not intended to represent a complete medical exam.

Hands-On Exercise 21: Documenting a Visit for Headaches

Rosa Garcia visits her doctor's office complaining of headaches for the last 5 days.

Step 1

If you have not already done so, start the Student Edition software.

Locate the Medcin icon shown at the beginning of the chapter, as Figure 3-1. If you do not see it on the computer desktop, click on the Start button, and look in Programs or All Programs

Step 2

When the Student Edition ... field either your name or student ID.

114   Chapter 3 | Learning Medical Record Software

Note

Throughout the remainder of this book, red or blue circles will be printed in the text as a visual cue to instructions to click on a red or blue button to select a finding.

> ! **Alert**
>
> Some printers may close the dialog window before the printing ha~~~~ started. Th~~~~ do not exit~~~~ program u~~~~ have your ~~~~ in hand. Y~~~~ lose your v~~~~

Note

EHR

The acronym EHR is commonly used as shorthand for Electronic Health Records, and will be used in the remainder of this book.

▲ ▶ **Margin Notes and Boxes** boxes located throughout the chapters explain key terms, identify cautions, and emphasize points to remember.

◀ **Acronyms**
Acronyms and their definitions begin every chapter, providing learners with a quick reference.

ACRONYMS USED IN CHAPTER 3	
Acronyms are used extensively in both medicine and computers. The following are those which are used for the first time in this chapter.	
Dx	Diagnosis
Hx	History
Px	Physical Exam
Rx	Therapy (including prescriptions)
Sx	Symptoms
Tx	Tests (performed)

▲ **Learning Outcomes**
Each chapter begins with a list of learning outcomes that highlight the key concepts contained in that chapter.

A Real-Life Story

How I Learned to Stop Worrying and Love Forms

By Michael Lukowski, M.D.

Michael Lukowski is a specialist in obstetrics and gynecology. He has been practicing more than 20 years. He uses an EHR in his practice, enters his own data, and has designed his own EHR forms.

I started using forms right away. When the trainer told me about forms, I thought "this is the way to go." It slows you down if you have to search a lot. Forms gave me a discrete window into the database so that I could pick out things that I use day in and day out.

I try to put as much of my exam in as data points (findings) rather than just free-text. I use free-text only as a comment to a finding. To me the whole idea of this is to have retrievable information that I can analyze over time. So I always try to use the (nomenclature) database as my main way to construct a note and then add free-text to that if I have to. I find that I use less and less free-text because I can pick out findings that say pretty much what I need to say.

Workflow

Using forms I do what I have always done. My nurse puts in the vital signs; we do some simple lab tests like a hematocrit. The patient is sitting in the exam room when I go in. I sit down and talk with her. As we are talking, I am filling in her history using a tablet computer, just like I used to do with a paper chart. When I am done with that part of the exam, I call my nurse in and do the physical exam.

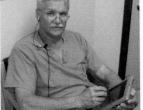

Photo by Richard Gartee.
Dr. Lukowski Enters Data in the Exam Room on a TabletPC Using a Form He Designed.

When the physical exam is finished, I leave and come back to my office. While the patient gets dressed, I finish filling out the rest of the encounter. The patient comes to my office once she is dressed and we talk a little bit more; I finalize her note and write any prescription. If the patient has a pharmacy that receives electronic prescriptions, I transmit them directly to the pharmacy. If the pharmacy does not, I print it on paper and the staff brings it to me to sign.

Forms

I use four forms: Gyn, Post-partum, Pre-op, and then one that contains all the procedures I do, which is still a work in progress, but it covers a lot.

I have a number of tabs within each form. For instance, the Gyn form starts with the intake page. My assistant fills in menstrual history, pap smear, mammograms, methods of birth control, and so on.

I move through the rest of the tabs except at the right end of the form, I use three different tabs for assessment so that I can have all the diagnoses I normally use available without searching.

190   Chapter 4 | Data Entry at the Point of Care

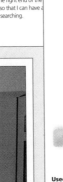

Diagnosis	Dx Hist	Family Hist
Cancer	✓ N	✓ N
Diabetes	✓ N	✓ N
Heart Attack	✓ N	
Hypertension	✓ N	
Migraine	✓ Y	✓ Y
Peptic Ulcer	✓ N	
Reflux	✓ Y	
Stroke	✓ N	

◀ **Real Life Story** Each chapter features a Real Life Story told by a doctor, nurse, administrator, physician assistant or patient about their experiences with Electronic Health Records. These vignettes help learners connect chapter content to real life in the clinic.

Visualizing the Electronic Health Record

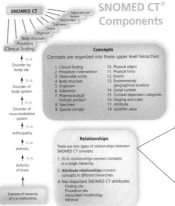

Used by permission of the College of American Pathologists.
▶ **Figure 2-4 SNOMED CT Components.**

◀▲ **Figures and Tables** Numerous figures throughout the text help learners visualize workflow scenarios and technical concepts. Photographs of healthcare providers using various types of EHR systems and medical devices make it easy to see the practical applicability in a medical office.

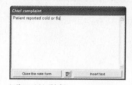

▶ Figure 4-34 Chief Complaint Dialog for Patient Reported Cold or Flu.

Step 4

In this exercise, the nurse will begin the visit by taking Kerry's Vital Signs.

Use the form labeled "Vitals," which you will select from the Forms Manager, invoked on the Active Forms tab (as you have done in previous exercises).

Enter Kerry's Vital Signs in the corresponding fields on the Form as follows:

Temperature:	**99**
Respiration:	**23**
Pulse:	**78**
BP:	**120/80**
Height:	**60**
Weight:	**100**

When you have finished, compare your screen to Figure 4-35 and, when it is correct, click on the Encounter tab at the bottom of the screen.

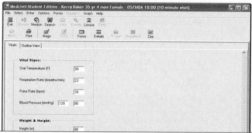

Chapter One Summary

Although Electronic Health Records have been called by various names for the last 30 years, the acronym EHR is currently used as shorthand for Electronic Health Records. By EHR, we mean the portions of a patient's medical record that are stored in a computer system as well as the functional benefits derived from having an electronic health record.

The drawbacks to nonelectronic records are numerous. Handwritten records often are abbreviated, cryptic, or illegible. Information cannot be easily accessed or shared. Nonelectronic charts must be copied and faxed or transported from one office to another. Finally, paper charts are not searchable, except by manually opening every chart and reading it.

The goal in creating Electronic Health Records is not necessarily to eliminate paper copies of records but to eliminate paper as the *only* copy of a patient's medical record. The EHR can help to improve patient health, the quality of care, and patient safety by providing access to complete, up-to-date records of past and present conditions. This enables EHR records to be used in ways that paper medical records cannot. These include Health Maintenance, Trend

▲ **Chapter Summary** Summaries at the end of each chapter synthesize key points for students.

Practice Opportunities

Testing Your Knowledge of Chapter 4

You may run the Medcin Student Edition software and use your mouse on the screen to answer the following questions:

1. How do you select a List?

2. How do you select Forms?

3. List three features Forms have that Lists do not.

4. Describe what the Prompt button on the toolbar does.

Write the meaning of each of the following medical abbreviations (as they were used in this chapter):

5. ROS _____

6. HPI _____

7. HEENT _____

8. URI _____

9. Sig _____

10. How do you indicate a "possible" diagnosis?

11. Auto-Negative (the Negs button) functions on what two tabs?

12. Describe how to record a test that was ordered and describe how to record a test that was performed.

13. What Entry Details field is used with a finding to indicate the patient's fever was "mild"?

14. How do you change the numbers on the List Size button and what do the numbers do?

15. You should have produced four narrative documents of patient encounters, which you printed. If you have not already done so, hand these in to your instructor with this test. The printed encounter notes will count as a portion of your grade.

▲ **Test Your Knowledge** Open-ended study questions at the end of each chapter allow learners to test their knowledge and think critically.

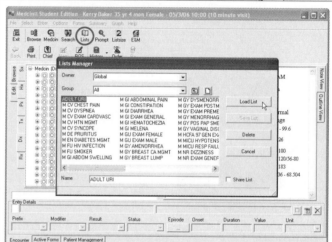

▲ **Hands-On Exercises** Over 50 step-by-step, Hands-On exercises allow the student to learn by doing. The majority are based on the companion Medcin® Student Edition software to provide a computer experience similar to an actual medical office. *Call-outs*: easy to follow step-by-step format, screen captures of the computer screens illustrate the steps of the exercise providing a ready reference for the student, designed to produce medically accurate exam notes.

Hands-On Exercise 28:
Timed Experiment for Extra Credit (optional)

Now that you have learned that the Lists and Auto Negative feature can help you enter EHR data more quickly, prove it to yourself with the following experiment.

Step 1
Look at the clock and write down the current time.

Step 2
Select the same patient, **Kerry Baker**, and create a New Encounter for the same date, but use a different appointment time.

Use the date **May 3, 2006**, the time **10:15 AM**, and the reason **10 Minute Visit**.

Steps 3–18
Turn back to the previous exercises (Hands-On Exercises 26 and 27) and repeats steps 3–18 exactly. Work carefully but as quickly as you can.

Step 19
Look at the clock and write down the time you finished.

◀ **Comprehensive Evaluations** Learners will test their mastery of the material through two comprehensive evaluations found at the mid-point and end of the text. Each evaluation includes both a written test and a hands-on exercise.

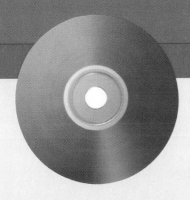

The Medcin® Student Edition Software

◆ Multi-user, allowing multiple students to work simultaneously, and it keeps each student's work separate. Print-outs from the exercises automatically include the student's login name or ID.

◆ Contains the entire Medcin nomenclature used in professional EHR systems. Medcin is the licensed core technology in many prominent EHR systems. Since 10 of the top 15 EHR systems for medical offices use the Medcin nomenclature as the technology underlying commercial EHR systems, students in most cases may apply skills they acquire in this course directly to an EHR application in their office. Those systems will not be identical to the student software, but they will seem very familiar to someone who has completed this course.

◆ All work is printed and no exercise requires saving. This allows students from multiple classes to share the same computer and avoids complications caused by saving and backing up student data, no exercise in the student edition requires the students to save.

◆ Since students can not save the work to resume later, each exercise been designed to be completed in a normal class time.

◆ The printers will use the standard Windows system and any compatible printer should work.

◆ For distance learning, the software allows the student to "Print to HTML" which will output the exercise document into a file that can be e-mailed or given to the instructor who may open and view the student's work with an ordinary web browser such as Microsoft Internet Explorer.

◆ Software distribution includes two options: one version will be for schools with networked computer labs, and the other will accommodate those schools that want each student to work individually with their own copy of the software, for example, distance learning or home study courses.

◆ All schools will receive software they can install on the school network and computer lab workstations. Schools may decide to use just the text book alone, or a version which is bundled with the software and installation instructions for students to install at home or at school.

Software Requirements

To complete the exercises in this book you will need access to the Medcin Student Edition software. If you are taking this course in a classroom the software will already be installed. If you are in a distance learning program or working independently, you will need to purchase the software CD (ISBN 0-13-178937-6). Follow the directions for installation included with the CD.

Minimum Workstation requirements:

Processor: 200 mHz Pentium

Windows XP, Windows 2000 (or later) with MDAC component installed

RAM: 64 megabytes (free not counting OS)

Number of colors: 256 (8 bit color)

Display size (pixels per inch): 800 x 600 (1024 x 768 recommended)

Internet Explorer 5.5 or later

Microsoft.Net Framework version 1.1 or later

You must have mouse with at least two buttons that perform the right and left click functions.

If you are installing the software on an individual workstation you will also need a CD-ROM drive and sufficient space on your hard drive.

About the Author

Prior to becoming a full-time author and consultant, Richard Gartee served as vice president of product development and subsequently as director of design strategy at Medical Manager Research & Development, Inc. His 20 years of experience in the design, development, and implementation of practice management and Electronic Health Records software date back to the earliest days of the field. He was involved in the development of leading medical software systems including The Medical Manager, Intergy, and Intergy EHR, among others.

Richard also served as a liaison to other companies in the medical computer industry as well as Blue Cross/Blue Shield plans, a U.S. Department of Commerce International Trade Mission, and various universities. He served as a voting member of two of the national standards groups currently guiding Electronic Health Record developments (ANSI X-12 and HL7 Standards groups discussed in Chapter 2). He has been a faculty member/speaker at TEPR, the Electronic Health Records conference, for over 10 years. He is the author of two previous textbooks on computerized medical systems.

Acknowledgments

This book was made possible by the contribution of many individuals and several of the most prominent commercial EHR vendors, whom I personally would like to thank and acknowledge here.

I first would like to thank Peter S. Goltra, David Lareau, and Roy Soltoff of Medicomp Systems, Inc. To provide the student a complete interactive learning experience that could be transferred to the real world, I needed computer software that used a standard that is prominent in the real world. The standard with the most practical application at the point of care is Medcin.

Peter S. Goltra is the father of the Medcin nomenclature. He is the founder and CEO of Medicomp Systems, which he established in 1978 to develop advanced documentation and diagnostic tools for use by physicians at the point of care. His honors include an award from the American Medical Informatics Association for contributions to the field of medical informatics.

Peter understood my vision for the book and software immediately and it was with his blessing that the Medcin software was made available to the student. He generously lent the resources of his busy company to enable the development of this project.

David Lareau is chief operating officer of Medicomp Systems, Inc. Before joining Medicomp in 1995, Mr. Lareau founded and served as CEO of a medical software and billing company and served as controller of one of the nation's largest distribution companies. In addition to his COO duties, David is the leading proponent of the Medcin nomenclature, having personally presented it to thousands of physicians, key EHR developers, and decision makers during his 10-year tenure.

David was fundamental to the development of the exercises in this textbook. He tirelessly provided his expertise and drew on his relationships with Medcin physician advisors to ensure the exercises were medically accurate and relevant to the student learning experience.

Roy Soltoff is the director of software development for Medicomp Systems. Mr. Soltoff has been involved in software development, starting with AT&T in 1964. He joined the Medicomp development staff in 1992 and has been responsible for significant advances in clinical user interface design.

Roy and I met at his offices to identify what the student would need, and then, over the course of the next few months, he single-handedly turned the Medicomp software into the Medcin Student Edition. When I was writing the book, Roy was always available to help me understand the software or better explain some nuance of the EHR to the student.

The medical content and EHR theory of the textbook were greatly enhanced by my acquaintance with Dr. Allen R. Wenner, M.D.

Dr. Allen R. Wenner, a physician, teacher, author, speaker, and expert on information technology, has practiced family medicine in Columbia, South Carolina, for 27 years. He works part time for Primetime Medical Software, Inc., a medical software publishing company. He currently serves on the Board of Medical Examiners for the State of South Carolina. He was an Assistant Clinical Professor of Family Medicine at the University of South Carolina for 19 years. He has taught thousands of physicians about information technology in health care in the United States, Asia, and Europe, and is widely quoted in trade journals and medical publications. He has been called "the EMR guru" by the editor of *Medical Economics*.

Allen, too, understood my vision for the book and contributed generously with his thoughts, theories, and real-life stories. His company allowed me to quote freely from his works and to use photos from his office and home to better help the student understand the practical application of his ideas. My thanks go to Allen, not only for all of his contributions to this project but also for his efforts to advance the adoption of electronic health records.

Whereas I am deeply appreciative of all the editors who assisted me with this book, I would especially like to acknowledge Joan Gill who, from our very first conversation, grasped what we were trying to accomplish and who cleared the path for me at every step of the way.

Two features of the book I thought would bring the real world into the classroom was the inclusion of real-life stories and photos illustrating the systems actually used in clinical settings.

My special thanks go to the many individuals who shared firsthand experiences in real-life stories and allowed them to be used in this book. Their unique perspectives help the student understand the relationship of the conceptual to the practical. I would like to thank Richard A. Gartee, Sharyl Beal, R.N., Alison Connelly, P.A., Michael Lukowski, M.D., Philip C. Yount, M.D., Allen R. Wenner, M.D., Michelle White (whose story was written by Julie DeSantis), and Primetime Medical (who contributed the real-life story of Mr. John Gould).

Many commercial EHR vendors and medical device manufacturers also assisted me by providing photographs of their systems in use. It was my belief that students could better visualize the material by seeing actual examples of real system applications. I thank them for allowing their copyrighted work to be reprinted herein. In alphabetical order:

Allscripts, LLC (special thanks for the extra efforts of Lisa Johnson for everything I needed and thanks to Judy Beckenbach for the screen captures)

EHS—Electronic Healthcare Systems (special thanks to Susan Majors for supplying pediatric forms which were modified for the well-child exercises in Chapter 7. Note that the EHS forms are superior to the edited versions I created for the book.)

GE Healthcare (special thanks to Derek Schoonover)

IMPAC Medical Systems (thanks to Julie DeSantis)

Medem, Inc. (special thanks for allowing students to use the **ihealthrecord.org** Web site)

Midmark Diagnostics Group (special thanks to Heather Childs and Glen Mizelle)

NextGen (special thanks to Karen Fretz who prepared exactly the screens I needed)

Primetime Medical Software & Instant Medical History (especially Dr. Allen Wenner)

Quest Diagnostics (special thanks to David Dickey)

RelayHealth Corporation (thanks to Briana Pompei)

WebMD, Inc. for use of **Medscape** screens (special thanks to Jennifer Meyers Newman for putting me in touch with all the right people, and to Dr. Jim O'Connor, M.D. of **Emdeon Practice Services** for his advice on asthma codes)

Welch Allyn (special thanks to Brent Murphy)

Also thanks to Michael Lukowski, M.D. for allowing me to reproduce his GYN form.

This book is a strong proponent of codified health records using national standards. My thanks to the organizations responsible for three of the key medical record coding systems, SNOMED CT, MEDCIN, and LOINC, for allowing me to reprint portions of their work. These are the College of American Pathologists, Medicomp Systems (mentioned previously), the Regenstrief Institute and the LOINC committee.

Reviewers

I also would like to thank the academic reviewers, who over the course of their summer vacation took time to read and review every chapter.

Robin Berenson, ABD, MS, JCTC
Faculty
Spartanburg Technical College
Spartanburg, South Carolina

Mary T. Boylston, RN EdD
Chair and Associate Professor
Department of Nursing
Eastern University
St. Davids, Pennsylvania

Leah Grebner, RHIA, CCS
Director of Health
Midstate College
Peoria, Illinois

Bonnie Hemp, BS, RHIA, CPHQ
Chair, Health Information Technology
Owens Community College
Toledo, Ohio

Linda Scarborough, RN, CMA, CPC, BSM
Health Care Management Technology Program Director
Lanier Technical College
Oakwood, Georgia

Lynn G. Slack
Medical Programs
ICM School of Business & Medical Careers
Pittsburgh, Pennsylvania

Marsha C. Steele, MEd, RHIA
Former Director, Health Information Technology
Henry Ford Community College
Dearborn, Michigan

Medcin Consulting Editors

Finally, I would like to recognize the work of the numerous doctors who consulted on the development of the Medcin nomenclature. These clinicians did not review the exercises in this book, but they did review the medical accuracy of the Medcin nomenclature that underlies this entire work. Therefore, I would like to acknowledge their work in the development and evolution of the knowledge base on which the Medcin Student Edition is based.

Medcin Consulting Editors

Robert G. Barone, M.D.
Clinical Assistant Professor of Ophthalmology,
Cornell University Medical College;
Attending Surgeon, The New York Hospital
New York, NY

J. Gregory Cairncross, M.D.
Professor, Departments of Clinical
Neurological Sciences and Oncology,
University of Western Ontario and London Regional
Cancer Centre
London, Ontario, Canada

Richard P. Cohen, M.D.
Clinical Associate Professor of Medicine,
Cornell University Medical College;
Associate Attending Physician
The New York Hospital
New York, NY

Bradley A. Connor, M.D.
Clinical Assistant Professor of Medicine,
Cornell University Medical College;
Adjunct Faculty, Rockefeller University;
Assistant Attending Physician,
The New York Hospital
New York, NY

David R. Gastfriend, M.D.
Assistant Professor in Psychiatry,
Harvard Medical School;
Director of Addiction Services,
Massachusetts General Hospital
Boston, MA

Stephanie M. Heidelberg, M.D.
Medical Director, Adult, Older Adult Programs,
American Day Treatment Centers, Fairfax, VA
Psychiatrist, Adult Day Treatment Program,
Northwest Mental Health Center, Reston, VA

Edmund M. Herrold, M.D., Ph.D.
Associate Professor of Medicine,
Director, Section of Biophysics and Biomechanics,
Division of Cardiovascular Pathophysiology
Cornell University Medical College
Associate Attending Physician
The New York Hospital
New York, NY

Allan N. Houghton, M.D.
Professor of Medicine and Immunology,
Cornell University Medical College;
Chair, Immunology Program,
Memorial Sloan-Kettering Cancer Center
New York, NY

Ralph H. Hruban, M.D.
Associate Professor of Pathology,
Associate Professor of Oncology,
The Johns Hopkins School of Medicine;
Director, Division of Cardiovascular-Respiratory Pathology
The Johns Hopkins Hospital
Baltimore, MD

Mark Lachs, M.D., MPH
Assistant Professor of Medicine,
Cornell University Medical College;
Chief, Geriatrics Unit,
Department of Medicine,
The New York Hospital
New York, NY

Fredrick A. McCurdy, M.D., Ph.D.
Associate Professor of Pediatrics,
Director of Pediatric Undergraduate Education,
University of Nebraska College of Medicine
Omaha, NE

Paul F. Miskovitz, M.D.
Clinical Associate Professor of Medicine,
Cornell University Medical College;
Associate Attending Physician,
The New York Hospital
New York, NY

Preeti Pancholi, Ph.D.
Staff Scientist, Department of Virology and Parasitology,
Kimball Research Institute
New York Blood Center
New York, NY

Louis N. Pangaro, M.D.
Associate Professor, Clinical Medicine,
Vice Chairman For Educational Programs,
Department of Medicine, Uniformed Services
University of The Health Sciences,
F. Edward Herbert School of Medicine
Bethesda, MD

William B. Patterson, M.D., MPH
Assistant Professor of Environmental Health,
Boston University School of Public Health
Boston, MA
President, New England Health Center
Wilmington, MA

Edward J. Parrish, M.D., M.S.
Assistant Professor of Medicine,
Cornell University Medical College;
Department of Medicine, Division
of Rheumatology,
The New York Hospital,
Hospital for Special Surgery
New York, NY

David Posnett, M.D.
Associate Professor of Medicine,
Cornell University Medical College;
Division of Immunology, Dept. of Medicine,
The New York Hospital, New York, NY

Calvin W. Roberts, M.D.
Professor of Ophthalmology,
Cornell University Medical College
New York, NY

Ronald C. Silvestri, M.D.
Assistant Professor of Medicine,
Harvard Medical School,
Director, Medical Intensive Care Unit,
Deaconess Hospital
Boston, MA

Michael Thorpe, M.D.
Musculoskeletal Radiology Fellow,
The Hospital for Special Surgery
New York, NY

Anshu Vashishtha, M.D., Ph.D.
Adjunct Faculty Member,
Laboratory of Bacterial Pathogenesis
and Immunology
The Rockefeller University,
Clinical Fellow in Allergy and Immunology,
The New York Hospital
New York, NY

H. Hallett Whitman, III, M.D.
Clinical Assistant Professor of Medicine,
Cornell University Medical College,
Clinical Affiliate, Hypertension Center,
The New York Hospital, New York, NY
Attending Physician in Internal Medicine and
Rheumatology, Summit Medical Group, Summit, NJ

E. David Wright, M.D.
Clinical Assistant Professor of Medicine,
Department of Dermatology,
University of Virginia Health Sciences Center,
Charlottesville, VA
Dermatology Associates, Inc.,
Attending Physician, Winchester Medical Center
Winchester, VA

Joseph Zibrak, M.D.
Assistant Professor of Medicine,
Harvard Medical School,
Associate Chief of Pulmonary and Critical
Care Medicine,
Beth Israel Deaconess Medical Center
Boston, MA

Electronic
Health Records

Electronic Health Records— An Overview

Learning Outcomes

After completing this chapter, you should be able to:

◆ Define electronic health records

◆ Explain why electronic health records are important

◆ Discuss what forces are driving the adoption of electronic health records

◆ Describe the flow of medical information into the chart

◆ Describe different methods of capturing and recording data

◆ Understand levels of electronic health record implementations

◆ Describe workflow of physician orders and results

◆ Explain why systems and devices should be able to exchange electronic data

◆ Compare electronic health records in an inpatient versus outpatient setting

ACRONYMS USED IN CHAPTER 1	
Acronyms are used extensively in both medicine and computers. Listed below are those that are used in this chapter.	
AHRQ	Agency for Healthcare Research and Quality
CAT	Computerized Axial Tomography
CDISC	Clinical Data Interchange Standards Consortium
CPRI	Computer-based Patient Record Institute
CPOE	Computerized Physician Order Entry, also Computerized Provider Order Entry
CT Scan	Computerized Tomography
DAW	Dispensed As Written
DICOM	Digital Imaging and Communications in Medicine
DUR	Drug Utilization Review
ECG	Electrocardiogram
EHR	Electronic Health Record
ER	Emergency Room
FDA	Food and Drug Administration
HHS	U.S. Department of Health and Human Services
HIPAA	Health Insurance Portability and Accountability Act
HIT	Health Information Technology, also Healthcare Information Technology
HL7	Health Level 7
ICU	Intensive Care Unit
IOM	Institute of Medicine of the National Academies
MRI	Magnetic Resonance Imaging
PET	Positron Emission Tomography
PHR	Personal Health Record
PSA	Prostate-Specific Antigen test

What Are Electronic Health Records

The concept of computerizing a patient's medical record has been around for about 30 years. It has been called by various names, including: Electronic Medical Records, Computerized Medical Records, Computer-based Patient Records, Longitudinal Patient Records, Electronic Chart, and other terms. All of these names referred to essentially the same thing, what is today called Electronic Health Records.

The IOM (which stands for the Institute of Medicine of the National Academies) sponsored studies and created reports over the last 15 years, which led the way toward the concepts we have today for electronic health records. In 1991, the IOM called for the creation of "an electronic patient record that resides in a system specifically designed to support users by providing accessibility to complete and accurate data, alerts, reminders, clinical decision support systems, links to medical knowledge, and other aids."[1] Originally, the IOM called this the

[1]R. S. Dick and E. B. Steen, *The Computer-based Patient Record: An Essential Technology for Health Care*, Institute of Medicine, Washington, DC: National Academy Press, 1991, revised 1997, 2000.

EHR

The acronym EHR is commonly used as shorthand for Electronic Health Records, and will be used in the remainder of this book.

"Computer-based Patient Record," but, by 2003, IOM renamed it the Electronic Health Record or EHR.

Like the diversity of names, there exists a diversity of definitions for the EHR as well. The IOM did not exactly define the contents of an EHR but, rather, put forth a set of eight core functions that an EHR should be capable of performing. According to the IOM report, the eight core functions are:[2]

◆ **Health information and data** A defined dataset that includes items such as medical and nursing diagnoses, a medication list, allergies, demographics, clinical narratives, and laboratory test results; providing improved access to information needed by care providers.

◆ **Result management** Computerized results can be accessed more easily (than paper reports) by the provider at the time and place they are needed.

Reduced lag time allows for quicker recognition and treatment of medical problems.

The automated display of previous test results makes it possible to reduce redundant and additional testing.

Having electronic results can allow for better interpretation and for easier detection of abnormalities, thereby ensuring appropriate follow-up.

Access to electronic consults and patient consents can establish critical linkages and improve care coordination among multiple providers, as well as between provider and patient.

◆ **Order management** Computerized Provider Order Entry (CPOE) systems can improve workflow processes by eliminating lost orders and ambiguities caused by illegible handwriting, generating related orders automatically, monitoring for duplicate orders, and reducing the time to fill orders.

CPOE for medications reduces the number of errors of medication dose and frequency, drug–allergy, and drug–drug interactions.

The use of CPOE, in conjunction with an EHR, also improves clinician productivity.

◆ **Decision support** Computerized decision support systems include prevention, prescribing of drugs, diagnosis and management, and detection of adverse events and disease outbreaks.

Computer reminders and prompts improve preventive practices in areas such as vaccinations, breast cancer screening, colorectal screening, and cardiovascular risk reduction.

◆ **Electronic communication and connectivity** Electronic communication among care partners, can enhance patient safety and quality of care, especially for patients who have multiple providers in multiple settings and must coordinate care plans.

Electronic connectivity is essential in creating and populating EHR systems with data from laboratory, pharmacy, and radiology, and other providers.

---

[2]Ibid.

E-mail and Web messaging have been shown to be effective in facilitating communication both among providers and with patients, thus allowing for greater continuity of care and more timely interventions.

Automatic alerts to providers regarding abnormal laboratory results reduce the time until an appropriate treatment is ordered.

Electronic communication is fundamental to the creation of an integrated health record, both within a setting and across settings and institutions.

◆ **Patient support** Computer-based patient education has been found to be successful in improving control of chronic illnesses such as diabetes in primary care.

Examples of home monitoring by patients include self-testing by asthma patients (spirometry), glucose monitors for diabetes patients, and holter monitors for heart patients.

Data from home monitoring can be merged into the EHR (as will be shown later in this chapter).

◆ **Administrative processes and reporting** Electronic scheduling systems increase the efficiency of health care organizations and provide better, timelier service to patients.

Communication and content standards are important in the billing and claims management area.

Electronic authorization and prior approvals can eliminate delays and confusion; immediate validation of insurance eligibility results in more timely payments and less paperwork.

EHR data can be analyzed to identify patients potentially eligible for clinical trials, as well as candidates for chronic disease management programs.

Reporting tools support drug recalls.

◆ **Reporting and population health** Public and private sector reporting requirements at the federal, state, and local levels for patient safety and quality, as well as for public health, are more easily met with computerized data.

The labor-intensive and time-consuming abstraction of data from paper records and the errors that often occur in a manual process can be eliminated.

The reporting of key quality indicators used for the internal quality improvement efforts of many health care organizations is facilitated.

Public health surveillance and timely reporting of adverse reactions and disease outbreaks are improved.

Later in this chapter, we will discuss initiatives by the U.S. government to encourage the development of health care information technology. It will become apparent how the IOM definitions of core functions influenced and were adapted into the framework proposed by the government.

Another early contributor to the thinking on EHR systems was the Computer-based Patient Record Institute (CPRI), which identified three key criteria for an EHR:

◆ Capture data at the point of care

◆ Integrate data from multiple sources

◆ Provide decision support

Finally, there was HIPAA, the Health Insurance Portability and Accountability Act passed by Congress in 1996. You will learn more about HIPAA in Chapter 2 and Chapter 8, but what is relevant here is that although the HIPAA security rule didn't define an EHR, it perhaps broadened the definition. The security rule established protection for *all* personally identifiable health information stored in electronic format. Thus, everything about a patient stored in a health care provider's system was protected and treated as part of the patient's EHR.

In *Electronic Health Records: Changing the Vision*, authors Waters, Murphy, and Hanken define the EHR to include "any information relating to the past, present or future physical/mental health, or condition of an individual which resides in electronic system(s) used to capture, transmit, receive, store, retrieve, link and manipulate multimedia data for the primary purpose of providing health care and health-related services."[3] The core functions defined by the IOM and CPRI broaden the definition even further, suggesting that the EHR is not just what data is stored but what can be done with it. The availability of complete and accurate electronic patient data facilitates the additional capabilities of EHR systems to use that data. While exploring the EHR, this book will provide examples of where and how this extended functionality is achieved.

Combining the work of IOM, CPRI, and HIPPA, we derive a working definition. In the broadest sense, EHR includes dental and other records about the patient as well, but this book will focus on patient care in a clinical setting. In the context of this book, we will use the following definition for **EHR—the portions of a patient's medical records that are stored in a computer system as well as the functional benefits derived from having an electronic health record.**

Although sometimes an EHR is referred to as a paperless chart, the goal in creating electronic health records is not necessarily to eliminate paper copies of the records, but to eliminate paper as the *only* copy of a patient's medical record. The EHR system strives to improve patient health care by giving the provider and patient access to complete, up-to-date records of past and present conditions; it also enables the records to be used in ways that paper medical records could not.

Why Electronic Health Records Are Important

Historically, a patient's medical records consisted of handwritten notes, typed reports, and test results stored in a paper file system. A separate file folder was created and stored at each location where the patient was examined or treated. X-ray films and other radiology records typically were stored separately from the chart, even when they were created at the same medical office.

---

[3]Gretchen Murphy, Kathleen Waters, Mary A. Hanken, and Maureen, Pfeiffer (Editors), *Electronic Health Records: Changing the Vision*, page 5, W.B. Saunders Company, 1999.

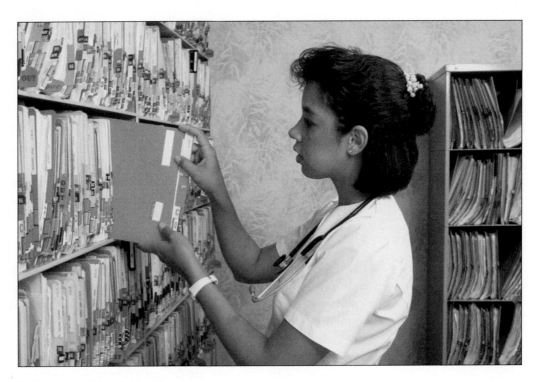

▶ **Figure 1-1 Filing Paper Charts.**

Here are some of the drawbacks to paper records: Handwritten records often are abbreviated, cryptic, or illegible. When information is to be used by another medical practice, the charts must be copied and faxed or mailed to the other office. Even in one practice with multiple locations, the chart must be transported from one office to another when a patient is seen at a different location than usual. Paper records are not easily searchable. For example, if a practice is notified that all patients on a particular drug need to be contacted, the only way of finding those patients is literally to open every chart and look at the medications list.

Certainly, the ability to find, share, and search patient records is a strong point for an EHR, yet there are other concepts that take the practice of medicine to levels which cannot be achieved with paper records. Four examples of this are: Health Maintenance, Trend Analysis, Alerts, and Decision Support. These will be covered in more detail in Chapter 7, but here is a brief overview of each.

Health Maintenance

The simplest example of health maintenance is a card or letter reminding the patient that it is time for a check-up. Dental and medical practices alike send these notices. In many offices today, this reminder is generated manually. At the patient's last visit, a staff member addressed a card to be mailed 6 months later, or entered a request in a computer. When the appropriate time had passed, the notices were printed by the computer or the cards were mailed. Because this is a manual process tied to the previous visit, it is usually used for one type of care, the return visit or annual check-up.

However, when a medical practice has electronic records, preventative screening can become more dynamic and sophisticated. Recommended tests and the intervals between them often vary by age and sex. Using the data in an EHR a computer can find patients over a certain age who are due for a mammogram, PSA, or other test and automatically generate reminders to them. Conversely, imagine a practice searching all of their paper charts to see who is due for a test.

Trend Analysis

When a health record is electronic, it is easy to compare data from different dates, tests, or events. Cumulative summary reports compare the values of test components from different dates. Effects of medication can be measured by comparing changes in dosage to changes in blood tests. A simple graphing tool can turn numeric data in the EHR into a powerful visual aid that would be impractical to create from a paper chart.

Alerts

An Alert is a term used in an EHR for a message or reminder that is automatically generated from the data. Alerts are usually based on programmed logic, rules about what message to use when two or more conditions are met. For example, an electronic prescription system generates an alert when two drugs known to have adverse interactions are prescribed for the same patient.

Decision Support

Decision support is not about "artificial intelligence" replacing a physician with a computer. Physicians have been trained to naturally assimilate diverse bits of information from physical exams and test results leading to a medical decision. Through long years of training, they also have become very accustomed to researching medical literature when they have an unusual case. As the name implies, decision support is about providing help just when the clinician needs it. There are many examples, but let us look at three.

Prescriptions It used to be simple for a physician to prescribe a drug. However, insurance plans changed all that, dividing drug formularies into lists of preferred drugs, nonpreferred drugs, and drugs they won't pay for. If the patient's insurance won't pay for it, the patient may not follow the physician's instructions. Yet, how would a physician using a paper chart prescribe according to each patient's insurance formulary? Electronic prescription systems support the physician by comparing the prescription with the insurance plan formulary and if necessary suggesting alternate brands that are therapeutically equivalent. Electronic prescriptions will be discussed again later in this chapter.

Note	**Drug Formulary**

Drug formularies were around long before pharmacy benefit managers developed preferred drug lists. Drug formularies are used to look up drugs by names or therapeutic class, provide an updated list of the drugs that are available in the inventory, provide information on costs, indications for use, treatment recommendations, dosage guidelines, and prescribing information. However, health insurance programs now use the term *formulary* for plan-specific drug lists.

Medical References Decision support also can mean quick access to medical references directly from the EHR. This can make access to evidence-based guidelines or medical literature as easy as clicking on a link in the chart.

Protocols One form of decision support can ultimately speed up documentation of the patient exam and improve patient care. Protocols, standard plans of therapy, can be established for different conditions. When a doctor has assessed a patient with a particular condition, the appropriate protocol can appear on the EHR screen and all therapies ordered in a click of the mouse.

Forces Driving toward EHR

Social changes as well as medical specialization have altered what needs to be done with patients' medical records. In an increasingly mobile society, patients relocate and change doctors more frequently, thus needing to transfer their medical records from all previous doctors to new ones.

Additionally, many patients no longer have a single general practitioner who provides their total care. Increased specialization and the development of new methods of diagnostic and preventative medicine require the ability to share exam records and test results that are important to the patient's continuity of care.

One of the strongest forces for social change in the last decade went unnoticed until recently in health care. This is, of course, the World Wide Web. Patients use the Web every day for all kinds of tasks. Consumers are becoming accustomed to being able to access very sensitive information securely over the Web. They are beginning to ask: If I can write checks and use Internet banking securely; if I can trade stocks and see my brokerage account; if I can check in for my airline flight and print my boarding passes; why can't I see my lab test result? Additionally, there are literally millions of health-related pieces of information on the Web. Patients are arriving at their doctors' office armed with questions and sometimes answers. Medical information previously unavailable to the average consumer is now as easy to access as searching Google®.

Health care organizations, medical schools, employers, and even the government have recognized the importance of computerizing the various components of the medical record. President George W. Bush has approved projects that will encourage medical practices to implement electronic health records.

In a speech to the American Association of Community Colleges, President Bush said "The 21st-century health care system is using a 19th-century paperwork system. Doctors use paper files to keep track of their patients. Pharmacists have to figure out the handwriting of a doctor. Vital medical information is scattered in many places. X-rays get misplaced. Problems with drug interaction are not systematically checked. See, these old methods of keeping records are real threats to patients and their safety and are incredibly costly."[4] (A real-life example of what the president was talking about is illustrated by the true story *Where's My Chart.*)

---

[4]Remarks by President George W. Bush, April 26, 2004, at the American Association of Community Colleges Annual Convention, Minneapolis Convention Center, Minneapolis, MN; White House Press Office, Washington, DC.

President Bush didn't just arrive at that conclusion. Visionary leaders in medical informatics have been making the case for EHR for a long time. However, the combination of several important reports caught the public's attention and set in motion economic and political forces that may eventually transform our medical records systems.

Health and Safety

In 1999 the IOM published *To Err Is Human: Building a Safer Health System.* The report stated, "Health care in the United States is not as safe as it should be—and can be. At least 44,000 people, and perhaps as many as 98,000 people, die in hospitals each year as a result of medical errors that could have been prevented, according to estimates from two major studies.

"Beyond their cost in human lives, preventable medical errors exact other significant tolls. They have been estimated to result in total costs (including the expense of additional care necessitated by the errors, lost income and household productivity, and disability) of between $17 billion and $29 billion per year in hospitals nationwide. Errors also are costly in terms of loss of trust in the health care system by patients and diminished satisfaction by both patients and health professionals.

"A variety of factors have contributed to the nation's epidemic of medical errors. One oft-cited problem arises from the decentralized and fragmented nature of the health care delivery system—or 'non-system,' to some observers. When patients see multiple providers in different settings, none of whom has access to complete information, it becomes easier for things to go wrong."[5]

These statements got the attention of the press and public. They also got the attention of 150 of the nation's largest employers. Employers who sponsored employee health insurance programs had become frustrated by the increasing costs of health insurance benefits for which they had little or no say about the quality of care. Following the release of the IOM report, these employers formed the Leapfrog group.

The largest member of the Leapfrog group, General Motors, publicized the dilemma by revealing that for every car it produced it was spending more on health benefits than on steel. Leapfrog created a strategy that tied purchase of group health insurance benefits to quality care standards. It also promoted Computerized Physician Order Entry (CPOE) as a means of reducing errors.

The IOM study focused on medical errors occurring in hospitals, but other studies showed an even larger number of medical errors in outpatient settings. A study by the Center for Information Technology Leadership found more than 130,000 life-threatening situations caused by adverse drug reactions alone. The study suggested that $44 billion could be saved annually by installing Computerized Physician Order Entry in ambulatory settings.

The response to the IOM report was swift and positive, within both government and the private sector. Almost immediately, the Clinton administration issued an executive order instructing government agencies that conduct or oversee

---

[5]*To Err Is Human: Building a Safer Health System,* Linda T. Kohn, Janet M. Corrigan, and Molla S. Donaldson (Editors); Committee on Quality of Health Care in America, Institute of Medicine, Washington, DC, 1999.

health-care programs to implement proven techniques for reducing medical errors, and creating a task force to find new strategies for reducing errors. Congress soon launched a series of hearings on patient safety, and in December 2000 it appropriated $50 million to the Agency for Healthcare Research and Quality (AHRQ) to support a variety of efforts targeted at reducing medical errors.

"The AHRQ already has made major progress in developing and implementing an action plan. Efforts under way include:

◆ Developing and testing new technologies to reduce medical errors.

◆ Conducting large-scale demonstration projects to test safety interventions and error-reporting strategies.

◆ Supporting new and established multidisciplinary teams of researchers and health-care facilities and organizations, located in geographically diverse locations that will further determine the causes of medical errors and develop new knowledge that will aid the work of the demonstration projects.

◆ Supporting projects aimed at achieving a better understanding of how the environment in which care is provided affects the ability of providers to improve safety.

◆ Funding researchers and organizations to develop, demonstrate, and evaluate new approaches to improving provider education in order to reduce errors."[6]

National Coordinator for Health Information Technology

On April 27, 2004, President George Bush signed an Executive Order establishing the position of the National Coordinator for Health Information Technology, to "develop, maintain, and direct the implementation of a strategic plan to guide the nationwide implementation of interoperable health information technology (HIT) in both the public and private health care sectors that will reduce medical errors, improve quality, and produce greater value for health care expenditures."[7] The Office of National Coordinator is under the U.S. Department of Health and Human Services (HHS).

On May 6, 2004, Secretary of Health Tommy Thompson appointed David J. Brailer M.D., Ph.D., as the National Coordinator. On July 21, 2004, Dr. Brailer delivered *The Decade of Health Information Technology: Delivering Consumer-Centric and Information-Rich Health Care*, a framework for strategic action outlining 4 goals and 12 strategies for national adoption of health information technology. The following are excerpts from the executive summary of the report:[8]

Readiness for Change

"There is a great need for information tools to be used in the delivery of health care. Preventable medical errors and treatment variations have recently gained attention. Clinicians may not know the latest treatment options, and practices

---

[6]Ibid.

[7]Executive Order #13335, President George W. Bush, April 27, 2004.

[8]*The Decade of Health Information Technology: Delivering Consumer-centric and Information-rich Health Care*, U.S. Department of Health and Human Services, July 21, 2004, Washington, DC.

vary across clinicians and regions. Consumers want to ensure that they have choices in treatment, and when they do, they want to have the information they need to make decisions about their care. Concerns about the privacy and security of personal medical information remain high. Public health monitoring, bioterror surveillance, research, and quality monitoring require data that depends on the widespread adoption of HIT."

Vision for Consumer-Centric and Information-Rich Care

"Many envision a health care industry that is consumer centric and information-rich, in which medical information follows the consumer, and information tools guide medical decisions. Clinicians have appropriate access to a patient's complete treatment history, including medical records, medication history, laboratory results, and radiographs, among other information. Clinicians order medications with computerized systems that eliminate handwriting errors and automatically check for doses that are too high or too low, for harmful interactions with other drugs, and for allergies. Prescriptions are also checked against the health plan's formulary, and the out-of-pocket costs of the prescribed drug can be compared with alternative treatments. Clinicians receive electronic reminders in the form of alerts about treatment procedures and medical guidelines. This is a different way of delivering health care than that which currently exists, but one that many have envisioned. This new way will result in fewer medical errors, fewer unnecessary treatments or wasteful care, and fewer variations in care, and will ultimately improve care for all Americans. Care will be centered around the consumer and will be delivered electronically as well as in person. Clinicians can spend more time on patient care, and employers will gain productivity and competitive benefits from health care spending."

Strategic Framework

"In order to realize a new vision for health care made possible through the use of information technology, strategic actions embraced by the public and private health sectors need to be taken over many years. There are four major goals that will be pursued in realizing this vision for improved health care. Each of these goals has a corresponding set of strategies and related specific actions that will advance and focus future efforts. These goals and strategies are summarized below."

Goal 1: Inform Clinical Practice Informing clinical practice is fundamental to improving care and making health care delivery more efficient. This goal centers largely around efforts to bring EHRs directly into clinical practice. This will reduce medical errors and duplicative work, and enable clinicians to focus their efforts more directly on improved patient care. Three strategies for realizing this goal are:

◆ **Strategy 1. Incentivize EHR adoption.** The transition to safe, more consumer-friendly and regionally integrated care delivery will require shared investments in information tools and changes to current clinical practice.

◆ **Strategy 2. Reduce risk of EHR investment.** Clinicians who purchase EHRs and who attempt to change their clinical practices and office operations

A Real-Life Story

Where's My Chart?

A 63-year-old man went to his doctor's office in Kentucky complaining of chest pains and tightness in his chest. He was immediately transferred to the local hospital, where a stress test and cardiac catheterization confirmed he had had a heart attack. He was hospitalized overnight.

Early retirement from his stressful job as well as a regimen of exercise, diet, beta blockers, aspirin therapy, and other medications proved successful. He moved from Kentucky to Florida and tried unsuccessfully to have his medical records concerning the previous heart attack transferred to his new doctor in Florida. The ECG and stress tests were repeated in Florida. Finally, after two years, the records from Kentucky arrived.

In subsequent years, he moved twice more but, wiser now, he took copies of his medical records with him. He continued a normal and active life until age 77, when he slipped in his workshop and broke his right knee. With his leg in a cast he was less active; a blood clot formed and broke free.

Three weeks after he broke his knee, he went to the doctor's office with what he described as very severe flu symptoms, extreme fatigue, a bad cough, and sharp pains in his back when he moved or coughed. The doctor sent him to the emergency room, where he was diagnosed with a *pulmonary embolism* in the lower lobe of the right lung. He was hospitalized and put on a therapy of blood thinners.

At age 79, he was continuing to lead an active lifestyle, but he was experiencing occasional sharp brief chest pain and brief dizziness. His doctor scheduled a stress test and cardiac catheterization at a cardiac center connected to the hospital. A blockage was discovered and a double bypass surgery was performed at the same hospital. The patient tolerated the surgery well and recovered quickly.

However, one of the veins used in the bypass operation had been harvested from the leg that had the previous broken knee. Three weeks after he was discharged, he passed out and fell. He was taken by ambulance to the ER at the same hospital where he had had his surgery and where he had been hospitalized for the previous pulmonary embolism. Here is what happened:

▶ When the ambulance crew arrived at the house, they took a medical history from the patient and his wife. They gave him oxygen and transported him to the hospital.

▶ When the ambulance arrived at the hospital, the nurses and ER staff again took a medical history from the patient and patient's family.

▶ The patient's primary care physician has a complete medical history of the patient including copies of his records dating back to his heart attack in Kentucky, but the hospital system does not connect with the physician's office system.

▶ The patient reported that he had just had surgery at the same hospital only 3 weeks before. The hospital system surely had his medical history, but the ER is on a different system and the ER doctors didn't have access to the records.

▶ Although the ER is in the same hospital as the cardiac lab, the ER doctors didn't have access to those records, either.

▶ The patient told the ER staff he thought the symptoms felt similar to his previous experience with a pulmonary embolism, but even though the ER is in the same hospital where the patient was hospitalized for a pulmonary embolism 2 years before, the ER doctors didn't have access to the records from his past condition.

▶ A CAT scan was ordered based on patient history of the embolism provided by a family member, not his medical record.

▶ After waiting in the ER for 14 hours, he was hospitalized with two pulmonary embolisms, one in each lung.

Seven days later, the patient was discharged from the hospital. He has fully recovered and is doing fine.

This is not the story of poor medical care or a bad hospital. The hospital is affiliated with a major teaching hospital and is as good as or better than most. This is a story of the unfortunate state of medical records. Paper records are not accessible and can take months to transfer. The lack of timely copies of existing records often causes tests to be reordered or the obvious conditions to be overlooked. Electronic records are better, more accessible, but even the most sophisticated systems do not necessarily have the infrastructure in place to communicate with other EHR systems even in the same community or, as in this case, not even in the same facility!

face a variety of risks that make this decision unduly challenging. Low-cost support systems that reduce risk, failure, and partial use of EHRs are needed.

◆ **Strategy 3. Promote EHR diffusion in rural and underserved areas.** Practices and hospitals in rural and other underserved areas lag in EHR adoption. Technology transfer and other support efforts are needed to ensure widespread adoption.

Goal 2: Interconnect Clinicians Interconnecting clinicians will allow information to be portable and to move with consumers from one point of care to another. This will require an interoperable infrastructure to help clinicians get access to critical health care information when their clinical or treatment decisions are being made. The three strategies for realizing this goal are:

◆ **Strategy 1. Foster regional collaborations.** Local oversight of health information exchange that reflects the needs and goals of a population should be developed.

◆ **Strategy 2. Develop a national health information network.** A set of common intercommunication tools such as mobile authentication, Web services architecture, and security technologies are needed to support data movement that is inexpensive and secure. A national health information network that can provide low-cost and secure data movement is needed, along with a public-private oversight or management function to ensure adherence to public policy objectives.

◆ **Strategy 3. Coordinate federal health information systems.** There is a need for federal health information systems to be interoperable and to exchange data so that federal care delivery, reimbursement, and oversight are more efficient and cost-effective. Federal health information systems will be interoperable and consistent with the national health information network.

Goal 3: Personalize Care Consumer-centric information helps individuals manage their own wellness and assists with their personal health care decisions. The ability to personalize care is a critical component of using health care information in a meaningful manner. The three strategies for realizing this goal are:

◆ **Strategy 1. Encourage use of Personal Health Records.** Consumers are increasingly seeking information about their care as a means of getting better control over their health care experience, and PHRs that provide customized facts and guidance to them are needed.

◆ **Strategy 2. Enhance informed consumer choice.** Consumers should have the ability to select clinicians and institutions based on what they value and the information to guide their choice, including but not limited to, the quality of care providers deliver.

◆ **Strategy 3. Promote use of telehealth systems.** The use of telehealth—remote communication technologies—can provide access to health services for consumers and clinicians in rural and underserved areas. Telehealth systems that can support the delivery of health care services when the participants are in different locations are needed.

Goal 4: Improve Population Health Population health improvement requires the collection of timely, accurate, and detailed clinical information to allow for the evaluation of health care delivery and the reporting of critical findings to public health officials, clinical trials and other research, and feedback to clinicians. Three strategies for realizing this goal are:

◆ **Strategy 1. Unify public health surveillance architectures.** An interoperable public health surveillance system is needed that will allow exchange of information, consistent with current law, between provider organizations, organizations they contract with, and state and federal agencies.

◆ **Strategy 2. Streamline quality and health status monitoring.** Many different state and local organizations collect subsets of data for specific purposes and use it in different ways. A streamlined quality-monitoring infrastructure that will allow for a complete look at quality and other issues in real-time and at the point of care is needed.

◆ **Strategy 3. Accelerate research and dissemination of evidence.** Information tools are needed that can accelerate scientific discoveries and their translation into clinically useful products, applications, and knowledge."

Building the EHR

What organizations and leaders are saying is needed is a health record that is accessible from multiple locations within a given practice, capable of being transferred electronically to another health care provider and imported into the other system. To make this possible, the structure of the record will have to follow a standard which other systems can understand. The content also will have to be in a standard "codified" vocabulary, so that the provider receiving the record is certain as to the meaning of the content.

Medical vocabulary used in an EHR should be codified because there are often multiple medical terms for the same thing; additionally, medical records may contain a mix of medical terms and layman terms (such as symptoms and patient history). By assigning a code to each medical concept and using the same code for all synonyms of that concept, it becomes possible to exchange medical records between systems.

Using a standard codified vocabulary in an EHR system does not hinder the user, who typically sees only the medical terms, not the underlying codes. It does make the EHR records electronically searchable and improves the accuracy of the searches because it can find every instance of a medical event, regardless of the way the provider entered it. The development of standardized systems of codes used for medical terms will be covered in Chapter 2.

However, capturing and codifying the medical record is a task that requires not only computers and software, but changes also in the way providers work. To understand this, let us compare the workflow in a medical office using paper charts with a medical office using an EHR system.

Flow of Medical Information into the Chart

Dr. Lawrence Weed, M.D., father of the "problem-oriented chart," defined a structure for documenting a patient visit using four components, with the acronym SOAP. This is the style of chart typically used today. The four components are:

Subjective

Objective

Assessment

Plan

The following example will illustrate the workflow in a primary care medical practice using paper charts (see Figure 1-2). (Primary care includes specialties such as family physician, pediatrician, and internal medicine.)

1. An established patient phones the doctor's office and schedules an appointment.

2. The night before the appointment, the patient charts are pulled from the medical record filing system and organized for the next day's patients.

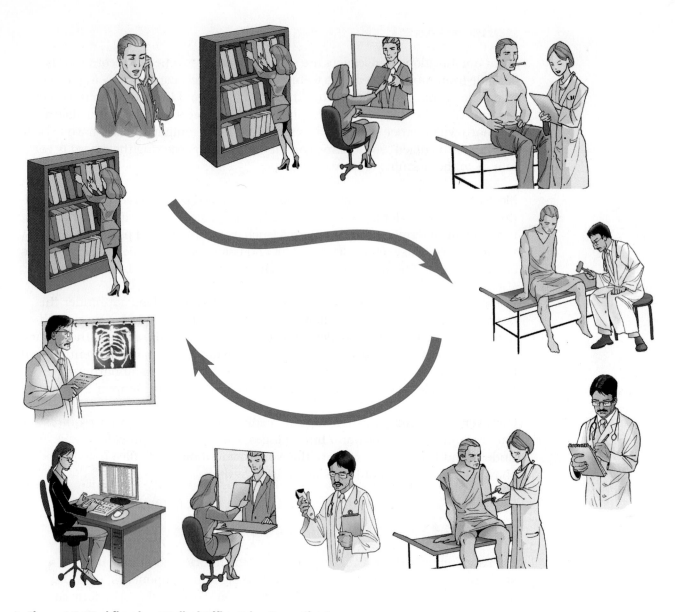

▶ **Figure 1-2 Workflow in a Medical Office Using Paper Charts.**

3. On the day of the appointment, the patient arrives at the office and is asked to confirm that insurance and demographic information on file is correct.

The patient is given a clipboard with a blank medical history form and asked to complete it. The form asks the reason for today's visit and asks the patient to report any previous history, any changes to medications, new allergies, and so on.

4. Patient is moved to an exam room and is ask to wait.

Subjective—the patient is asked to describe in his or her own words what the problem is, what the symptoms are, and what he or she is experiencing.

A nurse takes vital signs, reviews the form the patient completed, and may ask for more detail about the reason for the visit, which usually is called "the chief complaint." The nurse writes down the vital signs and chief complaint on a form that is placed at the front of the chart along with the updated patient form.

The doctor or other health care provider enters the exam room and discusses the reason for the visit and reviews the symptoms. The physician asks the patient to undress for the physical exam, and often leaves the room so the patient may do so.

While the patient is getting undressed, the clinician typically goes to another exam room and sees another patient.

5. When the physician returns, he or she performs the physical exam.

   Objective—the clinician performs a physical exam and makes observations about what he or she finds.

   Assessment—applying his or her training to the subjective and objective findings, the clinician arrives at a decision of what might be the cause of the patient's condition, or what further tests might be necessary.

   Plan of Treatment—the clinician prescribes a treatment, medication, or orders further tests. Perhaps a follow-up visit at a later date is recommended. A note will be made in the chart of each element of the plan.

6. If medications have been ordered, a handwritten prescription will be given to the patient or phoned to the pharmacy. A note of the prescription will be written in the patient's chart.

   The doctor marks one or more billing codes and one or more diagnosis codes on the chart and leaves the exam room.

7. If lab work has been ordered, a medical assistant will obtain the necessary specimen and send the order to the lab.

8. At many practices, the physician creates the exam note from memory, either handwriting in the chart or dictating the subjective, objective, assessment, plan, and treatment information.

9. When the patient is dressed, the patient will be escorted to the check-out area. The nurse or staff may give the patient education material or medication instructions.

   If x-rays or other diagnostic tests have been ordered at another facility, the office staff may call on behalf of the patient and schedule the tests.

   If a follow-up visit has been indicated, the patient will be scheduled for the next appointment.

10. The dictated notes are later transcribed and returned to the doctor to review before being permanently stored in the chart.

11. If lab, x-ray, or other diagnostic tests have been ordered, the results and reports are subsequently sent to the practice either by fax or on paper a number of days later. When received, they are filed in the patient's chart and the chart is sent to the clinician for review. They are reviewed by the physician, then filed in the paper chart.

12. The paper chart is filed again. Note that the chart may have to be refiled and pulled each time a new document, such as the transcription or lab report, was added, which required the doctor's review.

One obvious downside to this process is accessibility. If the patient chart is needed for follow-up visit or by another provider, it is not likely that it has been returned to the file room while it is pending dictation or while the provider is reviewing test results.

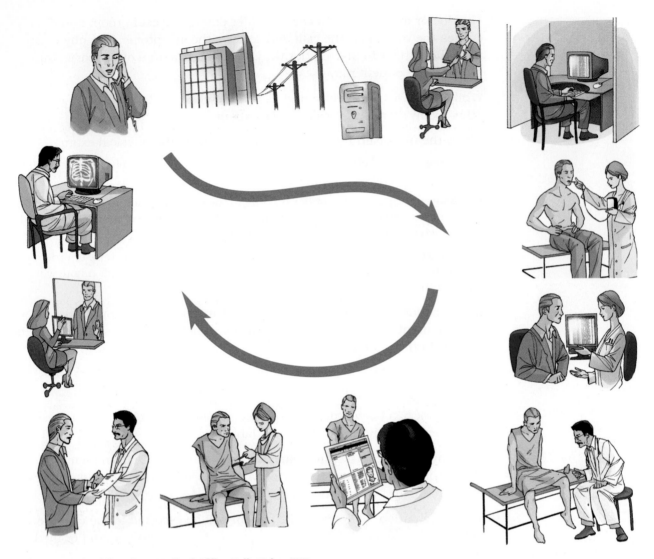

▶ **Figure 1-3 Workflow in a Medical Office Fully Using EHR.**

Flow of an Office Fully Using EHR

In the workflow just described, much of the chart may have been captured with pen on paper. This section will describe a visit to an office that fully uses the electronic capabilities that are available today in EHR systems including patient participation in the process and the capabilities of the Internet (see Figure 1-3).

1. An established patient phones the doctor's office and schedules an appointment.

2. The night before the appointment, the medical office computer electronically verifies insurance eligibility for patients scheduled the next day.

3. On the day of the appointment, the patient arrives at the office and is asked to confirm demographic information on file is still correct.

4. A receptionist, nurse, or medical assistant asks the patient to complete his or her medical history and the reason for today's visit using a computer in a private area of the waiting room. The nurse enters the patient's age, sex, and reason for the visit, makes sure that the patient understands how to use the system, and then leaves. The patient completes a computer-guided questionnaire concerning his or her symptoms and medical history.

Internet Alternative

As an alternative to steps 1 and 4, patients increasingly are able to request an appointment and receive a confirmation via the Internet or e-mail. Additionally, medical offices using software such as Instant Medical History (discussed in Chapter 7) can allow patients using the Internet to complete the history and symptom questionnaire from home before coming to the doctor's office.

5. When the patient has completed the questionnaire, the system alerts the nurse that the patient is ready to move to an exam room.

   The nurse measures the patient's height and weight and records them in the EHR. Using a modern device, vital signs for blood pressure, temperature, and pulse are taken and wirelessly transferred into the EHR.

6. **Subjective**—the nurse and patient review the answers the patient has provided. Where necessary, the nurse edits the record to add clarification or refinement.

   The nurse initiates the second computer screening, covering the history of the present illness, which also can be completed by the patient.

   The physician enters the exam room and discusses the reason for the visit and reviews with the patient the information already in the chart. The physician asks the patient to undress for the physical exam, and often leaves the room so the patient may do so.

   While the patient is getting undressed, the clinician typically goes to another exam room and sees another patient.

7. When the physician returns, he or she performs the physical exam.

   Objective—the clinician typically makes a provisional diagnosis mentally before performing the physical exam. This is often useful in allowing the clinician to select a list or template of findings to quickly record the physical exam in the EHR.

   The EHR presents a list of problems the patient reported in past visits that have not been resolved. The physician reviews each, examining additional body systems as necessary, and marks the improvement, worsening, or resolution of each problem.

   Assessment—applying his or her training to the subjective and objective findings, the clinician arrives at a decision of one or more diagnoses, and decides if further tests might be warranted.

   Plan of Treatment—the clinician prescribes a treatment, medication, or orders further tests using the EHR.

8. If medication is to be ordered, the physician writes the prescription electronically. The prescription is compared to the patient's allergy records and current drugs. The physician is advised if there are any contraindications or potential problems. The prescription is compared to the formulary of drugs covered by the patient's insurance plan and the physician is advised if an alternate drug is recommended (thereby avoiding a subsequent phone call from the pharmacist to revise the prescription). The prescription is then transmitted directly to the patient's pharmacy.

   A built-in function of the EHR accurately calculates the correct Evaluation and Management code used for billing. The billing code is confirmed by the physician and automatically transferred to the billing system.

When the visit is complete, so is the exam note. The physician can sign the note electronically at the conclusion of the visit.

9. If lab work has been ordered, a medical assistant will obtain the necessary specimen and the order is sent electronically to the lab.

10. When the patient is dressed, he or she is given patient education material and medication instructions.

Because of the efficiency of the EHR system, the physician has more personal time with the patient for counseling or patient education. In many systems, the provider can display and annotate pictures of body areas for patient education and print them so that the patient can take them home.

In some practices, the patient is given a copy of the exam notes for the current visit. Allowing the patient to take away a written record of the visit enables better compliance with the doctor's plan of care and recommended treatments. However, this is only possible when using an EHR, because the note is ready at the end of a visit instead of waiting on dictation and transcription.

11. The patient is escorted to the check-out area.

If x-rays or other diagnostic tests have been ordered at another facility, the office staff may call on behalf of the patient and schedule the tests.

If a follow-up visit has been indicated, the patient will be scheduled for the next appointment.

12. If lab tests were ordered, the results are sent to the doctor electronically, are reviewed on screen, and are automatically merged into the EHR.

If x-rays or other diagnostic tests have been ordered, the results and reports are subsequently sent to the practice electronically but as text reports. The reports and even corresponding images can be reviewed by the physician and included in the patient's EHR.

Note

Doctors Say

"Documenting an encounter at the point of care is the most efficient method of practicing medicine because the physician completes the medical record at the time of a patient's visit. Dictation time is saved (a primary care physician dictates for more than 50 minutes in an 8.2-hour workday), and the need for personal dictation aides is eliminated. Thus, point-of-care documentation is less expensive than traditional dictation with its associated high cost of transcription. In addition, the physician can sign the note immediately. Patient care is improved because the patient can leave with a complete copy of the medical record, a step that stimulates compliance. The delivery process is improved with point–of–care documentation because referrals can be accomplished with full information available at the time that the referral is needed. For these benefits to occur, the clinical workflow changes to improve efficiency, increase data accuracy, and lower the overall cost of health care delivery."[9]

—John W. Bachman, M.D.
—Allen R. Wenner, M.D.

[9]Allen R. Wenner and John W. Bachman, *Transforming the Physician Practice: Interview with a Computer, Healthcare Information Management Systems, 3rd Edition,* Edtors: Ball, Weaver and Kiel, Copyright © 2003 Springer, New York, NY.

Accessibility is not a problem in the EHR system because there is no chart to "refile." Multiple providers can access the patient's chart, even simultaneously; for example, a physician could review the previous lab results before entering the exam room, even if the nurse was currently entering vital signs in the chart.

Transition to an EHR

Having compared the two workflow scenarios, we see the immediate advantages of the EHR for the patient and clinician. But there is a period of transition for a practice and the necessity of following a strategy for moving from paper charts to EHR. Essential to every practice is the workflow of the provider. The primary concern will be, "What is the impact on the workflow of the provider?"

Think about the workflow of the office that used paper charts. One strategy is to determine if any of the information is already available electronically. The next step is to determine how much of the EHR can be implemented before impacting the provider workflow. In light of this, consider the following questions about the first workflow:

◆ What was the nurse or physician doing at the time of the patient interaction?

◆ Could they have recorded this data in a computer?

◆ Could they have saved time later?

◆ Could the data be entered by someone other than the person seeing the patient?

The patient completed a form concerning any previous history, any changes to medications, new allergies, and so on.

◆ Could the patient have used a computer, or could the form have been designed to be read by a computer?

◆ Could the patient have completed the information before the visit?

The nurse recorded various health measurements (vital signs) in the exam room.

◆ Could the nurse have recorded the "chief complaint" or the vital signs in a computer instead of on a paper chart?

◆ Were any of the instruments used capable of transferring their reading to a computer system?

During the physical exam, the physician made observations and an assessment. This was later dictated from memory, subsequently transcribed by a typist, and finally reviewed and signed by the physician.

◆ Is the time it would take to record the observations and assessment in the exam comparable to the time it takes to dictate and review the notes later?

The physician prescribed medications and ordered tests.

◆ Would the time spent entering the prescriptions on a computer justify the benefits of electronic prescribing?

◆ Are results available electronically from laboratories the medical practice uses?

◆ Would ordering a test electronically improve the matching of results to orders when the tests were completed?

Finally, the big question:

◆ How can the medical practice transition to an EHR with the least impact on the daily operation of the practice?

Levels of EHR Implementation

Today, many medical practices are in the process of selecting and implementing an EHR, but when doing so, patient care must continue and the flow of the office must not be disrupted. The implementation of an EHR in a busy physician practice is often accomplished in steps. Therefore, it may be desirable to look at the components that make up an EHR and implement them in parts rather than as a whole.

It also might be useful to look at the paper records and measure the type of documents within them. This will allow the practice to predict the amount of the chart that can be computerized before the clinician's time becomes a major factor. The contents of a medical chart might include the following:

◆ Exam notes from each previous patient visit or exam

◆ The patient's previous injury, disease, surgery, immunizations, and medical history

◆ Medications that the patient is currently taking as well as allergy history

◆ Results of lab or diagnostic tests, pathology reports

◆ Reports from specialists who saw the patient for specific conditions

◆ X-rays, CAT scans, or reports from radiologists who interpreted them

◆ Problem list (acute conditions for which the patient was recently seen as well as chronic conditions such as high blood pressure, diabetes, or heart disease that are monitored nearly every visit, and can affect decisions about medications and treatments for even unrelated illness)

◆ Vital signs (functional measurements recorded at nearly every visit, such as height, weight, blood pressure, temperature, pulse, and respiration rate)

Figure 1-4 illustrates some of the various components that might be found in a paper chart at three hypothetical medical practices. The percentage of each component reflects number of sheets of paper various styles of charting will accumulate.

The blue stacks represent a primary care practice with providers who handwrite their notes in a paper chart. The maroon stacks represent a primary practice whose providers dictate their notes, have them transcribed, then filed in the chart. The yellow stacks represent a radiology practice whose providers dictate and have their radiology reports transcribed. For purposes of the comparison, the radiologists' reports are graphed at the same position as a primary care doctor's exam notes.

Two factors will vary the quantity and importance of each component: first, the clinician's current style of charting, and, second, the type of medical specialty. For example, primary care physicians might have more pages of lab reports

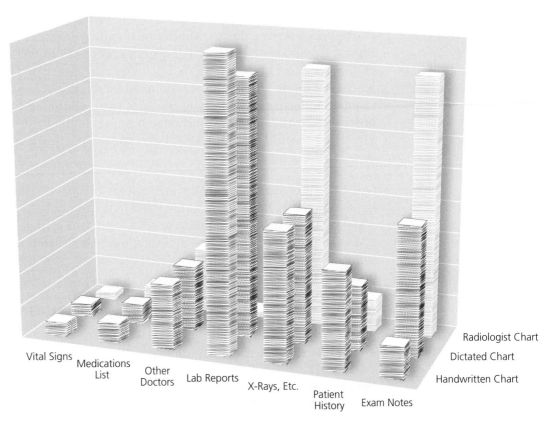

Vital Signs

Medications List

Other Doctors

Lab Reports

X-Rays, Etc.

Patient History

Exam Notes

Radiologist Chart

Dictated Chart

Handwritten Chart

▶ **Figure 1-4 Ratios of Pages in a Paper Chart by Provider.**

and patient history information than radiologists who hardly ever order lab tests. Conversely, radiologists' files will almost entirely be made up of diagnostic reports and images, such as x-rays. These are, of course, extreme comparisons, but they illustrate that the ratio of the chart will vary by specialty.

Even within the same type of specialty, in this example primary care, the number of pages can vary by the style of documentation. In most cases when clinicians dictate their notes it increases the number of pages because there is one or more pages for each visit transcribed.

Alternatively, many providers who handwrite their charts record multiple visits on a single page until the page has been filled up. In those practices, the lab reports will vastly outnumber the pages of exam notes because a lab report always consists of one or more pages, but the handwritten notes do not. In Chapter 5, you will learn the importance of completely documenting the patient visit to support the claim for billing. Because of this need for richer, more complete documentation, more and more practices are moving away from the handwritten chart.

Building the EHR in Steps

The challenge is to develop a strategy for building an EHR. This helps the provider by making the most important data available with the least impact on the workflow. One method is to examine the typical paper chart in a practice to determine the ratio of different pages of chart content. As illustrated earlier, the type of practice will determine the importance of various components in the EHR.

The components representing the largest portion of the chart, requiring the least change for the doctor, should be computerized first. For example, Figure 1-4 shows that paper lab orders and result reports represent a significant percentage of the paper in a primary care practice. Because it is the medical assistant or phlebotomist who most likely already completes the laboratory requisition form when drawing the specimen, changing to an electronic lab order and result system would have minimal impact to the ordering provider. The benefit would be that a very large portion of the chart would be computerized almost painlessly.

One benefit of starting with the lab system is that the numerical data that makes up many lab results lends itself to trend analysis, graphs, and comparison with other tests. The ability to review and present results in this manner gives the providers an immediate, tangible benefit from an EHR. Not only is the practice eliminating paper, but also it allows the provider to realize the trending potential of an EHR relatively early in the transition process.

Although the long-term goal is a uniform, codified, and searchable health record accessible from multiple locations,

◆ Which of these is the most important short-term goal?

For discussion purposes, assume that accessibility to records from multiple locations was a priority.

Figure 1-4 shows that the next largest portion of the patient chart is the doctor's dictated and transcribed exam notes (one page for each visit). If possible, word processing files of previous exam notes should be merged into the EHR.

If dictation is transcribed at the practice, the word processing files may still be available. If transcription is done off site, the transcription company may still have the files. In any case, the practice should request that all future transcriptions be returned with an electronic file.

Because transcribed notes are created in a computer, if the practice can obtain the files and merge them in the EHR the patients' records will be more accessible. Although, as text files, the dictated notes are not codified medical records, once merged into the EHR they become available from any location of the practice, as opposed to paper printouts, which are restricted to the location of the file folder.

There is also the question of what to do with the paper records created before the introduction of the EHR. In addition, the practice is likely to continue to receive referral letters and reports from specialists outside the practice on paper; what should be done with these?

Many practices choose to bring paper documents into the EHR as scanned images. Although document images do not offer the benefits of a codified medical record, they do provide widespread accessibility and a means to a complete electronic chart. Most document management systems allow various ID fields and keywords to be associated with the document images in the EHR. This adds a search capability to the electronic document files. Figure 1-5 shows an example of a document scanner used with an EHR system.

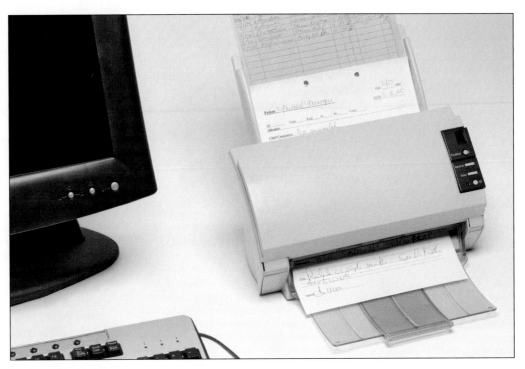

Courtesy of Allscripts, LLC.

▶ **Figure 1-5 ImpactMD Document Scanner.**

The process of scanning old charts as a means of building accessible historical records in the EHR can be daunting for established practices where hundreds of thousands of old charts may exist. The strategy for these practices is to only scan charts of patients who are scheduled to be seen. Thus, if the practice sees 100 patients a day, only 100 charts are scanned, not the thousands that are looming in the file room. This method also increases the likelihood that the chart the provider wants is already scanned in the system as the provider is most likely interested in upcoming patients and those recently seen.

Finally, consider the portion of the chart allotted for x-rays and other diagnostic images. Many of these files initially are in electronic format (x-rays are sometimes digital images first, then subsequently printed to film). Many EHR image systems will store and retrieve these images as easily as document images.

Using the example steps above, up to 80% of the chart has been converted to electronic files with almost no impact on the primary care provider's time with the patient. However, to move to a true EHR, the provider must eventually begin to put data into the system as well.

Comparing the EHR in an Inpatient versus Outpatient Setting

As we have just seen, different portions of the chart have more emphasis in different medical specialties. Primary care physicians record extensive information about the complete physical exam, whereas cardiologists mainly record the results of diagnostic procedures such as ECG, stress tests, and others.

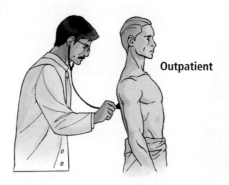
Outpatient

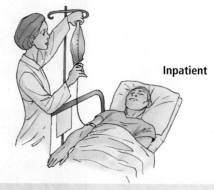
Inpatient

Most physician offices have a single chart for the patient. Notes for each visit, test results, and any other reports are added to the chart.	Most hospitals start a new chart each time a patient is admitted. Information from previous stays in the hospital is linked to the patient ID, but the current chart contains only information related to the current stay.
The quantity of data in an outpatient chart is relatively low by comparison.	The quantity of data in an inpatient chart is likely to be much larger. Vital signs are taken and nurses' notes are added numerous times per day; dietitians, respiratory therapists, and other providers add to the chart; there are typically many more orders for labs, medications, and so on.
The central element in the chart is the physician's exam note.	Physician exams tend to be brief; the main focus of the chart is the physician orders and nurse's notes indicating the patient's response.

▶ **Figure 1-6 Comparison of Outpatient versus Inpatient Charts.**

In addition to the type of specialty, the content of the EHR is affected by the type of facility. Whether the patient is being examined in a doctor's office, being treated in the Emergency Room, or is an inpatient at a hospital affects not only the kind of data but the quantity as well. Compare the differences between an outpatient and an inpatient medical record in Figure 1-6.

Any chart is likely to reflect the goals of the practice. The goal of hospital care is to improve and stabilize the patient to the point where the patient can be discharged. The goal of the primary care practice is to manage the long-term health of the patient. Therefore, the outpatient chart is concerned with trends in the patient's health that span months or years. The inpatient chart is focused on changes that occur in hours and days.

In addition to the items listed earlier, the principle difference between the inpatient and outpatient EHR is the system itself. As you have learned earlier in this chapter, data in the EHR comes from many sources. In most systems designed for physician's offices, the data typically is received and stored by the EHR software in one electronic medical record system. Most hospitals have a large number of departments using many different computer systems. The hospital EHR does not necessarily merge the data from these systems into its database. Often the hospital EHR allows the clinician to view data in these other systems through an interface but does not necessarily store the data in a single EHR.

Although the exercises in the chapters of this book use software simulating the implementation of an EHR in physician offices, the information and exercises may be applicable to nurses and medical assistants in both inpatient and outpatient settings.

Methods of Capturing and Recording Data

Earlier in the chapter, we discussed how data of three chart components could be made a part of the EHR: electronic lab orders and results, transcription files of exam notes saved as EHR text records, and scanned images of documents identified and assigned keywords as they are imported into the EHR. Also, radiology studies, if available as a digital image, can be directly incorporated into the EHR.

Now consider the remaining chart components that were previously identified in Figure 1-4 and how they might be captured into the EHR. These include vital signs, history, problems, and medications.

Vital signs are numerical in nature and therefore eminently applicable to trend analysis and graphing. These are especially useful for creating growth charts in pediatric practices and assisting patients with weight loss for adolescents and adults. Some of the equipment manufactured to take blood pressure readings, temperature, pulse, and respiration can automatically transfer the reading to an EHR. Unfortunately, this level of automation typically is found in hospital and ICU systems. The average medical office uses common instruments such as a scale, a thermometer, a blood pressure cuff, and so on. The measurements are manually taken and recorded by a medical assistant. Certainly, the medical assistant can enter the data in the computer, instead of writing it on a sheet of paper. The alternative is to update the office with portable equipment that interfaces to the EHR, as discussed at the end of this chapter and again in Chapter 6.

In addition to the vital signs, the nurse or medical assistant also talked to the patient about the reason for the visit, and possibly reviewed allergy or medication information. Using an EHR, the nurse or medical assistant can initiate an exam record for today's visit and enter the chief complaint, update any allergy records, and make note of any medications the patient may report using (purchased over the counter or prescribed by another practice). This uses the time of a nurse or medical assistant to build the EHR note but still does not impact the clinician's time.

There are a few EHR systems designed to allow a patient in the waiting room to complete a patient history form on a computer instead of a paper form on a clipboard. The patient-entered data is reviewed by the doctor during the exam and merged into the EHR. In Chapter 6, you will learn more about this type of system. Generally, however, this capability is rare. In most systems today, the patient information is keyed into the EHR by someone on the doctor's staff, either the medical assistant or a trained clerical person, not the patient. It is important to note that in a system in which the patient enters data in the waiting room, the patient is not working directly in the practice's EHR and the system is secure.

The patient's problem list (acute conditions for which the patient was recently seen as well as chronic conditions such as high blood pressure, diabetes, etc.)

may be able to be generated automatically from patient history and past visits, then simply updated by a nurse or doctor each time the patient is seen. You will learn more about problem lists in Chapter 6.

The first real requirement for the provider to enter data comes with medications. The law requires that only certain licensed providers can write prescriptions. This means that if the prescription is going to automatically get into the EHR as part of the workflow the provider is going to have to do it. Clinicians were long accustomed to scribbling an order on a prescription pad and handing it to a staff member or patient. However, drug interaction checking, insurance pharmacy benefit formularies, and better patient records are all reasons for doctors to change to electronic prescribing. In addition, writing prescriptions with the computer automatically builds an important record of the patient's current medications and makes renewing prescriptions for chronic patients much faster. Electronic prescriptions will be covered in Chapter 7.

The core of the true codified EHR comes when the provider begins to record the actual exam itself in a medical records program instead of dictating and transcribing it later. This phase takes more of the provider's time to enter the information in the computer. This is a point at which many EHR systems fail to be adopted by every physician in the practice. This can create mixed results in the EHR, if some physicians enter data while others persist with dictation/transcription.

Although some physicians see the time spent entering the EHR as a reasonable trade-off for the time spent dictating and reviewing transcriptions, others refuse, and continue in their old methods. If early in the implementation word processing files from transcriptions have been incorporated as text EHR records, physicians who continue to dictate will not create a problem because their records are part of the EHR. Although these text records are not codified like those created by the clinicians entering data, they are at least accessible.

Another approach that some practices have take is to create a new staff position called a medical scribe. This person's job is to enter the data in the EHR as the physician conducts the exam. The position replaces that of a medical transcriber.

Entering observations and findings as medical data into an EHR has many additional advantages for the provider than just the elimination of transcription. One of these is the correct calculation of billing and diagnosis codes. Government and private insurance claims have strict rules about what (evaluation and management) billing codes are allowed based on the documented level of an exam. Most EHR systems have built-in functions that help the provider select the correct billing code based on the data entered in the exam note. Many of these systems can automatically transfer the codes to the billing system when the exam is completed. This subject will be covered in Chapter 5.

Another important feature is the ability for the provider to view and incorporate information from a previous visit to update it in the current exam. Because frequently patients are seen in follow-up visits to previous exams, this can be a real time-saver for the provider. These and other benefits will become more evident later when you will begin working with the EHR in Chapter 3.

Workflow of Physician Orders and Results

As you learned earlier in this chapter, Computerized Physician Order Entry or CPOE is viewed by IOM, Leapfrog, and others as one of the key features of an EHR that can improve quality of care, patient safety, and clinician efficiency. Central to the process of health care is the ordering clinician. All types of treatments and care events are the result of physician orders. Examples include labs, x-rays, other diagnostic tests, medications, therapy, and even devices such as a wheelchair or eyeglasses.

In this section, we will look at the workflow surrounding several types of orders, and the effect of an EHR on the process. This book will generally refer to these as physician orders, even though it should be recognized that licensed nurse practitioners, physician assistants, and other qualified health care providers are permitted to write prescriptions and orders as well.

Lab Orders and Reports

In the simplest example, the physician wants additional information about the patient's health that can be obtained by analyzing the patient's blood. The physician "orders" a blood test. Implied within that order is a request for a nurse, phlebotomist, or other medical personnel to draw a sample of the patient's blood.

The test may be performed at a lab within the medical office or at an outside reference laboratory. The specimen may be drawn at the medical office and sent to the laboratory or the patient may be directed to the laboratory to have his or her blood drawn there.

If the clinician's diagnosis or plan of treatment is dependent on the outcome of the test, then timeliness is important. In such a case, the patient cannot be treated until the doctor receives and reviews the results. Although many of the steps are the same, electronic lab orders enable the provider to begin treatment sooner because the provider is aware of the results sooner. The following discussion compares an electronic and paper lab order and results. The workflow of an electronic lab system will be discussed further in Chapter 6.

Comparison of Lab Order and Results Workflow

1 The clinician's order for a blood test is transferred to a uniquely numbered *laboratory requisition*, which records information about the patient, the clinician, and the test to be performed.

The requisition form will require additional information, including when the patient last ate, what suspected diagnosis the physician is trying to rule out. Patient demographic information, date of birth, and insurance information must be provided for the lab to get paid for the test.

Certain tests may not be covered by the patient's insurance and the patient must sign an acknowledgment that he or she has been advised that the test will not be covered by his or her insurance.

Electronic	**Paper**
The electronic requisition is entered in a computer.	A paper requisition form supplied by the reference laboratory is used.
The patient's demographic and insurance information is populated automatically.	The patient's demographic and insurance information is copied by hand, onto the form, with inherent risks of a mistake when copying by hand.
The electronic order system compares the test codes on the order to coverage rules for the patient's insurance and automatically alerts the user if a signed patient acknowledgment is required.	Advance notice to the patient whether his or her insurance will pay for the test relies on either a call to the lab, a call to the insurance plan, or the medical assistant's memory.

2 The specimen of the patient's blood is drawn. Labels are attached to the sample to ensure it is clearly identified by patient and requisition when it is processed by the lab.

If the blood is drawn at the medical office but the test is not performed there, the sample is picked up by a courier and transported to the reference lab.

Electronic	**Paper**
Labels are generated by the computerized requisition system. The labels include the patient name, ID, and requisition number.	The paper form is accompanied by uniquely numbered labels. The medical assistant will write the patient name and ID on the labels.
The requisition is transmitted electronically to the lab system computer and contains the information required to process the test.	The paper requisition is delivered to the lab with the sample or brought by the patient. It is keyed into the lab system computer by a lab employee. There is an inherent risk of a typing error.

3 Blood tests are most often performed by automated equipment that communicates results to the lab computer system assigning values to codes for each component of the test. The lab system computer then compiles the results into a report that includes the information from the original requisition, test codes, codes for each component of the test as well as standard reference ranges for each associated with the actual value measured with the component. Additional notes, such as whether the value is considered outside the reference range (high or low) and whether the results were verified by repeat testing, also are merged into the report data.

4 When the report is complete it is sent back to the ordering clinician. Note: There also usually is a paper copy of the report printed by the lab even when an electronic order is used.

Electronic

The results are returned electronically and merged into the patient's EHR.

The clinician will be alerted that the results are ready.

Paper

A printed copy of the results will be faxed, mailed, or sent by courier to the practice.

A staff person at the doctor's office will file the paper copy in the patient's chart and make the doctor aware that the report has arrived.

5 The clinician will review the results of the test and take appropriate action.

Electronic

The clinician will review the results on screen, with access to other components of the EHR. This allows easy comparison of current results with previous tests and graph trends.

The clinician can then order the treatments or follow-up tests and send messages to the staff or the patient about the results.

Paper

The clinician will review the results in the paper chart. To compare results with any previous tests, the clinician will thumb through the pages of the chart.

The doctor will handwrite notes, or leave voice mail for his staff, who will call the patient.

Status From the beginning of the order to completion of the review by the clinician, there is the issue of order status. If too much time elapses between when the patient needs the test and an action is taken based on the test results, the patient's condition could deteriorate.

To determine how much time has elapsed, the medical office must know which patients have tests pending results and when they were ordered. The office is then in a position to follow up on the test by calling the lab or the patient.

Electronic

Orders are tracked in an EHR from the moment they are entered in the system. A report of pending orders is always available. As described in step 4, the clinician is notified as soon as results are ready.

Because the lab system received the requisition electronically, the lab can inform the medical office that the patient has not shown up (when an order has been in their system too long).

With an electronic order system, the patient's results are usually available the same day or the next morning.

Paper

In most practices, a copy of the order is in the paper chart. Unless a separate list is maintained of the tests ordered, and when results are received, the clinician never knows that a test is lost.

When the patient is sent to an outside lab with a paper requisition in hand, neither the lab nor the medical office knows if the patient fails to show up.

Medication Orders

The most common type of order is for medication. Drug prescriptions are commonly written by hand on a prescription pad and given to the patient to have filled at a pharmacy. Information about the medication is recorded in the chart by hand or the prescription is copied and filed in the paper chart. Alternatively, a member of the doctor's staff may phone the prescription to the pharmacy or the doctor may give the patient samples of drugs provided by the pharmaceutical company. In any case, the information is noted in the patient's chart.

When the patient goes to the pharmacy to have the prescription filled, the pharmacist will enter the information in the pharmacy computer system. The patient's insurance or Medicare may require that a generic or less costly drug be substituted for a brand-name drug on the prescription. Unless the physician has indicated DAW or "Dispense As Written" on the prescription, it is very likely that the pharmacist will substitute a medically equivalent drug for the one prescribed by the physician.

The pharmacy computer system is also likely to perform two other functions: "formulary compliance checking" and "drug utilization review" or "DUR."

Formulary compliance was discussed earlier in this chapter as an example of decision support. Formulary lists are usually per insurance plan, and because there are so many different plans, the pharmacy system usually checks the formulary by electronically communicating with an intermediary company called a pharmacy benefit manager.

Drug utilization review (DUR) is also performed via a computer system. The computer compares the prescription about to be filled with other prescriptions the patient is currently taking to determine if harmful interactions could occur when two or more medicines are combined. DUR is also capable of checking for potential errors where the dose in the prescription is too large or too small. If allergy information about the patient is available to the DUR system, warnings also can be given where allergic reactions might occur.

If either the formulary checking or the DUR indicates any problem with the prescription the pharmacist must contact the prescribing provider. Often the call from the pharmacist comes when the physician is with another patient, so a message is left and the call is returned at a later time. This creates a delay for the patient and pharmacist and consumes extra time for the physician who has to return the phone calls.

Prescriptions recorded and issued via computer have several advantages over the paper chart method. First, the physician issues the prescription and records it in the chart in one step. Second, the prescription can be transmitted electronically from the physician's computer system to the pharmacy, saving time for the patient, eliminating the need for the doctor's staff to call in the prescription, and reducing errors caused by handwritten prescriptions. Finally, the DUR and formulary compliance checking can be performed by the doctor's computer at the time the prescription is written. This allows any problems with the prescription to be corrected prior to sending it to the pharmacy. This drastically reduces phone calls back to the prescribing physician from the pharmacy, saving everyone time.

DUR is a very important feature that reduces the patient's risk of adverse drug reactions. DUR works best when all of the known drugs and allergy information is available and current. Therefore, an EHR should be able to record not only prescriptions issued by the physician's system but also medications prescribed elsewhere. These are usually reported by the patient during the nurse's interview or during the exam. The current medications list should be updated each visit prior to the provider issuing any prescriptions.

The electronic prescription component of an EHR can provide additional benefits to both the clinician and the patient. Because each medication is automatically recorded in the medications list as the prescription is created, a current and recent medications list is available to the clinician when writing the prescription. This reduces prescribing errors.

EHR systems also shorten the time it takes to write a prescription by maintaining a list of prescriptions the clinician writes frequently. This speeds up the writing of prescriptions for common ailments seen at the practice. Physicians of patients with chronic diseases frequently write renewals for existing prescriptions; with EHR systems, they perform this task with a few clicks of the mouse. Additional time is saved because all FDA-approved drugs are listed in the computer, eliminating the need to use a drug reference book to find an uncommon drug. Electronic prescriptions will be covered in Chapter 7.

Radiology Orders and Reports

When diagnostic information is needed, the physician may order an x-ray, CAT scan, PET, MRI, mammogram, or other diagnostic test. Most of these orders are not transmitted electronically today unless the x-ray or other device is located in the same facility as the ordering physician. Even then, it is common for these orders to be handwritten or verbal. Except for x-rays, most radiological studies must be scheduled ahead of time. Often, the physician's staff schedules an appointment with a diagnostic facility on behalf of the patient.

Once the x-ray, CAT scan, or other study has been completed, a radiologist interprets the results. Increasingly, these images are stored and read in a digital format. The radiologist uses a computer system with much higher resolution than standard computer screens to view the images. Special software not only displays the image but also allows the radiologist to manipulate it, zooming in and out, changing the contrast, reversing the image colors, and offering many other capabilities that help the radiologist.

While looking at the image, radiologists dictate a report, describe what they see, its size, location, and any other comments. Because the radiologists are using the computer controls to manipulate and control the image, their observations are seldom keyed into an EHR program. It is standard practice for a radiologist's report to be dictated, then typed by a medical transcriber. However, some radiology practices use speech recognition software, which converts the human voice into typed reports.

When the report is complete, and reviewed by the radiologist, it is sent to the ordering physician. Radiology reports are almost always originated in an electronic text format at the radiologist's office, and are usually sent on paper as a letter or fax.

Radiology reports are seldom available as a codified EHR record, but some medical offices may scan the paper reports as document images in the patient's EHR. Radiological observations that are codified are those related to the size and stage of tumors.

Within most hospital systems and between some medical offices, electronic text files of the reports also may be available. Copies of the images studied by the radiologist also are sometimes sent to the ordering physician. These images are usually in an electronic format, although x-rays may be sent as film. Electronic transmission of images uses a national standard called DICOM. Electronic orders, results, and other data may be communicated between the hospital system using another standard, called HL-7. Both DICOM and HL7 are discussed in the next section.

Electronic Data Interchange between Systems and Devices

Throughout this chapter, we discussed populating the EHR with data from external sources. This section will provide a brief overview of standards that make the exchange of data possible.

National standards for transferring medical information between systems are important to the EHR because they enable the direct transfer of information into the EHR. Two of these are HL7 and DICOM. National standards provide rules for the structure of a message between two computers, and define some of the codes that are used to identify the information within the messages.

HL7

HL7 stands for Health Level Seven, a nonprofit organization that developed and maintains the leading messaging standard used to exchange clinical and administrative data between different health care computer systems. The "Level Seven" portion of the name refers to the highest level of data communications—the application level. The organization and the standard it developed are both referred to as HL7.

The organization, comprised of health care providers, institutions, government representatives, and software developers, uses a consensus process to arrive at specifications acceptable to everyone involved. The HL7 specifications are updated regularly and released as new versions.

As a part of this course, it is not necessary to delve into the specific structure or flow of HL7 messages, but it is helpful to understand its advantages and limitations. HL7 is the glue that holds large institutional systems together. It is not uncommon for various departments within a hospital to use completely different computer systems created by unrelated vendors. The simplest act of transferring patient information from the admissions office to the radiology department or hospital pharmacy would not be easy without HL7. If you work in a hospital, your hospital probably uses HL7.

Of course, HL7 goes much further than specifying the communication of patient admission, registration, and discharge information. It includes a wide range of clinical information messages. As such, it is the primary standard for the communication of orders, lab results, radiology reports, clinical observations such as vital signs, and many other types of clinical data maintained in the EHR.

HL7 specifications are independent of any application or vendor; therefore, applications that can send and receive HL7 messages can potentially exchange information. Therein lies its advantage and importance to an EHR system.

HL7 has been successful because it is very flexible both in its structure as well as its support for multiple coding standards. However, when a message is received the codes and terms used by the other system may not match those used by the EHR. Therein lies its disadvantage.

To overcome this problem, segments of the HL7 message that contain coded data also contain an identifier indicating which coding standard is being used. A special computer program called an HL7 translator is used to match the codes in the message with the codes in the EHR. The translator also can reconcile differences between HL7 versions from multiple systems.

Although HL7 is adaptable to many different systems, it takes a lot of work. When implementing an EHR, it is important to understand each system that will be added, will take additional time and expense. Health care today does not have a uniform standard for data or codification. For each application that is connected, someone must set up a cross-reference list to map medical codes from the sending system to corresponding codes in the EHR system. The development of national standards for medical coding will be covered in Chapter 2.

CDISC

A subgroup of HL7 is CDISC, which stands for Clinical Data Interchange Standards Consortium. CDISC originated as a special interest group of the Drug Information Association but became its own entity and formed an alliance with HL7. Although the focus of HL7 is to facilitate message standards for a broad range of health care, CDISC has a specific focus on clinical drug trials.

CDISC standards enable sponsors, vendors, and clinicians to acquire and exchange data used in clinical trials. Because the FDA is the agency to whom the final results are submitted, the standard is very focused on following the FDA requirements. However, the commitment of CDISC to HL7 will eventually make it easier to use EHR data in clinical trial studies. It is mentioned here because you may encounter CDISC if you work at a health care practice that participates in Phase IV clinical trials.

Thus far, we have discussed EHR standards that represent codified or text-based medical records; however, some components of the EHR are best represented by images. As the cliché goes, a picture is worth a thousand words.

DICOM

DICOM stands for Digital Imaging and Communications in Medicine. It is the standard used for medical images, such as digital x-rays, CT scans, MRIs, and ultrasound. Other uses include the images from angiography, endoscopy, laparoscopy, medical photography, and microscopy. It was created by the National Electrical Manufacturers Association and is the most widely used format for sending diagnostic images.

In addition to setting the standard for the communication from a piece of imaging equipment to a software application, the standard also defines the specification for a file that contains the actual digital image. A DICOM file includes a "header" that contains information about the image, dimensions, type of scan, image compression, and so on, as well as patient information such as ID number or name. DICOM-compatible software is required to view the image.

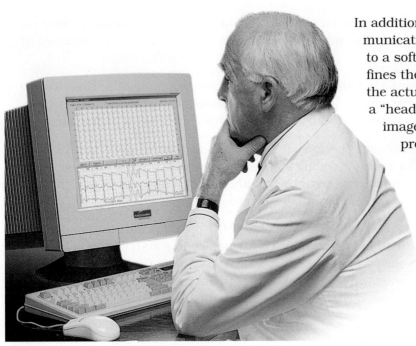

Courtesy of Midmark Diagnostics Group.

▶ **Figure 1-7 Doctor Reviewing Data from an IQmark™ Advanced Holter.**

Medical Devices

Medical devices can output important and useful medical information that can be received and stored as data in the patient's EHR. HL7 is often used to exchange demographic information between the device and the EHR system. However, the type of data and method of communicating between the device and EHR often are proprietary to the particular device.

Still, the advantage of having the data in the EHR is so strong as to warrant the additional interfaces. Many vendors of EHR systems recognize this and have developed relationships with one or more device manufacturers (see Figure 1-7). Some of these manufacturers include GE Healthcare, Midmark Diagnostics Group, and Welch Allyn. More information about these and other devices that send data to the EHR will be found in Chapter 6 and Chapter 9.

Chapter One Summary

Although Electronic Health Records have been called by various names for the last 30 years, the acronym EHR is currently used as shorthand for Electronic Health Records. By EHR, we mean the portions of a patient's medical record that are stored in a computer system as well as the functional benefits derived from having an electronic health record.

The drawbacks to nonelectronic records are numerous. Handwritten records often are abbreviated, cryptic, or illegible. Information cannot be easily accessed or shared. Nonelectronic charts must be copied and faxed or transported from one office to another. Finally, paper charts are not searchable, except by manually opening every chart and reading it.

The goal in creating Electronic Health Records is not necessarily to eliminate paper copies of records but to eliminate paper as the *only* copy of a patient's medical record. The EHR can help to improve patient health, the quality of care, and patient safety by providing access to complete, up-to-date records of past and present conditions. This enables EHR records to be used in ways that paper medical records cannot. These include Health Maintenance, Trend

Analysis, Alerts, and Decision Support. Codified records also make it easy to find, share, and search patient records.

Social changes driving the need for EHR include an increasingly mobile society in which patients move and change doctors more frequently. Additionally, patients today see multiple specialists for their care. This means their medical records no longer reside with a single general practitioner who provides their total care. Thus, the ability to share exam records and test results is important to the patient's continuity of care.

Patients using the Internet are asking, "Why can't I see my chart on the Web?" The Internet offers access to millions of pieces of health-related information, some of which patients are bringing to their doctor appointments.

Health care organizations, medical schools, employers, and even the government have recognized the importance of computerizing the various components of the medical record. Studies from the IOM and others have shown that a large number of deaths are occurring from preventable medical errors; many are related to not having access to the proper medical information. Leapfrog (a collation of employers) has made implementation of EHR a priority to improve health care.

President George W. Bush has approved funding and established the position of the National Coordinator for Health Information Technology under the Department of Health and Human Services, to "develop, maintain, and direct the implementation of a strategic plan to guide the nationwide implementation of interoperable health information technology . . .."[10] To meet the president's goals for an EHR, a uniform, codified, searchable health record that is accessible from multiple locations is needed.

By codified record, we mean a system of standard codes assigned to medical terms underlies the description that is visible to the user. Codes are used to unify synonyms for the same medical concept. Codes ensure the meaning of medical information is understood when it is transferred to another system. Searching codified medical records is more efficient and accurate because it overcomes the different ways clinicians may have stated the same medical concept.

Implementing an EHR requires changes in the way providers work. Many medical practices choose to implement the EHR in steps that incrementally increase the involvement of the provider over time so that the flow of the office and patient care can continue without being disrupted.

Implementation of EHR in levels usually consists of identifying portions of the chart that may originate as electronic data before being printed on paper. These may be available for import into the chart. Examples include electronic lab orders and results, word processing files from dictated exam notes that have been transcribed, and scanned images of referral letters and scanned pages of the old chart.

Population of the EHR from external sources requires the different systems to be able to communicate and effectively transfer data between. To accomplish this, national standards have evolved that allow data from disparate systems to be sent in a format that is comprehensible to the receiving system. Three of

---

[10]Executive Order #13335, President George W. Bush, April 27, 2004.

these are: HL-7, which is used for patient demographics, lab orders, results, radiology reports, and clinical observations; DICOM, which is used for diagnostic images such as x-rays and CAT scans; and CDISC, which is used to communicate information for clinical trials.

There also are medical devices that measure vital signs, ECG, and other diagnostic tests, which can send their data into the EHR. Interfacing and importing data from labs, other facilities, and medical devices adds significant content to the EHR system without manual entry of the data by the clinic staff.

Eventually, the clinician must begin using the system. Using the EHR will take more of the clinician's time than a paper system, but the benefits can far outweigh weigh the effort required. One example is electronic prescriptions, which also can include formulary decision support and DUR Alerts to the prescribing physician. Using electronic prescriptions can prevent errors and save the doctor phone calls later. Often, clinicians begin using the EHR system by writing prescriptions and then eventually move on to documenting the patient exam.

Testing Your Knowledge of Chapter 1

1. What does the acronym EHR stand for?

2. What is the definition of an EHR?

3. Explain the benefits of EHR over paper charts.

Give examples for the following terms:

4. Trend Analysis

5. Decision Support

6. Alerts

7. Health Maintenance

8. Describe what generally takes place from the time a patient checks in at a physician's office until the patient checks out.

9. Describe what points of the workflow are different between offices using a paper and an electronic chart.

10. Describe at least three differences between inpatient and outpatient EHR systems.

11. Describe the workflow associated with an Electronic Lab Order.

12. Name at least three forces driving the change to EHR.

13. What are the four goals of the Strategic Framework created by the Office of the National Coordinator for Health Information Technology?

14. Name some advantages of electronic prescriptions.

15. What is HL7?

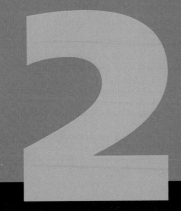

Chapter Two

Coding Standards

Learning Outcomes

After completing this chapter, you should be able to:

- Describe the importance of codified electronic health records

- Explain the government's influence on coding standards

- Have an understanding of prominent EHR code sets such as SNOMED CT, MEDCIN, and LOINC, as well as various nursing code sets

- Have an understanding of prominent billing code sets such as CPT-4, ABC, ICD-9CM, and ICD-10

- Explain how EHR code sets differ from CPT, ICD-9CM, and NDC codes

Acronyms are used extensively in both medicine and computers. Listed below are those that are used in this chapter.

ABC	Alternative Billing Codes
AMA	American Medical Association
ANA	American Nurses Association
CCC	Clinical Care Classification system
CDC	Centers for Disease Control
CDISC	Clinical Data Interchange Standards Consortium
CHCS II	Composite Health Care System—version 2 (Department of Defense)
CMS	Centers For Medicare and Medicaid Services (formerly HCFA)
CPT-4	Current Procedural Terminology—Fourth Edition
DICOM	Digital Imaging and Communications in Medicine
DOQ-IT	Doctors' Office Quality Information Technology (CMS project)
E & M	Evaluation And Management (codes)
EHR	Electronic Health Record
FDA	Food and Drug Administration
HCFA	Health Care Financing Administration (CMS predecessor)
HCPCS	Healthcare Common Procedure Coding System
HDL	High Density Lipoprotein
HHS	U.S. Department of Health and Human Services
HIPAA	Health Insurance Portability and Accountability Act
HL7	Health Level 7
ICD-9CM	International Classification of Diseases, Ninth Revision with Clinical Modifications
ICD-10	International Classification of Diseases, Tenth Revision
ICD-10PCS	International Classification of Diseases, Tenth Revision, Procedure Coding System
ICNP	International Classification for Nursing Practice
IHS	Indian Health Service
IOM	Institute of Medicine of the National Academies
LDL	Low Density Lipoprotein
LIS	Laboratory Information System
LOINC	Logical Observation Identifier Names and Codes
NASA	National Aeronautics and Space Administration
NANDA	North American Nursing Diagnosis Association
NCVHS	National Committee on Vital and Health Statistics
NHS	National Health Service (United Kingdom)
NIC	Nursing Interventions Classification
NLM	National Library of Medicine
NMDS	Nursing Minimum Data Set
NOC	Nursing Outcomes Classification

Acronyms are used extensively in both medicine and computers. Listed below are those that are used in this chapter.

OCR	Optical Character Recognition
PCDS	Patient Care Data Set
PMRI	Patient Medical Record Information
PNDS	Perioperative Nursing Data Set
SNOMED	Systemized Nomenclature of Medicine
SNOMED CT	Systemized Nomenclature of Medicine Clinical Terms
SNOMED RT	Systemized Nomenclature of Medicine Reference Terminology
UMLS	Unified Medical Language System
VA	U.S. Department of Veteran Affairs
WHO	World Health Organization

The Value of Codified Electronic Health Records

Chapter 1 defined the EHR as the portions of the patient's medical record stored in the computer system as well as the functional benefits derived from having an electronic health record. This section will explore:

1. Three ways patients' medical records are stored in computer systems

2. How the form they are stored in enables or encumbers the expanded functions recommended by the IOM and others.

Forms of EHR Data

There are three ways that patient records can be stored:

Digital images—this category includes scanned documents, diagnostic images, digital x-rays, and even annotated drawings or sound recordings.

When this type of data is imported into the EHR, it is usually cataloged with key words and a description that can be used to locate the item later. For example, if the paper chart is scanned in the computer, the person scanning the documents might catalog the images of the pages by date and type of report (lab, letter, exam note, etc.) and the source (name of the doctor or lab).

Text—the second type of data includes word processing files of transcribed exam notes and text reports. It is obtained principally in the EHR by importing text files from outside sources. The text files are typically cataloged with date, time, and perhaps keywords. For example, the text file of an exam note also might be cataloged with a description of the reason for the office visit.

Discrete data is the third form of stored information in an EHR. Data in this form is the easiest for the computer to use. It can be instantly searched, retrieved, and combined in different ways.

Discrete data in an EHR may be subcategorized into **fielded** data and **coded** data.

Fielded data assigns each piece of information its own place in the medical record called a "field." The meaning of the information is inferred from its position in the record.

For example, a record of the patient's medical problem might look like this:

"knee injury," "20060331," "improved," "20060428"

The fields in this example are surrounded by quotation marks. The computer would be programmed to look for the name of the problem in the first field, the date of onset in the second field, the status of the problem in the third field, and the date of the last exam in the fourth field.

Fielded data is the most common way to store information in computers and EHR systems. It is fast and efficient and uses very little storage space.

The downside of fielded data is that only software programmed with the particular order of the fields will know the meaning of the data. For example, another system that stored the same information but in different fields would not understand the data. This example underscores the importance of national standards such as HL7 discussed in Chapter 1. HL7 enables different applications to send and receive fielded data independently of how each application might store it internally.

Coded data is fielded data that goes a step further. By associating a code for each medical term and storing the appropriate code in the medical record, ambiguities about the clinician's meaning are eliminated.

Continuing with the example of knee injury, providers at two other clinics might have phrased the problem differently:

1. "twisted his knee"
2. "knee trauma"

A search of medical records for "knee injury" might not find the records created by these other two clinicians. When an EHR uses an underlying coding system in addition to the text description, the computer can find and match the desired information regardless of the clinician's choice of words. When a code is stored in the medical record in addition to the text description, the record is considered codified.

Limitations of Types of Data

An EHR with any form of data offers improved accessibility over a paper chart, but as more of an EHR is codified the computer can do more with it. The form the data is stored in determines to what extent the computer can use the content of the EHR to provide additional functions, which improve the quality of care.

Scanning images of old charts and other documents makes them available to providers at multiple locations. But even though there is some information in the indexed description of the item, the actual contents of the page can only be known by displaying the image and looking at it.

Text files (if they are available) can provide information that is more useable by the computer than scanned images of the same documents. Several key differences:

Text data	**Image data**
Many different applications can open and display text files.	Images usually require a special viewing application to display the image.
Text information can be dynamically reformatted to display on devices with different size screens.	Images can be zoomed in or out to improve readability but cannot usually be reformatted to fit a different device.

The content of the text also can be searched by a computer, for example, to determine which exam notes contain a specific medical term or phrase.	The content of an image cannot be searched by a computer.

Although text files can be searched, the time required to do is usually too long to make it useful for real-time alerts, health maintenance, or other functions recommended by the IOM in Chapter 1.

Discrete codified data is required to achieve extended functionality in the EHR. Because coded data is nonambiguous, the computer can use it for health maintenance, orders and results, trend analysis, decision support, administrative processes, and population health reporting. When an EHR is codified using a recognized coding standard, data exchange is also facilitated, because a receiving system using the same codes will correctly interpret the content.

To illustrate the advantage of codified data we will compare the ability to use the results of laboratory reports stored in the three types of data discussed earlier.

Comparison of Lab Results

Most medical practices use lab tests to measure the level of certain components present in specimens taken from the patient. When the same test is performed over a period of time, changes in the results can indicate a *trend* in the patient's health. The clinician compares the results from several lab reports. How easy it is to make the comparison depends on how the lab report is stored in the EHR.

Figure 2-1 shows an example of lab tests received on paper and scanned as an image into a document storage and retrieval system. Scanning images makes the report accessible at multiple locations for multiple providers. However, the computer cannot "read" the images to locate, for example, "patients with total cholesterol greater than 200." To compare previous results for even one patient, the clinician would have to locate and view those reports in the same way as reading them on paper.

Figure 2-2 shows a similar set of test results stored in a text file (similar to a word processing document). Text files can be searched with a sophisticated software program to determine which reports contained the name of the test. This would allow a clinician to quickly find which lab reports to compare, but the search would only find the exact test named in the search. For example, in Figure 2-2, the lab named the test "Total plasma Cholesterol," but a search for "total cholesterol" might not find this report because the names do not match precisely.

Next, look at the tests in Figure 2-2; notice the arrangement of the result values and the normal ranges into columns. Were the columns created by tab characters or were multiple spaces inserted in each line to make the columns line up? It is impossible to tell by looking at the report, but the fact that the answer might be "either" makes it impractical for a computer to determine where the result values begin and end. Real-time uses for text data in an EHR are generally limited by the form of the data to searching and viewing.

```
QUEST DIAGNOSTICS INCORPORATED
CLIENT SERVICE 813.972.7100

SPECIMEN INFORMATION
SPECIMEN:      TP016756T
REQUISITION:  0005290
LAB REF NO:

COLLECTED:  02/08/2003   10:00
RECEIVED:   02/08/2003   14:02
REPORTED:   02/08/2003   08:48
```

```
              PATIENT INFORMATION        ┌─────────────────────────────────┐
              Patel Raj                   │ REPORT STATUS  Final            │
                                          └─────────────────────────────────┘
              DOB: 05/06/1949  Age: 54    ORDERING PHYSICIAN
              GENDER: M                   DR.RICE
              SS: 654-98-7526
              ID: PATID-10                CLIENT INFORMATION
                                          97504017
                                          EMAXX TEST ACCOUNT
                                          MINDY SMITH
                                          4225 E FOWLER AVE
                                          TAMPA, FL 33617-2026
```

Test Name	In Range	Out of Range	Reference Range	Lab
LIPID PANEL				
TRIGLYCERIDES		150 H	<150 MG/DL	TP
CHOLESTEROL, TOTAL	195		<200 MG/DL	TP
HDL CHOLESTEROL	40		>OR=40 MG/DL	TP
LDL-CHOLESTEROL	98		<130 MG/DL (CALC)	TP
CHOL/HDLC RATIO	4.9		<5.0 (CALC)	TP
PROTHROMBIN TIME WITH INR				TP
INTERNATIONAL NORMALIZED RATIO (INR)	2.7			

```
              SUGGESTED THERAPEUTIC RANGES USING INR
              FOR STABLY ANTICOAGULATED PATIENTS:

                  ROUTINE ORAL ANTICOAGULANT THERAPY                = 2.0- 3.0

                  ORAL ANTICOAGULANT THERAPY FOR PATIENTS WITH
                  THROMBOEMBOLIC EVENTS ON STANDARD DOSES OF
                  COUMADIN AND THOSE WITH MECHANICAL HEART VALVES    = 2.5- 3.5

                      INR REFERENCE INTERVAL APPLIES TO PATIENTS
                      NOT ON ANTICOAGULANT THERAPY:                    0.9- 1.1

                  SUGGESTED INR THERAPEUTIC RANGE FOR ORAL
                  ANTICOAGULANT THERAPY (STABLY ANTICOAGULATED
                  ANTICOAGULANT THERAPY (STABLY ANTICOAGULATED
                  PATIENTS)

                      ROUTINE THERAPY:                                 2.0- 3.0

                      RECURRENT MYOCARDIAL INFARCTION
                      OR MECHANICAL PROSTHETIC VALVES:                 2.5- 3.5
```

PROTHROMBIN TIME		25.0 H	9.0-11.5 SECONDS	

```
Patel, Raj - TP016756T
```

▶ **Figure 2-1 Scanned Image of Paper Lab Report.**

```
Raj Patel: M: 4/25/1928:

Doctor's Laboratory
3/10/2006 11:30AM

Tests
Blood Chemistry:                        Value           Normal Range
Total plasma cholesterol level          215 mg/dl        140 - 200
Plasma HDL cholesterol level             40 mg/dl         30 - 70
Plasma LDL cholesterol level             98 mg/dl         80 - 130
Total cholesterol/HDL ratio             5.4               4 - 6

Hematology:                             Value           Normal Range
INR                                     2.1              25 - 40
```

▶ **Figure 2-2 Results of Two Lab Tests in the Form of a Text File.**

Improved functionality of the EHR is achieved when the lab reports are received as codified data, in a standard format. This enables the computer to store the results by their test code, and the values of the results in their own fields. When data is stored in this manner the clinician can, of course, view the report in a format similar to the two previous examples. However, because the results are coded, the clinician can simultaneously compare values from several tests performed over a period of time.

Figure 2-3 provides an example of how data from multiple lab tests can be quickly extracted and graphed for the clinician. The value of the total

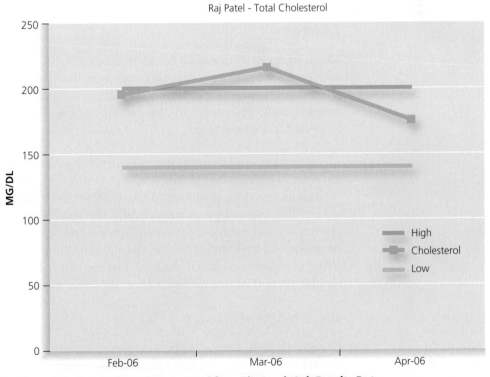

▶ **Figure 2-3 Graph of Total Cholesterol from Electronic Lab Results Data.**

cholesterol results over a 3-month period of time is trended with the green line. The reference ranges of normal values (High 200, Low 140) are shown in the graph as red and blue lines. Using a graph the clinician can easily see the trend of this patient's total cholesterol.

Lab tests are a good example of codified data because virtually every reference lab and every Laboratory Information System (LIS) codifies their tests and the components within the tests. (HDL and LDL are examples of components within the Total Cholesterol test, shown in the previous figures.)

Today, some labs use proprietary codes created by the lab, whereas other labs use codes based on a standard coding system called LOINC. LOINC stands for Logical Observation Identifier Names and Codes and will be discussed later in this chapter.

The benefit of codified data in the EHR is apparent from the lab results example. However, if the practice received results from multiple labs and the codes were not alike it would not be possible for the clinician to compare the results from two different labs on the same graph. Here then is the key point of this chapter:

EHR data stored in a machine-readable, codified form adds significant value, but using a national standard code set instead of proprietary codes to codify the data will better enable the exchange of medical records between systems, improve the accuracy of the content, and open the door to the functional benefits derived from having an electronic health record.

When EHR is stored as codified data using a set of standard codes, additional benefits can be realized. Two examples of expanded functionality to be gained from lab results are alerts and health maintenance.

Alerts

Alerts in an EHR are automatic messages to the clinician or other staff person. Alerts may simply be a warning message that pops up on the screen while the user is performing a particular action, or an alert can be an e-mail message automatically generated by the system. Some alert systems even have the ability to dial a doctor's pager.

Alerts are generated when the computer is programmed with a rule that looks for certain conditions. In lab tests, the computer can examine the value of test results as the data is stored in the EHR. If the values of specific components exceed the amount programmed into the rule, an alert is generated. Codified results are necessary for the computer to recognize which components should be examined and which rule is to be used. The lab results should be codified using a uniform national standard to ensure that the alert system can identify similar tests that are received from multiple labs.

Health Maintenance

Early detection, through preventative screening, helps patients live healthier lives. Preventative care systems, also known as health maintenance systems, generate reminders to the patient or clinician when tests are due. Using a sophisticated set of rules, the computer compares a list of the tests recommended for patients of a certain age and sex to the patient's medical history. It also calculates the time since the test was last performed and compares that to the recommended interval for repeat testing. If the system determines a test is due, a reminder is generated.

It would be difficult to create standardized rules for the preventative care system if the tests were not coded using a standardized coding system. It would be impossible to examine that data at all if labs were stored an image or text file of the tests. Health maintenance is one of the many functions of the EHR that requires codified computer data using a national standard.

This example illustrates how lab data can extend the functionality of the EHR. However, preventative care screening guidelines are not limited to lab tests; other examples include mammograms, hearing, and vision screening, as well as elements of the physical examination. To fully extend the EHR requires not only codified lab data but the rest of the medical record as well. This includes patient history, symptoms, chronic problems, previous exams, surgeries, medications, treatments, and other information.

Standard Coding Systems

Within medicine, there are many different words to describe the same symptom, condition, or observation. Additionally, clinicians often use short abbreviations to document their observations in a patient's chart. This makes it difficult to compare notes from one physician to another. To realize the full benefits of an EHR, it is necessary to record clinical information in a codified format instead of a text record. The more that the medical record can be codified, the more useful the data becomes to the clinician.

It is relatively easy for a medical practice to obtain and store lab results as computer data because the tests and components originate as codified data when a laboratory system processes the tests. However, other information in the medical record does not necessarily start out as codified. To capture this information as codified data requires a change in the process the clinician uses. It also requires adoption of a coding system.

To create an EHR that is able to receive, create, and compare medical information from numerous sources, it is necessary to adopt a coding system that is used by other providers, in other words, a national standard. The remainder of this chapter will examine the evolution of several prominent medical code sets, their applicability to the EHR, and the influence of governments on the adoption of national standard code sets.

Government Influence on Coding Standards

Although manufacturing and financial industries have created and voluntarily adopted standards of their own, the health care field has been slow to agree on and accept standard systems. As a result, the government has had more influence on the acceptance and adoption of national standards in health care than in other industries.

In the last two decades, it has often been the selection of a code set by the Centers for Medicare and Medicaid Services (CMS), its predecessor the Health Care

Financing Administration (HCFA), or the Food and Drug Administration (FDA) that forced the health care industry to some standard. The strongest government influence occurred when Congress included an Administrative Simplification Subsection in the 1996 Health Insurance Portability and Accountability Act (HIPAA).

Among other things, the HIPAA subsection required that nearly all participants in the health care system used standardized transactions and use standardized code sets within those transactions. The act went further by designating the National Committee on Vital and Health Statistics (NCVHS), an advisory panel within the U.S. Department of Health and Human Services (HHS), as the entity that would select national standards for HIPAA.

The U.S. government continues to influence the health care industry by taking leadership roles in other ways as well. In May 2004, then Secretary of the Department of Health and Human Services Tommy G. Thompson announced the adoption by federal agencies of national standards. A fact sheet from HHS reads: "HHS, with the Departments of Defense and Veterans Affairs, has worked aggressively to adopt health information standards for use by all federal health agencies. As part of the Consolidated Health Informatics initiative, the agencies have agreed to endorse 20 sets of standards to make it easier for information to be shared across agencies and serve as a model for the private sector."[1]

The largest of those projects, the U.S. Department of Defense's Composite Health Care System II (CHCS II), will serve as a rigorous test of concepts that can be applied to EHR systems in the private sector. The system enables physicians to record patient visits, test results, and diagnoses using a standardized nomenclature. It is being installed in 139 military medical centers.

Another agency leading by example is the Indian Health Service (IHS), which is implementing an electronic health record system for Native American Indians that permits the patients' health records to be accessed at any tribal health care facilities where they seek care. The IHS system also has been adopted by NASA.

CMS is funding a 2-year special study that is intended to demonstrate improvements in care to Medicare beneficiaries resulting from the use of Electronic Health Records in primary physician offices. The Doctors' Office Quality Information Technology (DOQ-IT) project aims to provide implementation, education, and quality improvement assistance for small to medium-sized physician offices migrating from paper charts to an EHR.

Similar government influence has occurred in the United Kingdom, where the National Health Service invested approximately £3.2 billion in a national electronic patient file. The EHR is intended to cover each British citizen from the cradle to the grave. The initiative includes information exchange between hospitals and general practitioners, as well as the participation in development of an international coding standard (discussed later).

---

[1]Department of Health and Human Services press office Fact Sheet, May 6, 2004.

Comparison of Prominent EHR Code Sets

Each code set that becomes a national standard does so because it was designed for a particular purpose and became widely adopted. Some code sets are used for billing and provide precise shorthand that identifies the exact service performed. Other code sets are classification systems used to codify medical records for research and analysis. A code set designed specifically to record medical observations is often referred to as a clinical "*nomenclature.*"

Nomenclature (from the Latin *nomenclatura*—a list of names) is a system of names used in a field of science, typically created by a recognized group or authority. In an EHR, the term is used for organized lists of medical phrases and codified to help to standardize the way clinicians record information. EHR nomenclatures are sometimes called clinical vocabularies or clinical terminologies. Using an EHR nomenclature provides consistency in patient records and improves communication between different medical specialties.

> **Note**

> ### Early Medical Nomenclature
>
> **How about Latin? For several centuries, European and American doctors were required to read and write Latin. The anatomical body, diseases, drugs, and organisms were given Latin names. A physician from any region could describe a medical finding with a precision that could be understood by any other physician.**

How EHR Nomenclatures Differ from Other Code Sets

EHR nomenclatures differ from other code sets and classification systems in several ways. They are designed to codify the details and nuance of the patient–clinician encounter. EHR nomenclatures are different from billing code sets in this aspect. For example, a procedure code used for billing an office visit does not describe what the clinician observed during the visit, just the type and complexity of the exam. EHR nomenclatures need to have a lot more codes to describe the details of the exam; for this reason, they are said to be more granular.

EHR nomenclatures have hundreds of thousands of codes to represent not only procedures and diseases but also the symptoms, observations, history, medications, and a myriad of other details. The level of granularity determines how fine a level of detail is represented by a code in the nomenclature.

However, too much granularity can make a code set difficult to use at the point of care. The point of care is when both the clinician and patient are present. Extremely granular code sets, called reference terminologies, are impractical for a clinician to use in an exam. Designed for data analysis, these code sets often are applied to the medical records after the fact for a specific research project.

To balance the need for granularity with the practical requirements of point of care documentation, EHR nomenclatures use the concept of "*findings*" or codified observations, which are medically meaningful to the clinician. Although some systems of clinical vocabulary are just "data dictionaries" that are used to standardize medical terms, EHR nomenclatures precorrelate those terms into clinically relevant *findings*.

For example, a clinical vocabulary will have the terms: eye, arm, leg, chest, nostril, left, right, red, yellow, radiating, discharge, and pain. These terms could be combined in many ways, some of them meaningless. *Findings* are less granular than individual terms but combine those terms in ways that are clinically relevant. For example, "chest pain radiating to the left arm" uses one coded *finding* to record five clinical terms as a meaningful symptom.

Findings are often linked to other findings, whereas codes in classification code sets are usually only related to the root code of the group the code is in.

For example, the *finding* abdominal pain is related to more than 550 diagnosis codes, whereas a specific diagnosis code for peptic ulcer is not related to any other diagnosis code.

Conversely in an EHR nomenclature the diagnostic finding peptic ulcer is related to 168 other findings (one of which is abdominal pain).

Linked or indexed findings in an EHR nomenclature enable clinicians to quickly locate related symptoms, elements of the physical exam, assessments, and treatments when documenting the visit.

EHR users tend to locate findings by the description, not by the code. EHR nomenclature code numbers are typically invisible to the user. In contrast, billing codes for procedures and diagnoses may be very familiar to the clinician. Procedure codes may be preprinted on encounter forms, and the clinician may write diagnosis codes on orders and encounter forms. But for findings in an EHR, the clinician neither knows nor cares what the code numbers are.

A feature unique to EHR nomenclatures is that they often include internal cross-references to other standard code sets. These tables help the EHR to communicate with other systems. Code sets not designed for an EHR do not typically contain a map to other code sets with their structure.

The following sections will provide a brief history and purpose of several of the most prominent coding standards you are likely to encounter or use in an EHR.

SNOMED CT®

SNOMED stands for Systemized Nomenclature of Medicine; CT stands for Clinical Terms. SNOMED CT is a medical nomenclature developed by the College of American Pathologists and United Kingdom's National Health Service. It is a merger of two previous coding systems, SNOMED and the Read codes.

The nomenclature had its origins in 1965 as Systemized Nomenclature of Pathology. It was subsequently expanded in 1974 and renamed SNOMED to reflect the inclusion of terms for a broad array of medical specialties. In 1993, further enhancement created a multidimensional, structured nomenclature for indexing medical diagnoses and treatments.

The granular nature of the coding system originally designed for pathology made it difficult to use in a real-time environment. In 1999, SNOMED RT was developed in conjunction with Kaiser Permanente to provide "a unified clinical terminology for health states, disease states, treatments, and outcomes." RT stands for Reference Terminology.

Meanwhile, in the United Kingdom, clinical codes were developed by Dr. James Read and were purchased for distribution by the U.K. National Health Service. The Read codes were subsequently renamed Clinical Terms Version 3. In 1999 an agreement was reached to combine the U.S. and U.K. coding systems into a unified global standard known as SNOMED CT, which had its first release in 2002.

Being international makes it unique among coding systems used in the United States. Not only is the nomenclature the result of a merger of U.S. and U.K. code sets, but also the nomenclature has been used in Germany, Iceland, the Netherlands, and Australia. SNOMED CT is also available in a Spanish language version.

In the United States, NCVHS recommended SNOMED CT as the general core terminology to support the patient medical record information. The NCVHS said: "The breadth of content, sound terminology model, and widely recognized value of SNOMED CT qualify it as a general-purpose terminology for the exchange, aggregation, and analysis of patient medical information. The broad scope of SNOMED CT itself and the inclusion within it of concepts from other important healthcare terminologies (including nursing) allow SNOMED CT to encompass much of the patient medical record information domain."

SNOMED CT includes cross-references to map SNOMED CT to other standard code sets discussed later in this chapter. These include: LOINC, ICD-10, ICD-O3, OPCS-4, CTV-3, SNOMED RT and includes nursing code sets: PNDS, NIC, NOC, NANDA, Clinical Care Classification, and the Omaha System.

SNOMED CT Structure The SNOMED CT Core terminology contains over 364,400 health care *concepts*, organized into 18 hierarchical categories. The data structure of SNOMED CT is complex. Concept names, descriptions, and synonyms number more than 984,000.

SNOMED Concepts have descriptions and Concept IDs (numeric codes). The concepts are arranged in the following hierarchies:

◆ Finding

◆ Disease

◆ Procedure and intervention

◆ Observable entity

◆ Body structure

◆ Organism

◆ Substance

◆ Pharmaceutical / biological product

◆ Specimen

◆ Physical object

◆ Physical force

◆ Events

◆ Environments and geographical locations

◆ Social context

◆ Context-dependent categories

◆ Staging and scales

◆ Attribute

◆ Qualifier value

SNOMED CT has approximately 1,450,000 semantic relationships in the nomenclature. There are two types of relationships between SNOMED CT concepts: *Is-A* relationships and *Attribute* relationships.

Is-A relationships connect concepts within a single hierarchy. For example, the disease concept Bronchial Pneumonia *Is-A* Pneumonia (also a disease concept).

Attribute relationships, however, connect concepts from two different hierarchies. For example, the disease concept Bronchial Pneumonia has the associated *Attribute* Inflammation (which is from a different hierarchy, morphology.)

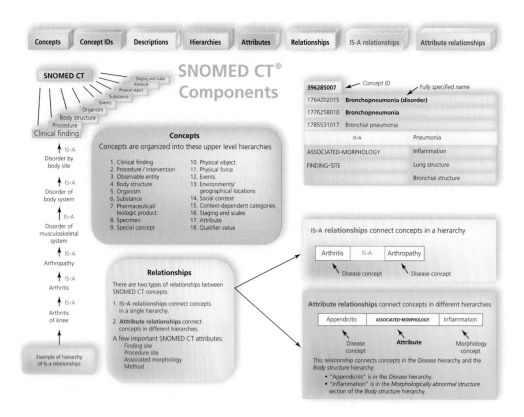

Used by permission of the College of American Pathologists.

▶ Figure 2-4 SNOMED CT Components.

SNOMED CT is often referred to as a "reference terminology." It provides very granular coding that normalizes data for research and reporting. Its structure provides millions of semantic links based on a term, word, or concept. Figure 2-4 illustrates many of the components of SNOMED CT, and provides examples of several ways in which relationships are defined. The concept IDs shown in the upper right portion of the figure are an example of SNOMED CT codes.

SNOMED has not historically been used for point-of-care exam notes. Since its selection as a core terminology by NCVHS, several commercial EHR software companies have stated they will incorporate SNOMED CT.

MEDCIN®

MEDCIN is a medical nomenclature and knowledge base developed by Medicomp Systems, Inc. in collaboration with physicians on staff at the Cornell, Harvard, Johns Hopkins, and other major medical centers. Development began in 1978 and the system was released in 1986. In 1997, the nomenclature codes and individual data elements were published as a national standard.

MEDCIN has been selected by NCVHS as an enabling standard because it enables the physician to create a complete electronic record at the time of the exam. NCVHS groups recommended coding standards into core standards and enabling standards.

A report to HHS Secretary Tommy Thompson stated: "The NCVHS asserts that compatibility of the core set of PMRI (Patient Medical Record Information) terminologies with these important related terminologies (specifically in the form of mappings) will enhance the value and accelerate the adoption of the PMRI terminology standards."[2]

MEDCIN includes cross-references to map MEDCIN to SNOMED CT as well as other standard code sets discussed later in this chapter. These include: ICD-9CM, CPT-4, LOINC, and RxNorm drug codes.

MEDCIN Structure The MEDCIN nomenclature consists of 270,000 clinical concepts or "*findings*" divided into six broad categories:

- Symptoms
- History
- Physical Examination
- Tests
- Diagnoses
- Therapy

Each finding has a numeric code up to seven digits in length.

MEDCIN differs from other EHR coding systems in that the nomenclature is not just a codified list of findings. The MEDCIN nomenclature is available in a "knowledge base" with a diagnostic index of more than 68 million links between clinically related findings. This "knowledge" enables an EHR system based on MEDCIN to quickly find other clinical "findings" that are likely to be needed; this in turn reduces the time it takes to create exam notes.

---

[2]NCVHS letter to the Secretary of Health and Human Services, November 5, 2003.

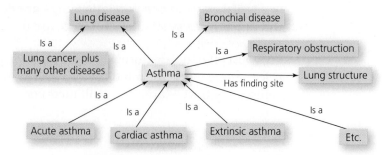

► Figure 2-5 SNOMED CT Links for the Term of "Asthma."

► Figure 2-6 MEDCIN Links
for the Term of "Asthma."

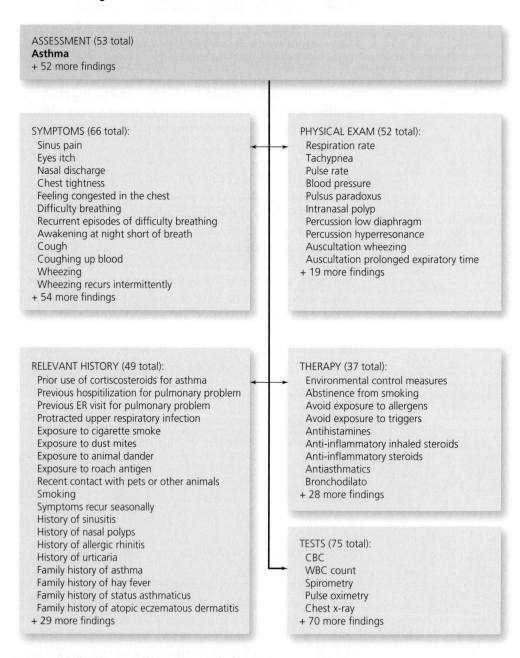

The purpose of the MEDCIN nomenclature and the intent of the design also differentiate it from other coding standards. Most of the other coding systems were designed to classify or index medical information for research or other purposes. MEDCIN was designed for point-of-care usage by the clinician so each "finding" represents a meaningful clinical observation or term.

This difference means a physician selects less individual codes to complete the patient exam note. For example, SNOMED CT has a code for "arm" and a code for "pain," MEDCIN has a "finding" for "arm pain." MEDCIN often has additional findings that infer important nuances, for example, the "finding" for "arm tenderness" might more accurately describe the patient's symptom than arm pain.

Figure 2-5 and Figure 2-6 compare the structure of SNOMED CT and MEDCIN using the finding for asthma. As you can see from the comparison, the MED-CIN knowledge base relates Asthma to 279 total direct links (only 70 are shown in Figure 2-6). Each of these has relevancy to point-of-care use for an asthma patient. SNOMED CT links include obvious links to asthma but not directly to the symptoms, tests, or therapy. Links in Figure 2-5 also connect to lungs and other lung diseases not related to asthma. Such associations are sometimes useful when coding records for research but can make it difficult for the clinician to use such a system while seeing the patient.

The MEDCIN knowledge base also includes 600,000 synonyms for findings allowing a finding to be looked up by several different terms. The MEDCIN knowledge base wraps each finding selected by the clinician with readable narrative text. EHR applications using the MEDCIN nomenclature can store medical information as coded data elements and still generate readable exam notes from the same data.

Many experts feel that for point-of-care documentation medical nomenclatures such as MEDCIN are the key to successful adoption of an EHR by clinicians. MEDCIN is used in many commercial EHR systems as well as the Department of Defense CHCS II system (discussed earlier in this chapter). Because of this, MEDCIN has been selected as the EHR nomenclature for the student exercises in this textbook. You will learn more about MEDCIN in subsequent chapters of this book.

LOINC®

LOINC stands for Logical Observation Identifier Names and Codes. LOINC is an important clinical terminology for laboratory test orders and results such as blood hemoglobin, serum potassium, and so on, as well as other clinical observations such as vital signs or EKG.

LOINC was created and is maintained by the Regenstrief Institute, which is closely affiliated with the Indiana University School of Medicine. LOINC was first released in 1995 and has become one of the standards designated by the U.S. government for the electronic exchange of clinical health information. By 2003, the LOINC database contained codes for more than 30,000 observations.

LOINC is important because most laboratories and other diagnostic services currently report test results using their own internal, proprietary codes. When an EHR receives results from multiple lab facilities, comparing the results electronically is like comparing apples and oranges. LOINC provides a universal coding system for mapping laboratory tests and results to a common terminology in the EHR. This then makes it possible for a computer program to find and report comparable test values regardless of where the test was processed.

Courtesy of Regenstrief
Institute Medical Informatics.

▶ **Figure 2-7 Scope of
LOINC Laboratory Terms.**

Laboratory LOINC scope	
Class	No. of terms
Antibiotic susceptibilities	1166
Allergy	2629
Blood bank	687
Chemistry	5681
Chemistry Challenges	1970
Coagulation	444
Cytology	49
Drug & toxicology	4900
Fertility	172
Flow cytometry cell markers	774
Hematology cell count	1386
HLA	346
Microbiology	7487
Molecular pathology	617
Pathology	158
Serology	947
Skin tests	38
Urinalysis	208

The LOINC terminology is divided into three portions, laboratory, clinical (non-laboratory), and HIPAA. The largest number of codes is in the laboratory section, which contains codes in 14 categories. Figure 2-7 shows a complete list of laboratory classes in LOINC and the number of terms in each class.

The second largest section of LOINC is the clinical section, which includes codes for vital signs, EKG, ultrasound, cardiac echo, and many other clinical observations.

A third section of LOINC has been created to categorize codes for a HIPAA claims attachment transaction. Claims attachments are used to provide additional information to support an insurance claim. Six types of attachments have been defined so far:

1. Laboratory reports

2. Nonlaboratory clinical reports

3. Ambulance transport

4. Emergency room visits

5. Medications

6. Rehabilitation

The wide acceptance of LOINC is due in part to its adoption by HL7 (discussed in Chapter 1). HL7 uses LOINC codes in its clinical messages. When HL7 was selected to write the HIPAA standard for claim attachments, LOINC codes were used. When the claim attachment contained laboratory or clinical results, the LOINC codes already existed, but for other types of attachments new codes had to be created.

Earlier in this chapter, we discussed trending lab results. To create a report comparing lab results from multiple labs, EHR systems must store lab data with the same coding standard. For this purpose, the LOINC standard is ideal.

The largest national laboratories, Quest and LabCorp have mapped their internal codes to LOINC and will include LOINC codes in their HL-7 messages. Many smaller labs are also sending LOINC codes. This means as results are received electronically they can be stored by the EHR using a standardized nomenclature. However, if a laboratory does not send LOINC codes, then the EHR system must do the mapping. To help with this, Regenstrief Institute provided a free software program called RELMA™, which has encouraged further adoption as a standard.

LOINC has been adopted as a standard coding system not only by national and regional laboratories but also by public health departments, the U.S. Centers for Disease Control (CDC), the Veterans Administration, and other standards organizations such as Clinical Data Interchange Standards Consortium (CDISC), which is used for clinical trial studies. LOINC is also being used in the Digital Imaging and Communication in Medicine (DICOM) standard for ultrasound messages. Both SNOMED CT and MEDCIN contain cross-references to LOINC codes.

UMLS®

UMLS stands for Unified Medical Language System® from the National Library of Medicine (NLM). Because students may find mention of UMLS elsewhere, it is included here. However, UMLS is not itself a medical terminology but, rather, a resource of software tools and data created from many medical nomenclatures including those described in this chapter. To quote the NLM, "The purpose of UMLS is to facilitate the development of computer systems that behave as if they 'understand' the meaning of the language of biomedicine and health."

Although UMLS is not a "standard" itself, it does serve as a repository for the coordination of many medical terminologies. UMLS was developed to index medical literature. It can be used to retrieve and integrate biomedical information and provides a cross-reference between medical vocabularies. UMLS began in 1986 and currently includes 30 medical terminologies and classification schemes.

Nursing Code Sets

Thirteen standards for nursing codes are recognized by the American Nurses Association today for use in the assessment, diagnosis, interventions, and outcomes of nursing care. Some of these are listed here.

NANDA Taxonomy II NANDA stands for the North American Nursing Diagnosis Association. Taxonomy means a system of classification. The Nursing Diagnosis code set standardizes 167 nursing diagnostic concepts. These identify and code a patient's responses to health problems or life processes that explain variance in patient outcomes that is different than the variance explained by disease diagnoses.

According to NANDA, Nursing Diagnosis represents "a clinical judgment about individual, family, or community responses to actual or potential health problems/life processes. Nursing diagnoses provide the basis for selection of nursing interventions to achieve outcomes for which the nurse is accountable."[3]

NANDA facilitates oral and written nursing communications and the process of assessing and treating the nursing diagnosis. It facilitates the development of

---

[3]NANDA Nursing Diagnosis: Definitions and Classifications 1992–1993, p. 5, by NANDA Staff, North American Nursing Diagnosis Association, Philadelphia, PA.

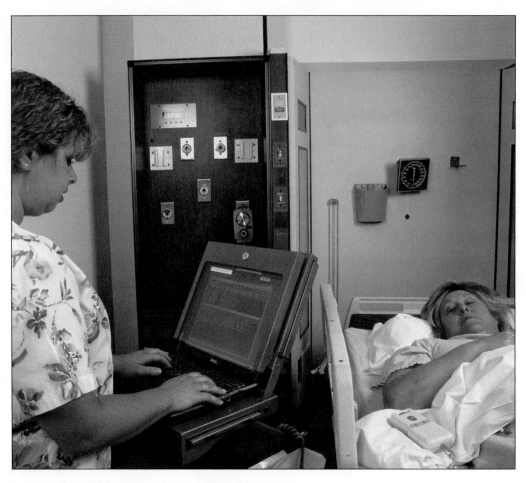

▶ Figure 2-8 Hospital Nurse Entering Chart in Computer.

computerized patient records and the collection, retrieval, and analysis of nursing data for education and research.

NIC NIC stands for Nursing Interventions Classification. It is a code set designed for documenting nursing interventions in any clinical settings. An intervention is defined as "any treatment, based upon clinical judgment and knowledge that a nurse performs to enhance patient/client outcomes." NIC was first published in 1992 and is updated every 4 years.

The system consists of numeric codes for 514 interventions that span all nursing specialties. The codes are grouped into 30 classes and 7 domains. The seven domains are: Basic Physiological, Complex Physiological, Behavioral, Safety, Family, Health System, and Community. NIC is used at the point of care to document care planning and nursing practices.

NOC NOC stands for Nursing Outcomes Classification and includes a comprehensive list of nursing outcomes. It is used to document the effect of nursing interventions on patient progress. Nursing Outcomes are the end result of care. NOC can be used to measure the quality of care, cost efficiency, and progress of treatment.

The system consists of numeric codes for 330 outcomes (311 individual, 10 family, and 9 community level outcomes). The codes are grouped into 31 classes and 7 domains. The seven domains are: Functional Health, Physiologic Health, Psychosocial Health, Health Knowledge & Behavior, Perceived Health, Family Health, and Community Health.

NIC and NOC codes were developed at the University of Iowa College of Nursing and are maintained by The Center for Nursing Classification and Clinical Effectiveness located there. NIC was developed by Gloria M. Bulechek and Joanne C. McCloskey. NOC was developed by Sue Moorhead, Marion Johnson, and Meridean L. Maas. The copyrights of both nursing classifications are owned by the publisher, Elsevier Science.

CCC Clinical Care Classification system (CCC) was developed by Virginia Saba at Georgetown University. It can be used to document patient care in hospitals, home health agencies, ambulatory care clinics, and other health care settings. Developed from government funded research, it was formerly known as the Home Health Care Classification system, but CCC is now considered applicable to clinical care as well as other health care services. The codes are alphanumeric, five characters long.

The CCC system provides standardized coding concepts for nursing diagnoses, outcomes, nursing interventions and actions in two interrelated taxonomies. CCC Nursing Diagnosis adds about 50 new concepts to NANDA. CCC Nursing Interventions codify 21 care components that cover the functional, health behavioral, physiological, and psychological aspects of patient care.

Omaha System The Omaha System is a standardized terminology recognized by the American Nurses Association. It has been in development since the 1970s and is one of the oldest systems for nursing documentation. It often is used in community base nursing such as visiting nursing associations.

The Omaha System is made up of three components: the Problem Classification Scheme, the Intervention Scheme, and the Problem Rating Scale for Outcomes. These are used to document the assessment, the interventions, and the outcomes.

The terms, codes, and definitions of the Omaha System are not copyrighted; however, it is usually implemented using two authoritative books that describe the system. Both books are written by Karen S. Martin, who has been involved with the development of the system since 1978.

The Omaha System is included in some of the standards discussed earlier in this chapter. These include the UMLS, SNOMED CT, and LOINC.

ICNP® ICNP stands for International Classification for Nursing Practice. It is the result of a project by International Council of Nurses, to create an organizing structure into which other nursing terminologies can be mapped. It was intended to facilitate the comparison of nursing data gathered from multiple systems. However, ICNP has evolved into a separate coding system attempting to unify other systems.

ICNP uses numeric codes to represent concepts in three areas: nursing diagnosis that ICNP calls Nursing Phenomenon, interventions that ICNP calls Nursing Actions, and outcomes.

A Real-Life Story

A Nurse's Notes

By Sharyl Beal, RN

Sharyl Beal is a Registered Nurse with a Master's degree in Nursing and a subspecialty in Nursing Informatics. She served as a nurse and a department head for 16 years. In her current position as Clinical Systems Analyst, she has been involved in creating and implementing electronic medical records for the nursing and ancillary departments at a 500-bed hospital in the Midwest.

Our hospital has successfully transitioned all nursing units to computerized patient charts. We rolled it out very slowly, one unit at a time, taking 3 years to implement all the areas. Today, all inpatient units are online including our behavioral health units. We don't print nursing reports, everyone works online. These are some of my experiences and observations from this project.

We did med/surg first because it is the broadest definition and fits the majority of patients. With that model in operation, we could go to the next unit and say "with this as a model what do we need to do to make it work for you." We did a fair amount of redesign as we added units, but sometimes they were minor things like adding descriptors that hadn't been necessary for another unit.

The first thing we did for each department was to spend considerable time flow-charting all their processes; how they get their patients, how they communicate about their patients, with whom, what it looks like. We created a "life in the day of" scenario for every skill level in the unit; then we designed their charting based on their patient population.

The last unit to go online was Behavioral Health. Behavioral Health was challenging because their charts contain more abstract observations describing mental reactions, emotional reactions, etc. But the most problematic unit was the Obstetrics Department.

OB charting is not difficult, but it is very meticulous. Our OB Department had a lot of rules and regulations about what had to be charted, and how it was to be worded. The hospital legal department had to review all of our designs before the nurses could begin using them, they then reviewed samples of what was actually being documented once the department went online. We had to do some redesign to let the nurses better describe things but we finally got it to everyone's satisfaction.

That was our design process; implementation was another matter. Our methodology of bringing one unit online at a time allowed us to provide plenty of support when the unit went online. I think that was key. Clinical Informatics personnel were scheduled in shifts that overlapped the nursing shifts. We were in the unit, with the nurses, 24 hours a day for the first 2 weeks. Whenever new users were struggling someone was right at their elbow to calmly guide them through, to make sure they were successful. Even with that level of support, there were some things that remained constant through the last unit of the rollout.

Nurses are very accustomed to being in control, confident in their expertise and their skills; when their department becomes computerized, all of a sudden everything they know has to be translated through the limitations of a computer. The most common reaction when we rolled out charting into a new unit was that the nurses were extremely apprehensive their first day of charting. The universal complaint was that they couldn't sleep the night before.

My experience was that at the end of the first day they were still not feeling good about it, but when they came back the second day they had figured out how to get through it and they had very few questions. By the third day, they were usually doing very well. They still didn't feel good about finding the information, but they knew they could do it.

The nurses' biggest fear was that they would spend all their time taking care of the computer instead of their patients. They verbalized that idea for months afterwards, but that really isn't reality. Research has repeatedly shown that nurses spend 50% to 70% of their time documenting. Nurses already spend an enormous amount of their work life documenting, but it takes them a long time to feel like they are spending less time on the computer than on their patients.

The real issue was that they felt like they were cut off from the information; they couldn't just flip open a chart and see something. They had to remember how to find it and that was time out of their day. I have had them cry; I have had them yell, venting their frustration. But the good part was that they were all in the same boat together so their peers readily understood what they were going through because they were all going through it together.

The nurses who had the easiest time transitioning were nurses who were accustomed to taking the time to write everything down as they went through their workday. The majority of nurses don't do that. Most nurses have notes stuffed in their pockets and tons of information in their head. They tend to store it up and write it all down when they come back from lunch at the end of their shift. When

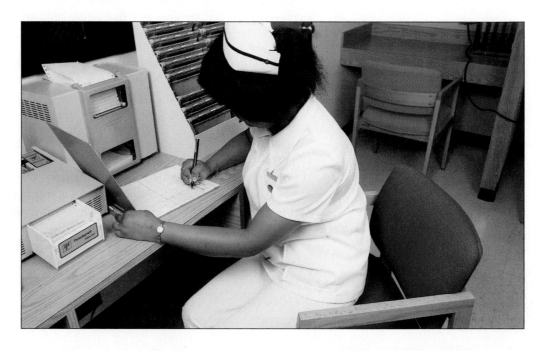

they try to follow that same model with a computer, but they are not yet comfortable with the computer, it is twice as hard because they have a lot to remember and they have to figure out what to do with it. Nurses who normally charted as their day progressed didn't have to remember as much so they seem to learn faster.

In nursing school you have to chart as it happens—the instructor is going to insist. This meant that nurses who just came out of nursing school had an advantage because they came to the job with good habits. Additionally, most of the new nurses grew up with computers and were more familiar with them.

We found that the ancillary departments, respiratory therapy, physical therapy, dietary, etc., were also easy to implement. Their documentation is much more concrete, limited in its focus, so it was much easier to adapt from paper to computer. They were almost self-sufficient from the very beginning.

The doctors, however, were another group. You have to spend time up front making sure the doctors can get the information, and most doctors cannot give up enough time in their day to learn a computer. The nurses trained for 8 hours for the computer but the doctors only for about 15 minutes. We balanced this by trying to be attentive to any doctor who came on the floor. We would often say, "Let me help you find the information. The nurses are now charting on the computer. As of today you are not going to find that information on a piece of paper. We don't print anything." The doctors have adapted to the readily available information so well that on the rare occasion when we have downtime, it is usually the physicians who are the most upset.

One thing I think is important is that the nursing leadership really dedicates time to learning the system so they are fully on board with why you are doing it and the benefits of it. Then when their staff is apprehensive or when the physicians are frustrated because the nurses haven't charted there is reinforcement from the management that computerized charting is an expectation.

The point was illustrated in two of the units we rolled out. In one unit, the leadership was very computer savvy and expected their staff to do well. They held reinforcing in-service programs every 10 days and they would have us talk about specific areas where they thought their staff was weak in charting. Because the nurse manager was so proactive, that whole area adapted very easily and as a result the physicians adapted very easily.

In another unit where the nurse manager was not very computer savvy the manager's apprehension was reinforcing to the staff. So it was very hard on our team to support them. Even though they have now been up a long time there is still a core group of people who just don't get it, because they don't have to get it.

One final benefit of an involved leadership is that it results in better charting. When we did the first units the implementation team spent a lot of time reading the documentation for quality, seeing if the nurses forgot to chart something, etc. However, as the rollout continued throughout the hospital, the implementation team couldn't really spend a lot of time reviewing. You really need the people who know the patient population of the unit, the leaders, the managers, or supervisors to be spending some time each day randomly selecting charts created by their nurses, reading them, and helping their nurses understand if they aren't doing it thoroughly enough. This not only improves the quality of the charts but also helps the staff get better at it quickly.

One factor that differentiates ICNP from other systems is that it has merged the two different taxonomies used for nursing diagnosis and nursing interventions into one classification, which can be used to represent diagnoses, interventions, and outcomes.

ICNP has only had limited implementation in the field, as Version 1 was just released in 2005.

NMDS NMDS stands for Nursing Minimum Data Set and is the result of conferences held at the University of Illinois College of Nursing in Chicago in 1977 and at the University of Wisconsin-Milwaukee School of Nursing in 1985. Originally developed by Harriet Werley and Norma Lang, it was, as the name suggests, an attempt to define the minimum set of basic data elements for nursing in a computerized patient record.

The NMDS includes the label and conceptual definition of those essential, specific elements that are used on a regular basis by the majority of nurses in types of settings. The elements are arranged into three categories: nursing care, patient or client demographics, and service elements.

The NMDS is intended to standardize the collection of essential nursing data and can be used to capture nursing data for comparison of patient outcomes.

PNDS PNDS stands for Perioperative Nursing Data Set and was developed by the Association of Perioperative Registered Nurses in the early 1990s. Like other nursing systems, it codifies nursing diagnoses, interventions, and outcomes, but this system is focused the special needs and level of detail required to document perioperative nursing.

PNDS is used by nurses in hospital perioperative settings to document the patient experience from preadmission to discharge. PNDS consists of 74 nursing diagnoses, 133 nursing interventions, and 28 nurse-sensitive patient outcomes. PNDS is being incorporated into SNOMED CT.

PCDS PCDS stands for Patient Care Data Set. The Patient Care Data Set was developed by Judy Ozbolt at the University of Virginia as a comprehensive catalog of terms used in patient care records at nine hospitals. PCDS was officially adopted as one of the standards by the American Nurses Association in 1998.

PCDS is different from the other classifications that have been previously described. Where CCC was based on home care nursing, the Omaha System on community based nursing, and PNDS on perioperative needs, PCDS has a much stronger acute care origin. PCDS also includes 200 more terms used by nurses in acute care settings than NANDA.

The system consists of terms for 363 problems, 311 goals, and 1357 patient care orders. PCDS is organized into 22 care components (the CCC components plus one as Immunology and Metabolism were divided into separate components). However, "the Patient Care Data Set has been developed primarily not as a classification system for clinical terms but as a data dictionary defining elements to be included in and abstracted from clinical information systems."[4]

---

[4]Multiple Attributes for Patient Care Data: Toward a Multiaxial, Combinatorial Vocabulary, Judy G. Ozbolt, Ph.D., R.N., 1997.

SNOMED CT As mentioned earlier, SNOMED CT incorporates several of the standard nursing code sets discussed here. It also may overlap the same concepts as several other nursing code sets, but it has not widely been adopted as a replacement for any of the existing nursing codes. It is hoped that will change.

Mary Kass, M.D., President of the College of American Pathologists, has stated "SNOMED CT facilitates efficiency and interoperability between the NANDA, NIC, and NOC mappings adding a critical dimension to the nursing documentation systems at the point of care—where it is needed most. These relationships help to increase the accuracy of clinical documentation and communication thus reducing potential medical errors associated with traditional paper records."[5]

How EHR Code Sets Differ from Billing Code Sets

Code sets that have been created or adapted for business purposes are not suitable for codifying electronic medical records. They are either too general—simply reporting a service that was rendered or a condition that was diagnosed—or in the case of drug codes they are too specific to be used for writing a prescription.

If you have worked in a medical facility you may already be familiar with several standard coding sets used for medical billing and pharmacy orders. Three of these are CPT-4, Current Procedural Terminology, ICD-9CM, International Classification of Diseases (ninth revision), and NDC, National Drug Codes. The following discussion of these and other billing code sets will cover the history, purpose, and importance of each. Examples will illustrate why these code sets are not used to code EHR data.

CPT-4®

CPT stands for Current Procedural Terminology. The numeral "4" represents the fourth edition of the coding system. CPT-4 codes are standardized codes for reporting medical services, procedures, and treatments performed for patients by the medical staff. CPT was created in 1966 by the American Medical Association to provide a uniform nomenclature that accurately identified medical, surgical, and diagnostic services.

Though originally shorter, the codes today are numeric, five digits long. A two-digit modifier is added for certain billing conditions. For example, when two surgeons are billing for the same surgery, a modifier is used to indicate the assistant surgeon.

In 1983, CPT-4 codes became standard for private insurance, Medicare, and Medicaid claims when it was adopted by the government as part of the Healthcare Common Procedure Coding System (HCPCS). CPT-4 expanded to include generic codes that covered almost any service that needed to be billed, but it did not include codes for billable supplies. Therefore, HCPCS II codes were created for billing supplies, injectable medications, and blood products.

---

[5]College of American Pathologists news release, January 25, 2005.

Subsequently, various state Medicaid programs as well as private insurance companies were allowed to add codes (designated HCPCS III) that were not part of CPT-4. These were often "local codes" used by only one plan or in one region. This created nonstandardization in the HCPCS code set.

Today, CPT-4 is the most widely accepted medical nomenclature used to report medical procedures and services to health insurance programs. CPT-4 is generally used in every medical office and ambulatory care setting because it is required for claim processing. Local codes have been eliminated from HCPCS and differences between state Medicaid codes have been resolved primarily because of HIPAA legislation that required the adoption of national standards. HCPCS and CPT-4 became designated code sets under HIPAA.

Note

E&M codes will be covered in depth in Chapter 5.

However, CPT-4 is not a very satisfactory nomenclature for an EHR. Its primary purpose is billing. As such, it provides a very uniform method of identifying a procedure or service but it does not provide much detail as to what occurred during that procedure. In the simplest example, certain CPT-4 codes are used to report patient examinations performed in hospitals, physician offices, and elsewhere. These are known as Evaluation & Management (E&M) codes, which are used to represent the extent to which the patient was examined and the amount of time the provider spent with the patient. However, no information can be gleaned from an E&M code as to which body systems were examined or what the findings were.

ABC

ABC codes are alternative medicine billing codes created to meet the need for codes to document and bill for alternative types of care which are not addressed by other coding standards. Providers such as acupuncturists, Ayurvedic doctors, behavioral health care workers, chiropractors, homeopaths, body workers, massage therapists, midwives, naturopaths, nurses, nutritionists, Oriental medicine practitioners, social workers, somatic educators, and others did not have sufficient codes to adequately describe their services.

ABC codes are similar in structure to CPT-4 codes but are not part of the CPT or HCPCS code sets. The codes are alphanumeric, five characters long, and allow a two-character modifier.

ABC codes are accepted as billing codes only by some payers. Because of a somewhat complex HIPAA rule, ABC codes are currently valid in HIPAA transactions with about 10,000 entities who registered to use them before May 29, 2003. They are valid in all paper transactions. ABC codes are expected to be adopted officially in 2006 as a subset of the existing HCPCS codes.

ICD-9CM

ICD stands for International Classification of Diseases, which is a system of standardized codes developed collaboratively between the World Health Organization (WHO) and 10 international centers. The coding system today evolved from the International List of Causes of Death, which was used by physicians, medical examiners, and coroners to facilitate standardized mortality studies. In 1948, WHO expanded and renamed the system to make it useful for codifying patient medical conditions as well.

The numeral "9" represents the ninth revision of the coding system, which has been revised about every 10 years from 1900 to 1979. By the time the ninth revision was published, the United States National Center for Health Statistics began to modify the statistical study with clinical information.

The letters "CM" stand for Clinical Modification. Clinical modifications provided a way to codify the clinical information about the health of a patient beyond that needed for statistical reports. In daily usage, the full acronym ICD-9CM is often just referred to as ICD-9.

With the addition of Clinical Modifications the codes became useful for indexing medical records, medical case reviews, and communicating a patient's condition more precisely. However, they took on even greater importance in 1989 when Congress made them mandatory on Part B Medicare claims. Other insurance programs followed suit, and ICD-9CM codes became required by insurance carriers to process (outpatient) claims.

ICD-9CM is currently published in three volumes. The first two volumes provide a listing and an index of diagnosis codes. The third volume, however, lists codes for hospital inpatient procedures.

The diagnosis codes are three characters, followed by a decimal point and up to two numerals. The first three characters of an ICD-9CM code identify the primary diagnosis; the two digits to the right of the decimal point further refine the diagnosis specificity.

Insurance billing allows for the use of multiple ICD-9CM codes for a single procedure, indicating one code as the primary diagnosis and additional codes as secondary conditions for which the treatment was done. Today, insurance reimbursement is tied to the proper use of ICD-9CM codes, in the proper order (of primary, secondary, etc.), and at the right level of specificity (number of decimal places).

The historical intent of the ICD was to classify similar causes of mortality and disease conditions into statistical reportable data. When it became required for insurance billing, the code set had to be further modified. The problem was if an ICD-9CM code was required for an insurance claim, but the patient was perfectly healthy, what code should be used? To solve this problem, ICD-9CM added a section of codes that start with the letter "V." These indicate nonillness conditions that can be used for billing.

If a coding system is already an international standard and already codifies most known medical conditions, why wouldn't it make a satisfactory system for an Electronic Health Record? When codifying medical information for statistical analysis or billing, ICD-9CM classifications are ideal. However, when recording medical findings about an individual, EHR data should be meaningfully specific. For example, a pediatrician might use the code "V20.20 Well-Child Check-up" when submitting a claim for a child's exam. Obviously, that code does not communicate anything about the child's size, growth rate, disposition, or demeanor.

Even when the ICD-9CM codifies details about a particular condition, the code may be too general for the EHR. An example of this is Asthma. The National

Institute of Health recommends that physicians classify patients with this condition as follows:

Asthma Mild Intermittent

Asthma Mild Persistent

Asthma Moderate Persistent

Asthma Severe Persistent

Each of these aspects of Asthma has specific criteria, but the ICD-9CM cannot express the important differentiations. Compare the IOM list with the ICD9-CM codes in Figure 2-9.

Code	Description
493.00	Extrinsic asthma, unspecified
493.01	Extrinsic asthma- with status asthmaticus
493.02	Extrinsic asthma, with (acute) exacerbation
493.10	Intrinsic asthma, unspecified
493.11	Intrinsic asthma- with status asthmaticus
493.12	Intrinsic asthma, with (acute) exacerbation
493.20	Chronic obstructive asthma, unspecified
493.21	Chronic obstructive asthma- with status asthmaticus
493.22	Chronic obstructive asthma, with (acute) exacerbation
493.81	Exercise induced bronchospasm
493.82	Cough variant asthma
493.90	Asthma, unspecified, unspecified
493.91	Asthma, unspecified- with status asthmaticus
493.92	Asthma, unspecified, with (acute) exacerbation

▶ **Figure 2-9 ICD-9CM Codes for Asthma.**

Another issue is that ICD-9CM codes do not distinguish between a code used to indicate the patient has a disease, or a clinician using the code to indicate that the diseased is "ruled out." In other words, there are no modifiers or qualifiers to the code. ICD-9CM codes will be discussed further in Chapter 5.

ICD-10

ICD-10 is the latest Revision to the International Classification of Diseases. It was released by WHO in 1992 and is used broadly in Europe and Canada. ICD-10 contains about twice as many categories as ICD-9 and uses more alphanumeric codes. Effective January 1, 1999, ICD-10 officially was implemented in the United States for reporting the cause of death on death certificates. It has not been implemented, and should not be used in place of ICD-9CM for reporting diagnosis on insurance claims.

Just as clinical modifications were added to ICD-9 codes to create ICD-9CM, work is now underway to add clinical modifications to ICD-10 to produce ICD-10CM. However, even when the work is completed, industry-wide transition to Revision 10 will require considerable time and effort. In the 20 years since the creation of ICD-9CM, nearly all medical practices and insurance plans have become computerized. Their systems contain coding and claim adjudication rules based on ICD-9CM, which will have to be modified before ICD-10 can be implemented as a standard. The clinical modifications in ICD-10CM will include only Volumes 1 and 2 (the diagnosis codes).

ICD-10PCS Hospitals use Volume 3 of ICD-9CM for coding inpatient procedures. It has been proposed that the Volume 3 procedure codes be replaced by a new Procedure Coding System called ICD-10-PCS. These procedure codes are not technically part of, nor derived in any way from, the ICD-10; only the name is similar. These codes were created by 3M Health Information Systems under a contract with Medicare. The ICD-10PCS codes are seven-digit alphanumeric codes and are intended to provide better codification of any underlying issues affecting a procedure performed.

There is some resistance to adopting the ICD-10PCS partly because it would have the same impact on computerized billing and claim systems, as discussed earlier. However, there is an even stronger concern by the AMA that ICD-10PCS would replace the CPT-4 codes, becoming the single coding standard for all procedures (inpatient and outpatient).

NDC and Other Drug Codes

NDC stands for National Drug Code. The NDC was originally created for out-of-hospital drug reimbursement under Medicare. However, in 1973 the FDA began maintaining a list of all drugs prepared or sold by registered drug companies. The NDC became the standard identifier for human drugs.

Each drug product listed by the FDA is assigned a unique 10-digit number. This includes all prescription and certain over-the-counter, insulin, domestic, and foreign drug products that are distributed in the United States. The 10-digit code is divided into three segments:

The first segment, the vendor or labeler code, is assigned by the FDA to the firm that manufactures, repacks, or distributes a drug product.

The second segment is the product code. It identifies a specific strength, dosage form, and formulation. The product codes are assigned by the firm.

The third segment, the package code, identifies package size. The package codes also are assigned by the firm.

NDC codes are used by the FDA for registration of drugs as well as by pharmacies and drug supply companies for ordering; however, the codes are not very useful for patients' charts or physicians to write prescriptions.

Whereas the CPT-4, and ICD-9CM codes are too general to adequately record detailed medical findings, the NDC has the opposite problem. Because the NDC is specific to a manufacturer, product, and even the size container in which the pharmacy purchases it, a physician cannot use the NDC to record a prescription.

Additionally, the lengths of the three segments which make up the NDC exist in three different configurations: 4–4–2, 5–3–2, or 5–4–1. In an attempt to normalize the numbers for their systems, some agencies treat the code as an 11-digit code instead of a 10-digit code by inserting a zero into the shortest of the 3 segments. Compare the two columns in Figure 2-10. Notice how the numbers were changed in the right column.

NDC Numbers	Modified NDC (Preceding Zero)
4444-4444-22	04444-4444-22
55555-333-22	55555-0333-22
55555-4444-1	55555-4444-01

▶ Figure 2-10 Comparison of NDC Codes and Modified.

Unfortunately, this attempt to normalize the lengths of the codes makes the drug codes "nonstandard." In fact, the modified codes would be invalid to a system that actually used NDC codes in their native form.

It is fair to say that the NDA drug codes, although useful in the drug business for inventory or FDA tracking, are not useful for prescription writing. Two federal projects are attempting to create codes more useful to the EHR. These are RxNorm and NDF-RT.

RxNorm RxNorm is a nonproprietary vocabulary being developed by the National Library of Medicine that represents drugs at the level of granularity needed to support clinical practice. RxNorm is available through the UMLS.

NDF-RT NDF-RT is a nonproprietary terminology being developed by the Department of Veterans Affairs (VA) that classifies drugs by mechanism of action and physiologic effect. NDF-RT is currently in use by the VA.

Proprietary systems of drug codes created by commercial businesses for their drug utilization review products are by far the most common drug codes found today in EHR systems. The companies include First Databank, Micromedex, MediSpan, and Multum. However, not one of them could be called a national standard because of the proprietary ownership of their code sets.

Conclusion

Does this mean that the Electronic Health Record does not use the CPT-4, ICD-9CM, or other standard codes? No, at this stage in the evolution of the EHR, dual coding systems are necessary. Today's EHR systems use complex cross-reference tables that allow the provider to record the patient's medical exam in accurate detail using an EHR nomenclature the EHR system then calculates CPT-4 and ICD-9CM codes for billing.

Similarly, prescriptions are often written for brand-name drugs. Then the pharmacy system matches it by generic name to the drug actually dispensed. It is not until the drug is dispensed that the NDC code is assigned (because the code is specific to the company that packaged the drug and the size of the package).

Nursing codes provide a clear example of the state of coding standards today. There are 13 different code sets officially recognized by the ANA. Most of the code sets cover the same aspects of nursing as the others, and many of them actually cross-reference one or more of the other nursing code sets.

A structured nomenclature as a codified standard is necessary to the evolution of a truly useful EHR. Human language, even medical language, has too many ways to say the same thing. Computers can provide timely alerts, trend analysis, health maintenance schedules, and interaction checking, to name only a few benefits of a true EHR. However, to do so, the symptoms, observations, drugs, interventions, outcomes, and all aspects of the chart must be recorded precisely, with consistent codes. If the medical record is codified using a standard EHR nomenclature, then it is possible to cross-reference the EHR codes to other code sets for billing or research studies.

Chapter Two Summary

The EHR was defined earlier as the portions of the patient's medical record stored in the computer system as well as the functional benefits derived from having an electronic health record. However, the form in which the the patient records are stored will affect the ability to achieve that extended functionality.

EHR data may be stored in several forms. The type of format the data is stored in determines to what extent the data can be used dynamically by the computer to extend the EHR. The forms of data are broadly categorized into three types:

1. Digital image data (provides increased accessibility)

2. Text-based data (provides accessibility, text search capability, and can be displayed on different devices)

3. Discrete data, Fielded and ideally Codified (provides all of the above plus the capability to be used for alerts, health maintenance, and data exchange.)

Increased benefits of an EHR can be realized when the information is stored as codified data. However, to receive and compare medical information from numerous sources it is necessary that the EHR codes adhere to a national standard.

Health care has been slow to develop and accept standard code sets. Often a code set has become a standard because a government organization such as CMS, HCFA, or the FDA has mandated its usage. A major change occurred with the passage of HIPAA, which mandated standardization and empowered the NCVHS to select standards for transaction formats and code sets.

Governments also influence standards by taking a leadership role such as adoption standards for federal agencies, or in the United Kingdom by codeveloping an EHR nomenclature.

Code sets are designed for a particular purpose:

Code sets used for billing use a code to identify the exact service performed.

Other code sets are classification systems used to codify medical records for research and analysis.

A code set designed specifically to record medical observations is referred to as a clinical "*nomenclature*." Using an EHR nomenclature provides consistency in patient records and improves communication between different medical specialties.

EHR nomenclatures differ from other coding standards in several ways:

♦ EHR nomenclatures precorrelate individual terms into clinically relevant "*findings*" or codified observations that are medically meaningful to the clinician.

♦ Reference Terminologies designed for research may codify each medical term, but these terms can combine in ways that are not clinically relevant; therefore, these nomenclatures are not easy to use at the point of care.

◆ Findings are often linked to other findings, which helps the clinician quickly locate associated information and shortens the time required to document the exam.

◆ EHR nomenclatures differ from billing codes in that EHR nomenclatures have the many more codes used to describe the detail of the exam such as the symptoms, history, observations, and plan. Billing codes tend to represent simply that the service was rendered.

◆ EHR nomenclatures tend to show findings by the name, not by the code. Typically, EHR code numbers are hidden, whereas diagnosis and procedure codes tend to be recognized and the code number used on orders and superbills.

◆ EHR nomenclatures often include cross-references to other standard code sets. Coding systems not intended for EHR do not typically contain a map to other coding systems.

Several of the most prominent coding standards you are likely to encounter or use in an EHR were discussed in this chapter.

SNOMED CT is a medical nomenclature developed by the College of American Pathologists and United Kingdom's National Health Service. It had its origins as a coding system for pathology and is often referred to as a "reference terminology." It provides very granular coding that normalizes data for research and reporting. SNOMED CT has been selected as a core terminology by NCVHS in the United States and by the NHS in the United Kingdom.

MEDCIN is a medical nomenclature and knowledge base used in many commercial EHR systems as well as the Department of Defense CHCS II system. It has been designated by NCVHS as an "enabling terminology."

MEDCIN differs from other EHR coding systems in that the nomenclature is not just a codified list of findings designed to classify or index medical information for research or other purposes. MEDCIN was designed for point-of-care usage by the clinician, so that each "finding" represents a meaningful clinical observation or term. The MEDCIN findings are linked in a "knowledge base." This enables a clinician to quickly find other clinical "findings" that are likely to be needed. This difference means a physician selects fewer individual codes to complete the patient exam note.

LOINC stands for Logical Observation Identifier Names and Codes. LOINC is an important clinical terminology for laboratory test orders and results because currently most laboratories and other diagnostic services report test results using their own internal, proprietary codes. When an EHR receives results from multiple lab facilities, LOINC provides a universal coding system for mapping laboratory tests and results to a common terminology in the EHR. This then enables a computer program to find and report comparable test values regardless of where the test was processed.

LOINC has become one of the standard code sets designated by the U.S. government for the electronic exchange of clinical health information.

UMLS is not itself a medical terminology but, rather, a "meta-thesaurus" created from many medical nomenclatures including those described in this chapter. It can be used to retrieve and integrate biomedical information and provide cross-references among selected vocabularies. It is maintained by the National Library of Medicine.

Nursing Codes Thirteen standards for nursing codes are recognized by the American Nurses Association today for use in the assessment, diagnosis, interventions, and outcomes of nursing care. Many of these are now incorporated into SNOMED CT. Nursing code sets discussed in this chapter include:

NANDA Taxonomy II facilitates oral and written nursing communication and standardizes 167 nursing diagnostic concepts. These can be used to codify a patient's responses to health problems, life processes, and patient outcomes. This facilitates codified nursing notes in the EHR and the collection, retrieval, and analysis of nursing data for education and research.

NIC is a code set designed for documenting nursing interventions (which are any direct-care treatment that the nurse performs on behalf of the patient). NIC is used at the point of care to document care planning and nursing practices.

NOC codifies nursing outcomes that are the end result of care. NOC can be used to measure the quality of care, cost-efficiency, and progress of treatment.

CCC or Clinical Care Classification system provides standardized coding concepts for nursing diagnoses, outcomes, nursing interventions, and actions. Originally developed for home health nurses, it can be used to document patient care in other health care settings.

Omaha System The Omaha System is one of the oldest systems of standardized terminology for nursing. It can be used to document nursing assessments, interventions, and outcomes.

ICNP stands for International Classification for Nursing Practice. It was intended to facilitate the comparison of nursing data gathered from multiple systems. It can be used to codify nursing phenomenon, nursing actions, and outcomes.

NMDS represents an attempt to define the minimum set of basic data elements for nursing in a computerized patient record. It is used to record nursing data for the comparison of patient outcomes.

PNDS is used in hospital perioperative settings to document the patient experience from preadmission to discharge. It is focused on the special needs and level of detail required to document perioperative nursing.

PCDS has been developed primarily as a data dictionary defining elements to be included in and abstracted from clinical information systems. It also is more oriented to acute care settings than the other nursing code sets.

CPT-4 codes are standardized codes for reporting medical services, procedures, and treatments performed for patients by the medical staff. They are part of the HCPCS codes required for CMS and private insurance billing. **HCPCS** codes extend beyond the CPT-4 codes adding codes for billing supplies, injectable medications, and blood products.

CPT-4 is the most widely accepted code set used to report medical procedures and services to health insurance programs. However, CPT-4 is not a very satisfactory nomenclature for an EHR. Although it provides a very uniform method of identifying a procedure or service it does not provide much detail as to what occurred during that procedure.

ABC codes were created to document and bill for alternative types of care that are becoming prevalent. ABC codes are similar in structure to CPT-4 codes but are not part of the CPT-4 or the current HCPCS code sets. ABC codes are accepted as billing codes only by some payers but are expected to be adopted officially in 2006 as a subset of the existing HCPCS codes.

ICD-9CM stands for International Classification of Diseases, Ninth Revision, Clinical Modification. The first two volumes of the codes are used for codifying diseases, injuries, health conditions, and causes of death.

The third volume of ICD-9CM is different because it lists codes for hospital inpatient procedures instead of diagnosis codes.

The historical intent of the ICD was to classify similar groups of mortality causes and disease conditions into statistical reportable data. The code set was adopted and modified to meet insurance billing requirements. Today insurance reimbursement is tied to the proper use of ICD-9CM codes, in the proper order (of primary, secondary, etc.), and at the right level of specificity.

ICD-10 is the latest revision. It is used in Europe but it has not been adopted in the United States, except for reporting the cause of death on death certificates. It should not be used in place of ICD-9CM for reporting diagnosis on insurance claims.

Clinical modifications must be made to create the U.S. version, ICD-10CM. This will include only diagnosis codes. A new Procedure Coding System, called ICD-10-PCS, will contain the inpatient procedures.

NDC codes are used by the FDA for registration of drugs as well as by pharmacies and drug supply companies for ordering; however, the codes are not very useful for patients' charts or physicians to write prescriptions. Two new systems RxNorm and NDF-RT have been suggested, but today most electronic prescription systems use proprietary codes created by commercial vendors for drug utilization review.

There are many standards of coding sets in use today. EHR nomenclatures map to many of those, especially codes used for billing. The fragmentation and duplication of code sets are part of the problem, but a codified EHR is superior to noncodified data. Examples in this chapter have shown that:

> **EHR data stored in a machine-readable, codified form adds significant value, but using a national standard code set instead of proprietary codes to codify the data will better enable the exchange of medical records between systems, improve the accuracy of the content, and open the door to the functional benefits derived from having an electronic health record.**

1. Name three forms of EHR data.

2. Name at least four medical code sets considered national standards.

3. Describe what influence the government has on the selection of standard code sets.

4. What does the acronym HIPAA stand for?

5. Which committee of the government has been designated to select national standards?

6. What is a nomenclature?

7. In an EHR, what is meant by the term "finding"?

8. Explain the difference between a "finding" and a billing code.

Each code set that becomes a national standard does so because it is designed for a particular purpose. Give a brief description of the original purpose of each of the following coding systems:

9. SNOMED CT

10. MEDCIN

11. LOINC

12. CPT-4

13. ICD-9CM

14. In the United States, should ICD-9CM or ICD-10 be used for insurance claims?

15. Describe the difference between an EHR nomenclature and a billing code set.

3 Learning Medical Record Software

Learning Outcomes

After completing this chapter, you should be able to:

- Start and stop the Student Edition software
- Navigate the screen
- Select a patient
- Create a new encounter
- Enter a Chief Complaint
- Enter vital signs
- Access the Symptoms, History, Physical Exam, Assessment, and Therapy tabs to select appropriate findings in each portion of the exam.
- Add Free text, prefixes, status, and results to findings
- Print a copy of the completed exam note

Introducing the Medcin Student Edition Software

In this chapter you will learn to document a patient visit using Medcin, one of the standard EHR nomenclatures discussed in Chapter 2. Special Medcin Student Edition software has been created for you to use with this course. It is similar to many commercial software packages that use the Medcin knowledge base for their EHR nomenclature.

The Student Edition software allows you select findings for symptoms, history, physical examination, tests, diagnoses, and therapy to produce medical documents typical of the physician exam notes created in a medical office. At the conclusion of certain exercises, you will print out your work and hand it in to your instructor.

Because the Student Edition is not a commercial medical record system, it will be different in some aspects from EHR systems you will encounter when working in a medical office. However, the concepts, skills, and familiarity with EHR systems you will acquire by practicing with the Student Edition software will transfer directly into the workplace.

As you have learned in the previous chapter, the Medcin nomenclature consists of 270,000 clinical concepts or findings, divided into six broad categories. The categories reflect the components of an outpatient encounter. The Medcin knowledge base connects these findings in a diagnostic index of more than 68 million links. One of the key challenges for clinicians using an EHR is to locate the findings applicable to the patient without spending too much time searching. The Medcin links provide the means to present clinically relevant information on demand at the point of care.

Exercises in this and subsequent chapters using the software will give you practical experience in creating electronic health records. Each set of exercises is designed to illustrate an EHR concept and will result in a documented exam note.

One goal of most EHR systems is to completely document the visit before the patient ever leaves the office. Once you have mastered the basics, you will learn in subsequent chapters to speed data entry through the use of forms, lists, and flow sheets. These capabilities are useful to document a patient visit during the course of the exam. Later, you also will learn how information from previous exams can be used during subsequent patient visits.

Understanding the Software

The following series of exercises are designed to allow you to become familiar with the Student Edition software, the Medcin nomenclature, and the screen navigation controls. Do not worry if you cannot complete all of them in one class period. A final version of the exercise is performed once you have become familiar with the concepts in this chapter.

Hands-On Exercise 1: Starting Up the Software

The Student Edition software should have been installed on your school's network computers or on your local workstation. Confirm with your instructor that this is the case, and then follow the steps below.

Step 1

Turn on the computer and wait for the Windows operating system desktop to appear on the screen. You may be required to log in; if so, ask your instructor for the correct log-in procedure.

Step 2

Locate the Medcin icon shown in Figure 3-1. If you do not see it on the computer desktop screen, click on the Start Button, and look in Programs or All Programs for the program named "MedcinSE."

Position the mouse pointer over the Medcin icon shown in Figure 3-1 and double click the mouse button. This will display the Student Edition login screen shown in Figure 3-2.

▶ **Figure 3-1 The Medcin Student Edition Icon.**

▶ **Figure 3-2 Student Edition Login Screen.**

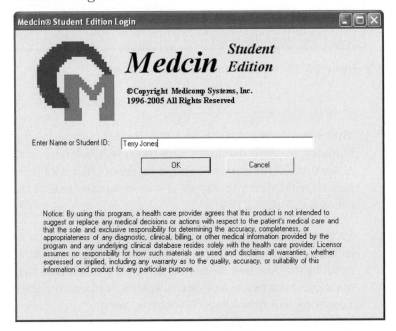

Step 3

Figure 3-2 shows the Medcin Student Edition log-in screen. The screen contains one data entry field and two buttons. The field is used for either the student's name or the student ID depending on the policy of the school. In the example, the student's name is Terry Jones. Do not type Terry Jones in the field; confirm with your instructor whether you should use your name or student ID.

Type either your name or student ID into the field.

When your name or ID is exactly as you want it to be, position the mouse pointer over the button labeled "OK," and click the mouse.

The button labeled "Cancel" is used to cancel the log in and close the window.

The main window of the Student Edition software will be displayed, as shown in Figure 3-3.

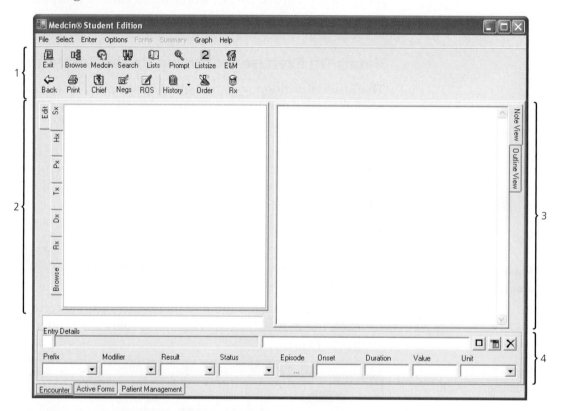

▶ **Figure 3-3 The Medcin Student Edition Window.**

Navigating the Screen

This section will explain how the screen is organized and discuss some of the features you will use later. The main window can be divided into four functional sections. These four sections interact with each other as you will learn in this chapter. Refer to Figure 3-3 and locate each of the sections indicated by the red numerals 1–4.

Section 1: The Menu Bar and Toolbar At the top of the screen, the words File, Select, Enter, Options, Forms, Summary, Graph, and Help are the Menus of functions in the Student Edition software. We call this the Menu bar. When you position the mouse over one of these words and click the mouse once, a list of functions will drop down below the word.

Once a list appears, moving the mouse pointer vertically over the list will highlight each item. In the Student Edition, highlight means a blue rectangle appears over the item. Clicking on the highlighted item will invoke that function. Clicking the mouse anywhere on the screen other than the list will close the list.

Also located at the top of your screen are two rows of icon buttons called a "Toolbar." The purpose of the Toolbar is to allow quick access to commonly used functions. Most Windows programs feature a Toolbar so you may already be familiar with the concept.

Toolbar buttons include a small picture called an icon intended to indicate the function of the button. Sometimes the pictures are intuitive, such as the image of a printer on the print button. Other times, the image is so obscure that memorization is really the only way to remember what it does. One solution is to include a label on the button, which is what the Student Edition does to help you quickly learn the function of each Toolbar button. Toolbar buttons will be introduced later in the chapter.

Section 2: The Medcin Nomenclature Pane The middle portion of the screen is divided into two window panes. The left pane (shown in Figure 3-3 with the numeral 2) is where the list of findings in the Medcin nomenclature will display. Because you have not yet selected a patient, the pane is empty. In the next exercise, you will select a patient and learn to navigate the Medcin Nomenclature Pane.

On the left of the nomenclature pane there are eight tabs. These look like tabs on file folders. These are labeled: Sx (symptoms), Hx (history), Px (physical examination), Tx (tests), Dx (diagnosis, syndromes, and conditions), and Rx (therapy). The tabs are used to logically group the findings into six broad categories. Two additional tabs labeled Browse and Edit will be explained as you use the software.

Section 3: The Encounter View Pane The right pane of the window (shown in Figure 3-3 with the numeral 3) will dynamically display the exam note as it is being created. When the clinician selects a finding from the nomenclature pane, the finding and relevant accompanying text are recorded in the exam note and displayed in the pane on the right.

Free-text also may be entered through the software, and it will appear in the exam note pane as well. This will become clearer during subsequent exercises. Because you have not yet selected a patient or an encounter, the pane is empty at this time.

There are two tabs on the right of this pane. The Note View tab displays the exam note exactly as it will be saved. The Outline View displays findings which have been selected as well as appropriate ICD-9CM or CPT-4 codes.

Section 4: Entry Details for a Current Finding The bottom portion of the screen (shown in Figure 3-3 with the numeral 4) consists of two rows of fields that allow the user to add detail to any finding in the exam note pane (discussed in section 3). Entry of data in these fields adds informational text to the finding in the exam note, and in some cases modifies its meaning.

For example, a patient reported symptom of "headaches" could be modified using the Entry Details field labeled "Status" to indicate the condition was "improving." The meaning of the finding could be altered completely by use of the Entry Details field labeled "Prefix" to indicate "family history of." This would indicate that the patient did not have this condition, but that it had been a problem for close relatives. Each of the fields in the details section of the screen will be covered in subsequent exercises in this book.

To actually see the interactions of the four sections of the screen, you need to select a patient and create a new encounter. The following exercises will show you how, but first let us discuss exiting the software.

Hands-On Exercise 2: Exiting and Restarting the Software

There are three ways to exit the Student Edition software; all perform the same function. In this exercise, you will practice exiting the software. You will then restart the program to continue with subsequent exercises.

At the top of your screen is a row of words called the Menu bar. Below it are two rows of buttons with icons, called the Toolbar. The first button in the Toolbar is labeled "Exit"; its icon looks like an open door. If you click on the Exit button, the Student Edition program will end and the window will close.

In the upper right corner of the window are three buttons that are standard to all Windows programs. These minimize, maximize, and close the window. The close button is red, with a large X. If you click on the close button, the Student Edition Program will end and the window will close.

Step 1

The first word in the Menu bar is *File*. Position the mouse pointer over the word *File* in the Menu bar at the top of the screen and click the mouse button once. A list of the functions on the File menu will drop down.

You will notice some of the items in the menu are listed in black text and some of them are in gray. Menu items in gray text indicate a particular function is not applicable to the current state of the exam note and are therefore not selectable. You may have noticed some of the buttons on the Toolbar also are gray; this is for the same reason.

Step 2

Move the mouse pointer vertically down the list until the *Exit* function is highlighted. Click the mouse on the word "Exit" to end the program.

Step 3

Start the Student Edition software again by repeating the first exercise, and logging in.

Hands-On Exercise 3: Using the Menu to Select a Patient

The first step in every encounter is to select the patient.

Step 1

Position the mouse pointer over the word *Select* in the Menu bar at the top of the screen and click the mouse button once. A list of the Select menu functions will appear (see Figure 3-4).

► Figure 3-4 Functions on
the Select Menu.

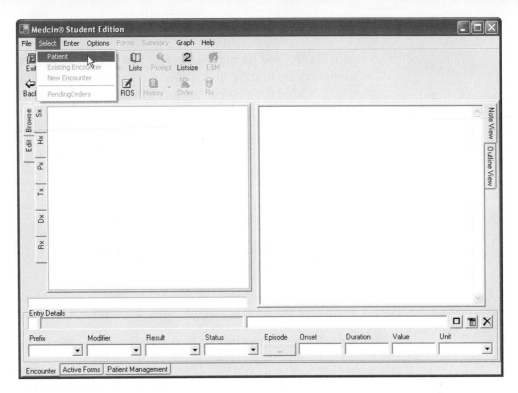

Step 2

Move the mouse pointer vertically down the list until *Patient* is highlighted.
Click the mouse on the word Patient to invoke the Patient Selection window
shown in Figure 3-5.

► Figure 3-5 Selecting Rosa
Garcia from the Patient Selection Window.

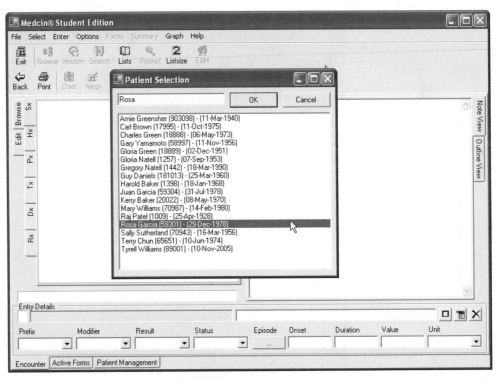

> **Note**
>
> **In most medical
> office software the
> patient locator
> window will have
> additional ways to
> sort and search the
> patient list, and
> may display more
> information about
> each patient.**

The Patient Selection window displays a list of all patients in the system, their first
name, last name, patient ID number, and date of birth. A field at the top of the window allows you to type the patient's name to quickly find someone in a large list.

Step 3

Find the patient named Rosa Garcia in the Patient Selection window by typing
"Rosa" in the field. When you start typing her name, the first name beginning

with an "R" will be highlighted as you continue to type the next alphabetical name will be highlighted. When Rosa Garcia is highlighted, click the OK button. Clicking the Cancel button will close the window.

An alternate method of selecting the patient in the locator window is to position the mouse pointer over the patient name and double-click the mouse. (Double-click means to click the mouse button twice, very rapidly.)

Step 4

Once a patient is selected, the patient's name, age, and sex are displayed in the title at the top of the window.

The Medcin Nomenclature (in the left pane) becomes active and the first group of findings (symptoms) is displayed.

The right pane containing the exam note is populated with the student's name or ID and the patient's name, sex, and date of birth.

Hands-On Exercise 4: Navigating the Medcin Findings

In this exercise, you will have an opportunity to become familiar with one way to navigate the Medcin nomenclature. In a subsequent exercise, you will learn to record the findings from the left pane into the exam note in the right pane. In this exercise, you will not yet record any findings.

Your screen should resemble Figure 3-6. If it does not, repeat the previous hands-on exercise.

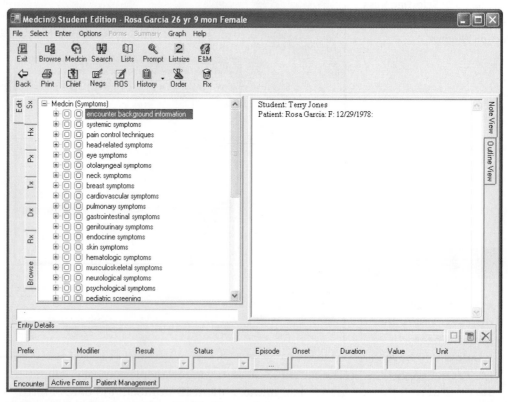

▶ **Figure 3-6 Left Pane Displays Medcin Nomenclature.**

Step 1

Look at the list of findings in the left pane. As mentioned earlier, the pane on the left of the screen is used to select findings to document the current patient encounter.

The Medcin Nomenclature consists of over 270,000 findings with 68 million relationships. To make it easy to find what you are looking for, the tabs on the left of the pane categorize findings into six broad groups that follow the order of a typical exam.

Chapter 1 described the standard order of medical exams in a SOAP format. The six tabs on the left pane make it easy to document in that format as follows:

Subjective	Sx	Symptoms
	Hx	History
Objective	Px	Physical Exam
	Tx	Tests (performed)
Assessment	Dx	Diagnosis
Plan	Rx	Therapy
		Tests (ordered)

In addition to the tabs, another feature that shortens the list of findings displayed in the nomenclature pane is to show only the main topics.

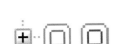

▶ **Figure 3-7 Buttons Used in the Nomenclature Pane.**

You will notice that most findings in the Medcin list are preceded by buttons. These are shown in Figure 3-7. The symbols on the buttons are a small plus sign, a larger button with a red circle, and a larger button with blue circle.

The small plus sign indicates there are more specific findings hidden from view that are related to the finding that is displayed.

Step 2

Locate the finding "head-related symptoms" in the nomenclature symptoms list, as shown in Figure 3-8. Position the mouse pointer over the small plus symbol and click the mouse button once.

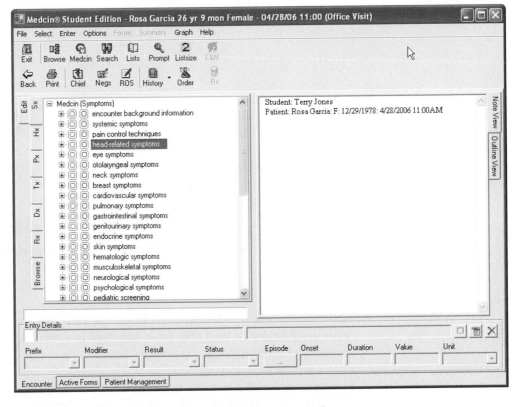

▶ **Figure 3-8 Locate the Finding "Head-Related Symptoms."**

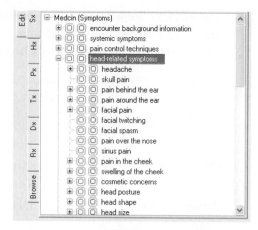

▶ **Figure 3-9 Expanded List of Findings for Head-Related Symptoms.**

Compare the left pane of your screen with Figure 3-9. The list should have expanded to reveal many additional head-related findings. Notice that the findings under "Head-Related Symptoms" are indented.

Notice also that some of the additional findings have small plus symbols as well, for example, "headache" and "pain behind the ear." This indicates even more specific findings are available for those items. Conversely, findings such as "skull pain," "sinus pain," and others no longer have the small plus. This means that there are not more specific findings for those items.

Step 3

Position the mouse pointer over the small plus symbol for the finding "headache" in the indented list, and click the mouse. The list expands further.

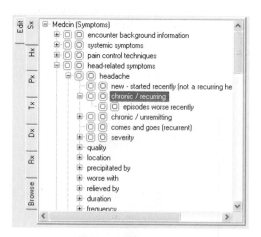

▶ **Figure 3-10 Fully Expanded List of Findings for Headache.**

Step 4

Notice that even the detailed the findings "chronic / recurring" and "chronic / unrecurring" still have small plus symbols indicating that further detailed findings are available.

Position the mouse pointer over the small plus symbol for the finding "chronic / recurring" and click the mouse. Compare your list to Figure 3-10.

This type of list is called a *Tree* because each indention of the list represents smaller branches of the finding above it. Look again at Figure 3-10; notice how each new level is indented further than the one above it. You may already be familiar with this concept because it is used in many other computer programs, including the Windows XP® Operating System.

Each time you clicked on the small plus symbol next to a finding in steps 2–4 the list grew. The terminology for this is to say that the tree has *expanded*. Also notice that a small minus sign replaced the small plus sign in the button next to the finding that has been expanded.

Step 5

Position the mouse pointer over the small minus symbol for the finding "head-related symptoms" and click the mouse button again. The expanded list of various types of head-related symptom findings will again be hidden from view. Your screen should once again look like Figure 3-8.

When you clicked on the small minus symbol for the main finding the number of findings for "head-related symptoms" was reduced back to one. The terminology for this is to say that the view of the tree is *collapsed*. These are the terms that will be used when working with Medcin lists for the remainder of this book.

Hands-On Exercise 5: Tabs on the Medcin Nomenclature Pane

Step 1

Position the mouse pointer over the Hx Tab (circled in red in Figure 3-11) and click the mouse once. The list will change to that shown in Figure 3-11. Notice that the currently selected tab has the appearance of being slightly raised from the others.

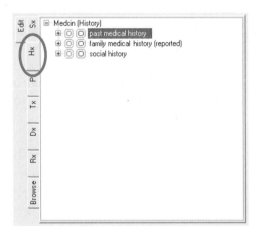

▶ **Figure 3-11 The History Tab (circled in red).**

Step 2

Position the mouse pointer over the small plus next to "past medical history" and click the mouse button to expand the list.

Step 3

Position the mouse pointer over the small plus next to "reported medications" and click the mouse button to expand the list. Click on the small plus sign next to the finding "recently stopped medication." Notice that this time there were too many findings to fit in the space allotted. A light blue scroll bar has appeared on the right side of the pane. You are probably familiar with the concept of scrolling a window.

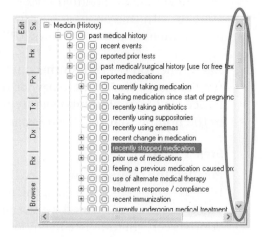

▶ **Figure 3-12 Expanded Past History (scroll bar is circled in red).**

Position the mouse pointer on the light blue scroll bar and hold the mouse button down while you drag the mouse in a downward motion. This action will scroll the list. Continue scrolling the list until you can see all the findings under "recently stopped medication," as shown in Figure 3-12.

Step 4

Position the mouse pointer over the Sx Tab and click the mouse once. The display will return to the previous list shown in Figure 3-8.

Step 5

Position the mouse pointer again over the Hx Tab and click the mouse once. Notice the list is expanded as when you left it. In most cases, the software will remember how much of the expanded tree was displayed in each tab as well as what finding was highlighted. This feature allows the clinician to easily go back to a previous tab to add another finding, and then return where he or she left off.

Step 6

Explore each of the remaining sections of the Medcin nomenclature pane, by clicking on each of the remaining tabs. Take a moment on each tab to look at the type of findings in each tab. Feel free to expand or collapse the list in any of the tabs.

Data Entry of the Examination Note

The main purpose of the EHR software such as those systems based on Medcin is to document the patient examination in a codified electronic medical record. This is done by selecting the finding from the Medcin nomenclature list in the left pane of the window. The finding and accompanying text are automatically recorded in the exam note displayed in the right pane of the window. The exam note portion of the screen is indicated by the numeral 3 in Figure 3-3.

Information is also added to the exam note by adding or modifying a finding using the Entry Details fields in the bottom portion of the window. The Entry Details section is indicated in Figure 3-3 with the numeral 4.

The following exercises are designed to let you explore the interactions of the four sections Student Edition window. During the course of these exercises, you will create your first patient exam note with the Medcin nomenclature.

Hands-On Exercise 6: Creating an Encounter

Clinician exam notes document a particular visit, exam, or other encounter between the patient and the provider. To maintain the associations of findings with the correct exam note, the EHR uses a unique record called an *encounter*. Until an encounter is selected or a new encounter is created, the software will not record findings. In this exercise, you will create a new encounter.

Step 1

The name of the patient Rosa Garcia should be displayed at the top of the Medcin window. If it is not, repeat Hands-On Exercise 3: Using the Menu to Select a Patient.

The Select menu (which you have used previously) also has functions to select an existing encounter or create a new encounter. In this exercise, you will create a new encounter.

Position the mouse pointer over the word *Select* in the Menu bar, and click the mouse button. Move the mouse pointer vertically down the list until the item *New Encounter* is highlighted. Click the mouse button.

Step 2

When you create a new encounter, a window is invoked that allows you to set the date, time, and reason for the visit. The month, day, year, and time will default to current date and time settings in your own computer. This means your initial screen will appear different from Figure 3-13.

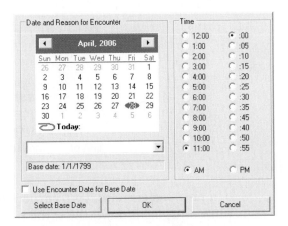

▶ **Figure 3-13 Date and Time of New Encounter—April 28, 2006 11:00 AM.**

Today's month and year are displayed in the calendar on the window. Today's date is circled in blue. Days that occur in the previous and subsequent months are in gray text.

It is important to set the date and time of the encounter to the date and time required by each exercise.

Setting the Date to April 28, 2006

Small gray buttons with left and right arrows are at the top of the calendar window. Clicking the button with the right arrow advances the calendar one month for each click of the mouse. Clicking the button with the left arrow takes the calendar backward one month for each click.

Click the buttons on the top of the calendar until the month April 2006 is displayed.

Position the mouse pointer over the 28th day and click the mouse button. The 28th will be highlighted with a blue oval.

The time is indicated on the right side of the window by white circles that have black centers. For example, in Figure 3-13, the circles next to 11:00 and :00 and :AM are each filled, indicating the time of the encounter will be **11:00 AM**.

Select the time by clicking your mouse in the circles next to 11:00 and :00 and :AM. Each of the circles should become filled in.

Step 3

The reason for the encounter is also set in this window. The encounter Reason field is located just below the calendar. To view a list of reasons, position the mouse pointer over the button with the down arrow in the right side of the field, and click the mouse. A drop-down list of reasons will appear as shown in Figure 3-14.

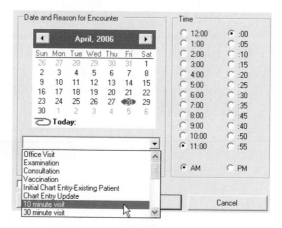

▶ **Figure 3-14 Select 10 Minute Visit from List of Reasons for Encounter.**

In a previous exercise, you learned to scroll a list by holding the mouse button while dragging it down the scroll bar. Using the same technique, you can scroll the list of reasons until you see the reason "10 minute visit." Highlight the reason by moving the mouse pointer over it. When the reason "10 minute visit" is highlighted, click the mouse button to select the reason.

Step 4

Compare your screen to Figure 3-15. Make certain you set the date, time, and reason correctly. If the date, time, or reason needs to be corrected repeat the previous steps.

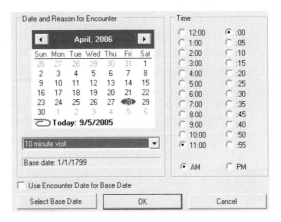

▶ **Figure 3-15 New Encounter for a 10 Minute Visit, April 28, 2006 11:00 AM.**

Locate the button labeled OK in the bottom of the New Encounter window, position the mouse pointer over the OK button, and click the mouse. The "date and reason for encounter" window will close.

Step 5

The encounter date, time, and reason "10 minute visit" should be displayed in the title of the window. The encounter date and time should be recorded in the exam note pane on the right side of the window.

Compare your screen with Figure 3-16; if your screen matches Figure 3-16, you are ready to proceed. If it does not, repeat steps 1–4.

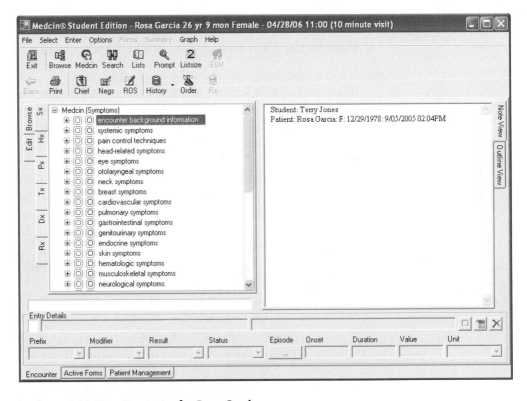

▶ **Figure 3-16 New Encounter for Rosa Garcia.**

The Student Edition software automatically calculates the patient's age based on the encounter date. Some of the features in the program use this information to present findings clinically relevant to the patient's age and sex, or information based on the patient's previous encounters.

Be careful to set new encounters to exactly match the date and time in the textbook exercises. Doing so will ensure that your screens and printed narrative documents match those in the book.

Hands-On Exercise 7: Recording Subjective Findings

Information is recorded in the exam note by clicking the mouse on the buttons adjacent to each finding (shown enlarged in Figure 3-17). Clicking on a button with the red circle will record the finding as it appears in the list and fill the circle red. Clicking on a button with the blue circle will record the finding in its opposite state and fill the circle blue.

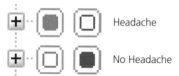

For example, clicking on the button with the red circle next to headache will record that the patient has a headache; clicking on the button with the blue circle will record that the patient has reported no headache.

When a finding is recorded in the exam note on the right pane, the description of the finding in the left pane also changes to match the selected state. For example, the finding Headache becomes "No Headache" when the blue button is selected, as shown in Figure 3-17.

▶ **Figure 3-17 Buttons Adjacent to Findings Fill with Color When Selected.**

For the remainder of this book, the buttons used to select findings will simply be referred to as the red button or the blue button.

A finding can be highlighted (surrounded with a blue background) without selecting either the red or blue button but by clicking on the description of the finding instead of the buttons. Highlighting a finding will be used in Chapter 4.

Step 1

Make sure that you have the Sx tab in the left pane selected. If you are uncertain, position the mouse pointer over the Sx tab and click the mouse once.

Using the skills you have acquired in a previous exercise, navigate the list of findings, and expand the tree of "head-related symptoms" until your list resembles the expanded tree shown in the left pane of Figure 3-18.

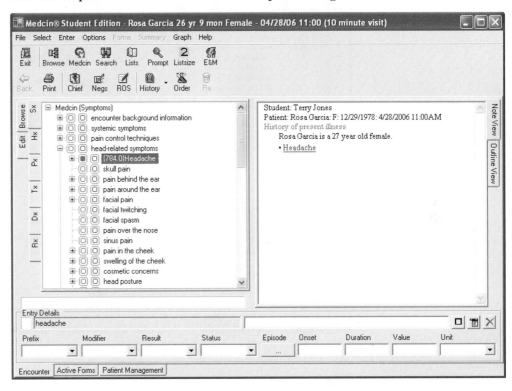

▶ **Figure 3-18 Expanded Tree for Head-Related Symptoms—Headache Finding Selected.**

Step 2

Position the mouse over the red button for the finding "Headache." Click the mouse button. Compare your screen to Figure 3-18.

The center of the button should turn red. This indicates that the finding has been selected. The word "Headache" should have also appeared on the right pane in the exam note.

Because this is the first time you have recorded a finding in the patient history section, a section title "History of Present Illness" and "Rosa Garcia is a 27 year old female" have been added to the exam note as well.

Section titles are dynamically added or removed by the software based on the findings selected. This creates a nice-looking exam note without adding empty sections. For example, if tests are not ordered, there is not an empty section of the note called "Tests."

Step 3

To further explore the operation of the red and blue buttons, position the mouse over and click on the blue button for headache instead. The center of the button should turn blue and the red button should return to its previous (cleared) state. Also the text in the exam note and the finding description will both change to "No Headache."

> **Note**
>
> Instructions to click a red or blue button refer to a Finding by its description before it is selected. Screen figures used for comparison show the description of a Finding as it appears after being selected.

Click on the red button to restore the finding back to "Headache." Make sure the button is red and the text in the exam note again reads "Headache."

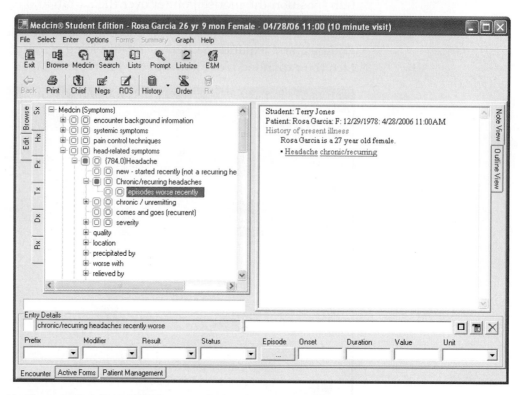

► **Figure 3-19 Selected Findings: Headache Chronic/Recurring and Worsening.**

Step 4

EHR information should be as specific as possible. If the patient indicates that her headaches are chronic, you will want to select a more specific finding.

Click on the small plus next to Headaches to expand the tree. Locate the finding Chronic/Recurring and click on the red button.

Did the circle turn red? Did the text change in the exam note?

Step 5

The patient further reports that her headaches have been getting worse.

Notice the small plus sign next to chronic/recurring, which indicates that there are more detailed findings available. Click on the plus sign to expand the tree.

Compare your screen to Figure 3-19.

Step 6

In the expanded list for chronic/recurring, click the mouse on the red button for "episodes recently worse."

Notice that the software changes the description of findings when you select them in this case the finding description changes to "chronic/recurring headaches recently worse." When the finding descriptions are too long, they are displayed truncated with an ellipsis (three dots), which indicates there is more to the description than will fit in the left pane.

Hands-On Exercise 8: Removing Findings

In Step 3 of the previous exercise you learned that you could change the state or meaning of a finding that was already recorded by simply clicking your mouse on the opposite color button. In that example, clicking on the blue button changed "headache" to "no headache" and clicking on the red button changed it back to "headache."

However, what if you accidentally clicked on the wrong finding? How would you undo it completely? In this exercise, you will learn how to remove findings from the exam note.

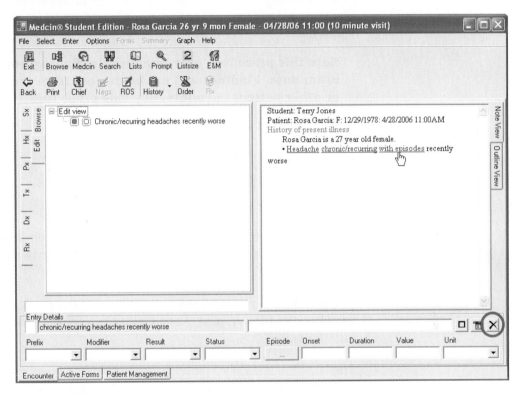

▶ **Figure 3-20 Edit Mode and Delete Finding Button (circled in red).**

Step 1

As mentioned previously, the left pane has two additional tabs, Edit and Browse. In this exercise, we are going to use the Edit tab.

Look at the exam note displayed in the right pane. Notice that findings in the exam note are underlined, surrounding text is black, and section titles are magenta.

Move your mouse pointer over the underlined finding "*with episodes*" in the exam note. The mouse pointer changes into the shape of a hand. While the hand is over the finding, click the mouse once. This will Edit the finding.

The nomenclature list in the pane on the left was replaced with an *Edit View* of the selected finding. The tabs on the left pane have also changed places; the Edit tab has moved to the next to the pane and the Sx, Hx, Px, Tx, Dx, and Rx tabs have moved to the outside row.

Step 2

Locate the button with an X in the lower right corner of the screen. (It is circled in red in Figure 3-20.) This is the Delete button, which is similar in appearance to the Delete button used in word processors, e-mail, and many other Windows programs. Position your mouse pointer over the Delete button and click once.

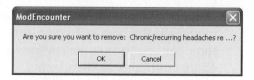

▶ **Figure 3-21 Click OK to Confirm Removing the Finding.**

A small window called a dialogue will appear (as shown in Figure 3-21). The dialogue is asking you to confirm your intention to remove the finding from the exam note.

Note this procedure only removes the finding from the patient's current exam note. Findings will not be deleted from the Medcin nomenclature or other patient encounters by this procedure.

Click on the OK button.

The finding "with episodes" and the text "recently worse" will be removed from the exam note. The left pane will remain on the Edit tab. This is normal.

Step 3

Practice removing findings by repeating steps 1 and 2 for each of the other two findings, headaches and chronic/recurring. The order that you remove them does not matter.

When you have removed the last finding for the section the section title "History of Present Illness" and "Rosa Garcia is a 27 year old female" will be removed automatically.

Step 4

Return the Medcin list to the left pane by positioning the mouse over the Sx tab and clicking once. This will swap the position of the outside tabs as well as re-display the Medcin nomenclature.

Hands-On Exercise 9: Recording More Specific Findings

In a previous exercise, you recorded a patient's symptom of chronic/recurring headaches by selecting three different findings from the list. There is nothing wrong with doing it that way if the natural flow of the exam progresses in that manner. For example, if when the patient reports having headaches, and the clinician asks if they are recurring, the patient says "yes," then the patient adds that they are getting worse.

However, if you have all of the information before selecting the finding, you can simply select the most specific finding and Medcin will add the surrounding text. In this exercise, you will record the same information about the patient's symptom by using only one finding.

Step 1

If your screen does not currently resemble Figure 3-16, repeat the necessary steps to select a patient, select a new encounter, select the Sx tab.

Expand the tree view of "head-related symptoms," "headache," chronic/recurring (clicking on small plus signs) until you can see the full list shown in Figure 3-22.

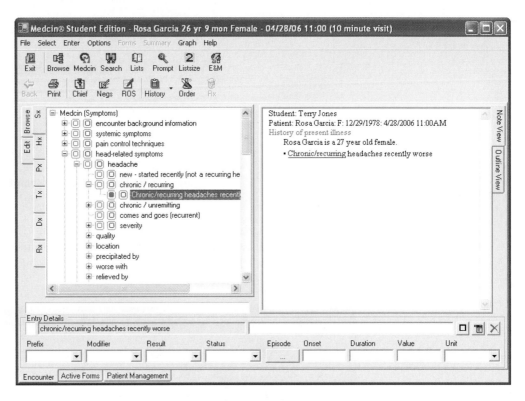

▶ Figure 3-22 Chronic/Recurring Headaches Recently Worse.

Step 2

Position the mouse pointer over the red button for the finding "episodes recently worse" (indented under "chronic/recurring") and click the mouse.

Compare your screen with Figure 3-22. Did the circle in the button turn red?

Compare the text of exam note in Figure 3-22 with the text in Figure 3-20. The two notes are different but medically equivalent. Additionally, in the codified EHR, Medcin has taken care of relating the underlying codes.

In the real-world application of electronic medical records, speed of input is important. Use whichever technique accurately documents the exam in the least amount of time. There is no reason to go back and delete the findings as we did in the previous exercise when they are correct. However, when an entire symptom or observation can be documented by selecting a single finding, do so, as you have in this exercise. The purpose of Hands-On Exercise 8 was to teach you how to remove findings when necessary.

Hands-On Exercise 10: Recording History Findings

The History tab is used to record the patient's past medical, surgical, family, and social history.

Step 1

Position the mouse pointer over the Hx tab and click the mouse once.

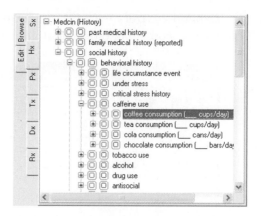

▶ Figure 3-23 Hx List—Coffee Consumption.

Step 2

Using the skills you have acquired in previous exercises, navigate the Medcin list, and expand the tree by clicking on the small plus signs next to "social history," "behavioral history," and "caffeine use." The left pane of the window should resemble Figure 3-23.

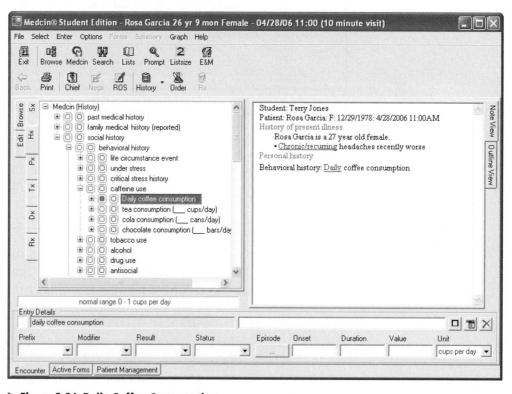

▶ Figure 3-24 Daily Coffee Consumption.

Step 3

Position the mouse over the red button next to the finding "coffee consumption (cups/day)." Click the mouse button. The circle in the button should turn red and "Behavioral History: Daily coffee consumption" should appear in the exam note pane on the right pane.

Compare your screen to Figure 3-24. Note that two new titles were added as well: Personal History and Behavioral History.

Adding Details to the Findings

In addition to the narrative text that the software automatically generates, you also can add further clarification to the exam note using *Entry Details* fields.

The section labeled "Entry Details" is located at the bottom of your screen. It was indicated in Figure 3-3 with the numeral 4. The Entry Details section consists of two rows of white boxes. These are the *Entry Details* fields.

The first row of fields contains the description of the currently highlighted finding, a note field for adding free-text about the current finding, and three buttons. You have already used the delete button (with the X) in a previous exercise. We will discuss and use the other two buttons in later exercises.

The second row contains the following fields: prefix, modifier, result, status, episode, onset, duration, value, and unit.

All of the fields in the Entry Details section apply to a single finding, the one currently selected.

In the following exercises you will learn to use the *Entry Details* fields. Notice the Entry Details fields as you select findings. In some cases, Medcin will automatically set one or more of the fields; sometimes you will set the field yourself.

Hands-On Exercise 11: Recording a Value

The value field can be used to enter a value about any type of finding. For example, the patient's weight could be entered for a finding of weight, or the result of a simple blood test performed in a doctor's office could be entered as a numeric value for the finding Hematocrit.

The unit field is related to the value field in that it describes the unit of measure for the value. In the two previous examples, the unit for weight would be pounds or kilograms, and the unit for the Hematocrit would be percent.

In this exercise, coffee consumption is measured in cups. So the value will be the number the patient consumed and the unit would be "cups per day."

Step 1

Make sure Daily Coffee consumption is the current finding. If you are beginning a new class, you will need to repeat the previous exercise to add the finding before proceeding.

Step 2

Locate the Value and Unit fields in the Entry Details section at the bottom of the screen. Notice that the Unit field already contains the words "cups per day."

Click your mouse on the value field and type the numerals **7–8**.

Press the Enter key on your keyboard.

Compare your screen with Figure 3-25. The text in the exam note should now read: "Behavioral History: Daily coffee consumption was 7-8 cups per day."

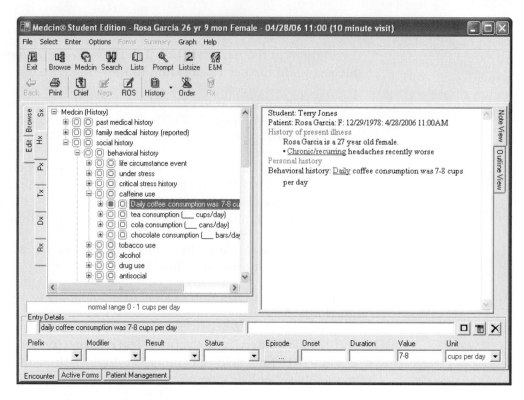

▶ Figure 3-25 Recording the Value 7-8 and Unit Cups Per Day.

Using Free-Text

In this exercise you will learn how to add your own text into the note. The term for this is "free-text," meaning that the text is not codified and might contain anything.

In contrast, the other Entry Details fields (prefix, modifier, result, status, episode, onset, duration, value, and unit) are stored as fielded data. This has the advantage of producing a uniform, searchable EHR throughout the medical practice.

Ideally, the less free-text used in the EHR, the better. Still, there are many times when free-text is appropriate, for example, adding a nuance to a finding that extends its meaning or entering text to more accurately portray the patient's own words.

Hands-On Exercise 12: Adding Free-Text

In this exercise, the patient reports she has recently stopped drinking coffee.

Step 1

Click on the small plus sign next to Daily coffee consumption to expand the list of findings. If you are beginning a new class, you will need to repeat the two previous exercises to add the finding before proceding.

Locate the finding "recently decreased" and click the mouse on the red button. Compare your screen to Figure 3-26.

► **Figure 3-26** Patient Reported Decreased Coffee Consumption.

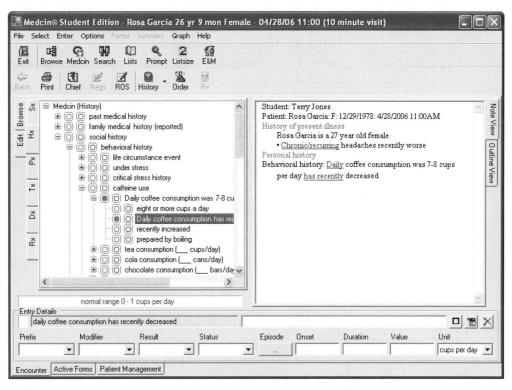

Step 2

Look at the Entry Details section at the bottom of your screen. There are two long fields in the first row. The gray field on the left contains the description that appears in the note and cannot be directly edited; the field on the right is used to add free-text to the currently selected finding.

► **Figure 3-27** Behavioral History with Additional Free-Text.

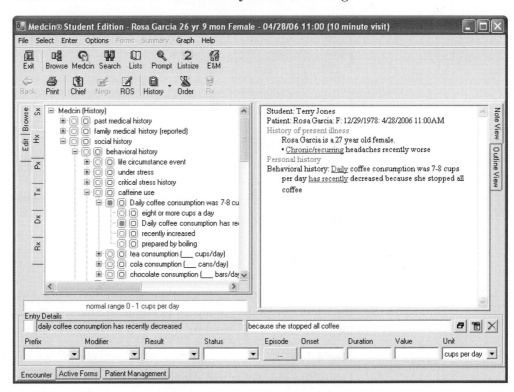

Click your mouse in the free-text field. Type "**because she stopped all coffee**" in the field and then press the Enter key on your keyboard. Compare your screen with Figure 3-27.

Hands-On Exercise 13: Recording Objective Findings

The Px tab is used to record the observations and results of the clinician's physical examination of the patient as well as measurements and vital signs recorded during the course of the visit.

Step 1

Position the mouse pointer over the Px tab and click the mouse once. The Physical Examination list will be displayed. Notice that the list is organized by body systems, essentially in the order you would perform a head-to-toe exam.

Step 2

Click on the small plus sign next to "Head" to expand the list. Locate the finding "evidence of injury" and click the mouse on the blue button. Compare your screen to Figure 3-28. The blue button should be filled in and the text "no head injury" should be recorded in the exam note on the right side of the screen.

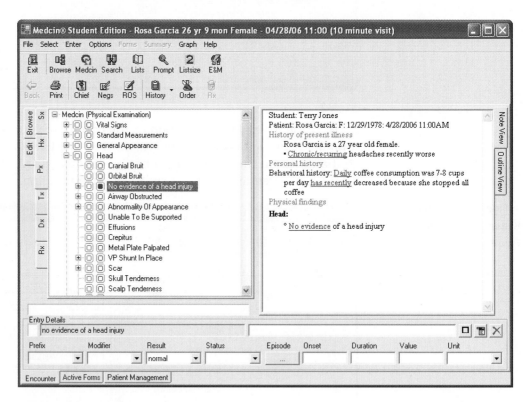

▶ **Figure 3-28 No Head Injury.**

Step 3

Look at the Entry Details field for *Result*. It was previously blank but now contains the word "normal." This is an example of how the EHR software can set the field for you based on the assumption that it is normal **not** to have a head injury.

Step 4

Using the mouse, scroll the list of physical examination findings until you see Neurological System. Expand the list by clicking on the small plus sign next to Neurological System.

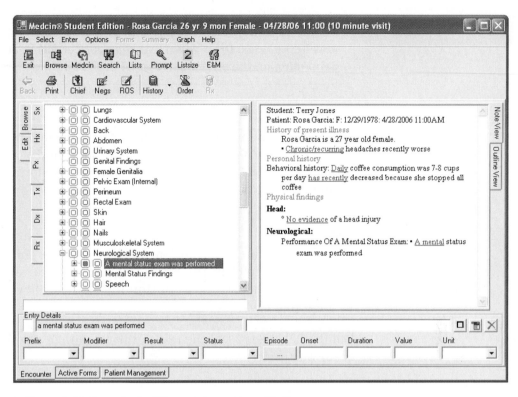

► **Figure 3-29 Neurological/Mental Status Exam Finding.**

Step 5

Locate the finding "A mental status exam was performed" and click the mouse on the red button. Compare your screen to Figure 3-29. The circle in the red button should be filled and the text should be recorded in the exam note.

Note that, except for the description of the finding, the Entry Details fields are blank. The software does not presume to know the result of the mental status exam.

Hands-On Exercise 14: Setting the Result Field

The prefix, modifier, result, status, and unit fields have buttons next to the field with an arrow pointing down. This type of button indicates there is a drop-down list of items you can use for that field. You have previously used this type of list to select the reason when creating a new encounter.

Step 1

Locate the Result field in the Entry Details section at the bottom of the screen. Click your mouse on the button with the down arrow in the field. A drop-down list of choices (as shown in Figure 3-30) will appear.

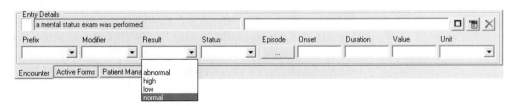

► **Figure 3-30 Drop-Down List for Result Field.**

Step 2

Position your mouse pointer on the result "normal" and click the mouse button. The field will display the word "normal," and the text in the exam note will change from "A mental status exam was performed" to "A mental status exam was normal."

Step 3

The first item in each drop-down list is a blank. The blank is selected whenever you want to clear the Entry Details field of a value. Practice this by clicking your mouse on the button in the result field and selecting the blank at the top of the list.

Did the field clear? Did the text in the exam note revert to "A mental status exam was performed"?

Step 4

Set the result back to "normal" by repeating steps 1 and 2. Your exam note should read "A mental status exam was normal."

Hands-On Exercise 15: Adding Detail to Recorded Findings

EHR software must be very flexible because additional observations or information from the patient could necessitate going back to any section at any time. In this exercise, you will add status information to the patient's reported symptom.

Step 1

Select the finding for edit by moving your mouse pointer over the words "Chronic/recurring" headache in the exam note. When the mouse pointer changes to a hand, click the mouse button. The Px tab in the left pane should be replaced by the Edit tab. This step of the procedure is the same one you used in Hands-On Exercise 8: Removing Findings.

Chronic/recurring headaches is now the current finding.

Step 2

Locate the Status field in the Entry Details section at the bottom of the screen. Click your mouse on the button with the down arrow in the status field. A drop-down list of phrases (as shown in Figure 3-31) will appear.

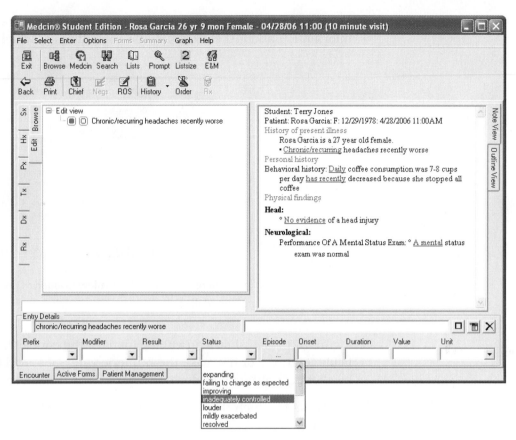

▶ Figure 3-31 Drop-Down List for Status Field.

Step 3

Position your mouse pointer on the status "inadequately controlled" and click the mouse button. The field will display a portion of the phrase, and the text in the exam note will change to "Chronic/recurring headaches recently worse which is inadequately controlled."

Hands-On Exercise 16: Adding Episode Detail to Findings

In addition to drop-down lists, another method of input allows you to quickly enter numerical data. In this exercise, you will add information about the frequency of the patient's headaches.

Step 1

The finding "Chronic/recurring" headache should still be selected for edit. If it is not, then repeat step 1 of the previous exercise.

Step 2

Locate the label *Episode* in the Entry Details section at the bottom of your screen. The Episode button located below the label has an ellipsis (three dots) on it. Click your mouse on the Episode button.

The Episode window shown in Figure 3-32 will be invoked. It is used to record information about the intervals and repetitions at which findings occur.

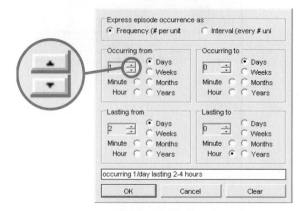

▶ **Figure 3-32 Episode Window (Numeric Controls Enlarged).**

Figure 3-32 also shows an enlargement of the control buttons for the numeric fields. Increase or decrease the numeric value of a field in the Episode window by clicking on the up or down arrow buttons next to the numeric field.

The units in which time is measured are set by clicking on one of the white circles next to Minutes, Hours, Days, Weeks, Months, or Years.

Step 3

Locate "Occurring from." Set it to 1 day by clicking on the up arrow button once and then clicking on the circle next to Days.

Step 4

Locate "Lasting from." Set it to 2 hours by clicking on the up arrow button twice and then clicking on the circle next to Hours.

Step 5

Locate "Lasting to." Set it to 4 hours by clicking on the up arrow button four times and then clicking on the circle next to Hours.

Step 6

Compare your screen to the Episode window in Figure 3-32, then click on the OK button.

Look at the exam note in the right pane. Does the text read "Chronic/recurring headaches recently worse occurring 1/day lasting 2–4 hours which is poorly controlled"?

Hands-On Exercise 17: Recording the Assessment

The assessment is the clinician's diagnosis of the patient's problem or condition.

Step 1

Position your mouse pointer on the tab "Dx" and click the mouse. The Diagnosis, Syndromes, and Conditions list should be displayed in the left pane of the window.

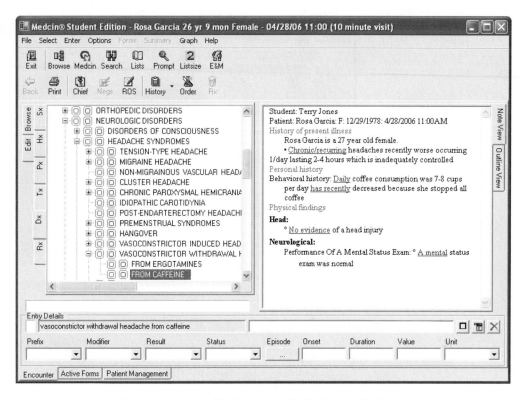

▶ **Figure 3-33 Dx Tab—Assessment: Withdrawal Headache from Caffeine.**

Step 2

Scroll the list downward until you see "Neurological Disorders." Click on the small plus sign to expand the list. Locate "Headache Syndromes" in the list and click on the small plus sign.

Locate "Vasoconstrictor withdrawal headache" and click on the small plus sign. Locate the finding "From caffeine." The expanded list of findings is shown in Figure 3-33.

Step 3

Position your mouse pointer on the red button next to "From caffeine" and click the mouse. The finding "Vasoconstrictor withdrawal headache from caffeine" should be recorded in the exam note under a new heading: "Assessment."

Hands-On Exercise 18: Recording Treatment Plan and Physician Orders

In Exercise 12, you added free-text to a specific finding. Medcin also has several special findings that are used as anchors for general free-text entry.

Additionally, when there are more than a few words of free-text to enter, a larger window may be useful as well. In this exercise, you will add a free-text finding and enter information through a special free-text window.

Step 1

Position the mouse pointer on the Rx tab and click the mouse button. The Medcin Therapy list will be displayed.

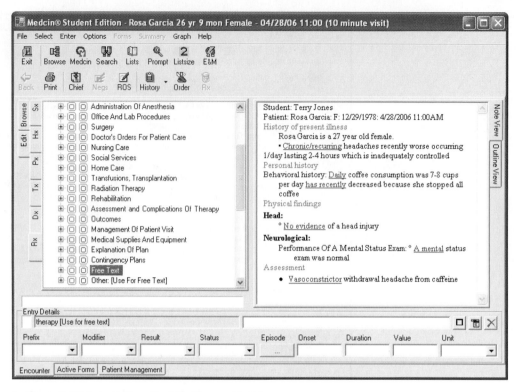

▶ Figure 3-34 Locate Free-Text Finding on Rx Tab.

Step 2

Scroll to the bottom of the list and locate the finding labeled "Free Text" as shown in Figure 3-34.

Click on the red button next to the finding "Free Text." The circle in the red button should be filled in and a new therapy section should be appear on the exam note, with the words "Free Text (therapy)."

Step 3

This time, instead of typing free-text into the Entry Details field, you will invoke a small window used for adding and editing finding notes. In the lower right corner of your screen are three buttons. You used the delete button (with the X) in previous exercises. In this exercise you will use the Finding Note button, which is circled in red in Figure 3-35.

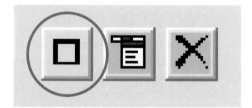

▶ Figure 3-35 Enlarged View—Finding Note Button (circled in red).

Position your mouse pointer on the Finding Note button and click the mouse. A small Finding Note window will be invoked as shown in Figure 3-36.

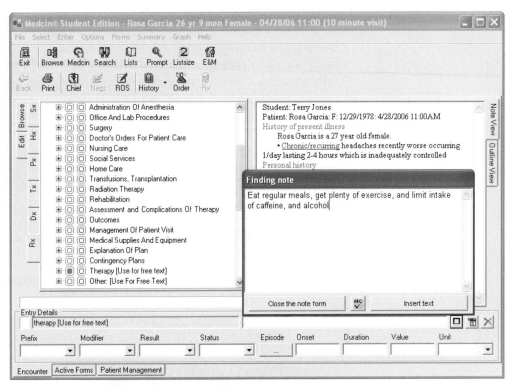

► **Figure 3-36 Finding Note Window Used for Free Text.**

Step 4

There are several advantages to entering free-text in this window as opposed to in the free-text field in the Entry Details section.

1. The area in the window is larger than the free-text field, making it easier to type longer notes.

2. The window includes a spell checker (the button in the center of the finding note window).

3. The Insert text feature allows frequently used text to be stored and inserted as free text whenever appropriate, saving time typing.

Type the following text into the Finding Note window:

"Eat regular meals, get plenty of exercise, and limit intake of caffeine, and alcohol"

When you have finished, click your mouse on the button labeled "Close the note form." This will add your text to the exam note.

Introduction to Using Forms

You may have noticed in the previous exercise that the finding note window was called a form. Forms make it convenient to enter findings or free-text without locating and selecting the finding from the nomenclature. When a form is used, the information is automatically recorded in the proper section of the exam note. In following two exercises, you will use forms to add information to the exam note.

Normally, the items in the next two exercises would have been recorded early in the exam; they were placed at the end of the exercises only because of the organization of the chapter.

Hands-On Exercise 19: Recording the Chief Complaint

Typically, the first thing recorded in the exam is a description of the patient's reason for the visit. This is called the "Chief complaint." You could locate the finding "Chief complaint" and then enter a free-text note, but because Chief complaint is a standard part of every exam, it is more efficient to provide a form for text entry.

Step 1

At the top of your screen are two rows of buttons called the Toolbar. The Toolbar was discussed at the beginning of the chapter and indicated in the section of Figure 3-3 with the numeral 1. The purpose of the Toolbar is to allow quick access to commonly used functions.

Locate the button labeled "Chief" in the second row of buttons on the Toolbar at the top of your screen. (See Figure 3-37.)

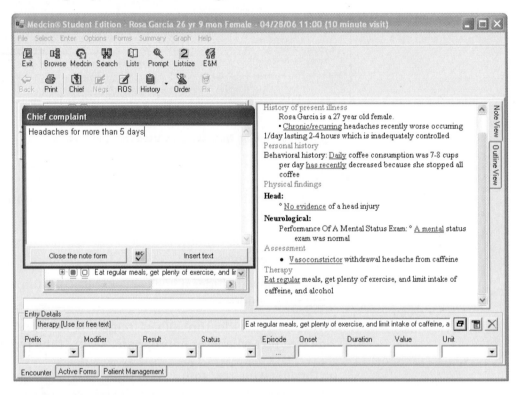

▶ **Figure 3-37 Chief Complaint Note Form Invoked from Toolbar.**

Step 2

Position your mouse pointer over the "Chief" button and click your mouse. The Chief complaint window will be invoked. This window will be similar to the finding note window in the previous exercise except that it will automatically record the text you enter into the proper section of the exam note with the finding for "Chief complaint" when you close the note form window.

Step 3

Type the following text into the finding note window:

"Headaches for more than 5 days"

When you have finished, compare your screen to Figure 3-37.

Position your mouse on the button labeled "Close the note form" and click the mouse. This will add a new section titled "Chief complaint" and the information you typed to the exam note in the right pane.

Hands-On Exercise 20: Recording Vital Signs

Forms are not limited to free-text. Many findings can be included on one form, and the form can contain specific Entry Details fields such as Result, Status, Value, and Unit.

One use of forms is to record Vital Signs (routine measurements of the body taken at nearly every medical practice). As you will see in this exercise, it is more efficient to enter numerical data using a form than to select findings one at a time and then enter data in the value field for each.

Step 1

At the bottom of the screen you will see three tabs, labeled Encounter, Active Forms, and Patient Management. All forms except the small free-text boxes used in previous exercises are accessed from the Active Forms tab.

Position your mouse pointer over the tab labeled "Active Forms" (circled in red in Figure 3-38) and click the mouse.

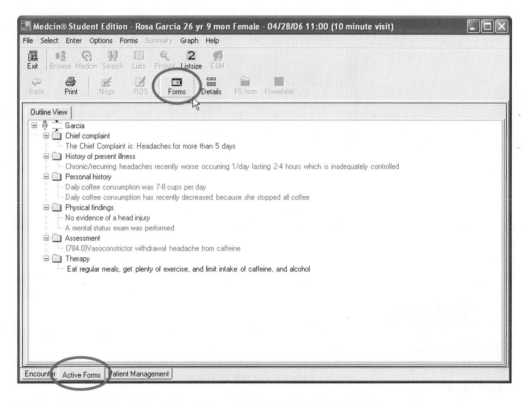

▶ Figure 3-38 Active Forms Tab and Forms Button (both circled in red).

When the tab changes, the familiar view of the Student Edition software will be replaced with an Outline View of the findings you currently have in your exam note. The Outline View presents the findings of the current encounter without the surrounding text. The findings are grouped in the order of the Medcin hierarchy. The Outline View will also show the ICD-9CM and CPT-4 codes for relevant findings as discussed in Chapter 2.

Because you may not have performed all the previous exercises in this class period, your Outline View may not have as much detail as shown in Figure 3-38.

Step 2

The Active Forms tab also has a slightly different Toolbar. Locate the button labeled "Forms" in the second row of buttons on the Toolbar at the top of your screen (also circled in red in Figure 3-38). Position your mouse pointer over it and click the mouse; this will invoke the Forms Manager window shown in Figure 3-39. The Forms Manager lists forms used in the Student Edition.

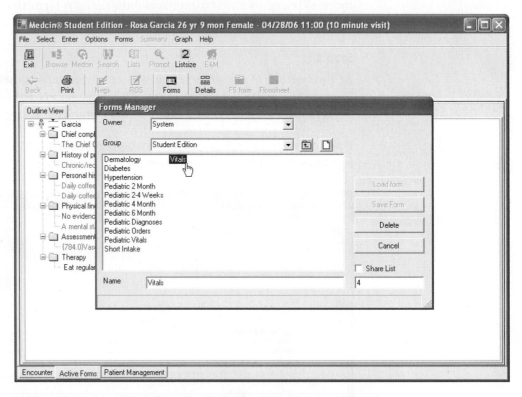

▶ **Figure 3-39 Select Vitals from the List in the Forms Manager Window.**

Locate and click on the form labeled "Vitals" in the Form Manager Window as shown in Figure 3-39. This should open the form shown in Figure 3-40.

Enter Ms. Garcia's Vital Signs into the corresponding fields. They are as follows:

Temperature:	**98.6**
Respiration:	**25**
Pulse:	**75**
BP:	**117/75**
Height:	**64**
Weight:	**140**

> **Note**
>
> **Systolic and Diastolic blood pressure readings are entered in two separate fields. Omit the "/" character when entering BP in the software.**

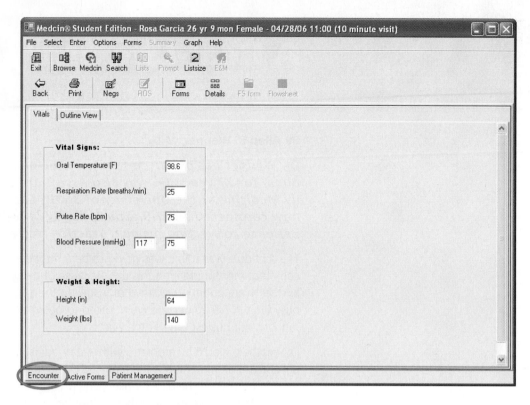

▶ **Figure 3-40 Vital Signs Form for Rosa Garcia.**

When you have entered all of the vital signs, compare your screen to Figure 3-40 and then click your mouse on the Encounter tab (circled in red) at the bottom of the screen.

The vital signs information will now be recorded in the exam note on the right pane under the Physical Findings section.

Step 3

Look at the results of the vital signs entry as they appear in the exam note. Also note the tab on the right pane labeled Outline View. This tab will display the same outline in the right pane, as was displayed on the Active Forms tab.

When you have finished looking at the note, exit the Student Edition software.

This completes the exercises that can be done separately.

A Real-Life Story

Paperless in Less Than a Day

By Allen R. Wenner, M.D.[1]

Dr. Wenner has practiced family medicine in Columbia, South Carolina, for 27 years. He was also Assistant Clinical Professor of Family Medicine at the University of South Carolina for 19 years. He is now considered an EHR expert, but here he shares his personal experience converting his own practice to Electronic Health Records.

The schedule was full. It was going to be a busy day. I had awakened 2 hours early that morning fearing this day. Because of delays in hardware installation and software updating, instead of installing the paperless system during our least busy time in December, we were forced to begin an electronic medical record in January, our busiest time of the year.

I knew there would be problems with a staff adjusting to the new workflow of a paperless environment, but the time had come to go to an electronic medical record or drown in the paper while being accused of Medicare fraud. There were many within the organization that did not believe it is possible to eliminate the majority of the paper in a medical office or comply with new HCFA documentation guidelines. I feared that we might get behind in the heavy patient schedule and the electronic medical record project would fail. If patients waited needlessly, the hope of converting to electronic medical record at this time would be lost. The project was already a year beyond my scheduled plan; so time was running out.

Because the project was to involve only a third of the clinic's patients, only brief training of three employees was completed. The training had occurred during breaks the previous day and was not well structured. It was anticipated that we would see only a few patients in the paperless environment the first day.

The change from paper chart to an electronic chart requires some familiarity with the software, but no amount of touching the keys can approximate the sensation when the patient arrives for care. As a sick patient begins his history, and the examination begins, the software cannot interfere.

The most difficult part of electronic medical record software is the new capability of software. Having multiple windows open in an electronic chart is like seeing several things at once. This is a stark contrast to the familiar one or two sheets that can be viewed in the paper record. Arranging the multiple windows in a way that is most appropriate for one's use in a real clinical examination requires time to think about and experience. On the first day of my actual use, the lack of familiarity with this new capability caused a decrease in my productivity as the information overwhelmed me. I felt lost at times not knowing what to do next. Disorientation is to be expected with any change this dramatic in the work process. All physicians will have difficulty making this leap just as I did that first morning. I felt lost and bewildered. I felt the uncertainty I first felt as a second-year medical student when I walked for the first time alone into an exam room with a live patient.

Before I arrived in the exam room, each patient completed a medical interview on the computer. I entered the room and the clinical examination began. Having a

---

[1]Allen R. Wenner, M.D., Primetime Medical, Inc. Used with permission.

documented medical history on each patient is like having a medical student examine the patient before you enter the room. It makes the job of gathering the data easier, faster, and better than having to do it entirely yourself. As I sat down, both the patient and I recognized a new format of the office visit—a triangle of the patient, the doctor, and the computer. As I confirmed the history and briefly edited the data that the patient had entered, the subjective note was completed without me dictating a word. Over half of my documentation was totally finished before I started the physical examination. Unhurried, for the first time I could ask my patients open-ended questions about how their illness was affecting their life. I could see quickly that, when all the pieces of the computer based paperless patient medical record functioned together, this would be a new world of health care delivery.

Next, I examined the patient. I entered the objective data for the physical examination in a documentation-by-exception fashion using hot keys. It was clear that this system was far faster, more complete, and better than any written or the dictated method that I had ever used. Again, everything was complete by the end of the exam with no dictation.

The subsequent thing I noticed on the computer screen was the appointment schedule online in real time. I had never seen it before. I never knew how many patients were actually waiting to see me, what time they had arrived, and why they were coming. It was immediately apparent that having the schedule of patients and their presenting complaints was helpful to the workflow. As patients arrived, I had the ability to order tests and procedures in advance of seeing them. This hastened workflow and saved the patient waiting time. Throat cultures were taken of all patients presenting with sore throats. I could look at the names and complaints of familiar patients and order studies from another exam room. This increased my efficiency.

The other remarkable part of the first morning was a consistency in the presentation of data. The nursing staff checked the vital signs and medications in a uniform fashion. Sometimes things were omitted or documented differently in the paper format by different staff members. The computerized format made everything the same. Because the medications were located in a consistent place on the screen, medication review was easier. This increased productivity slightly.

Laboratory, therapeutic, and radiological ordering were next in the workflow. Software streamlined this process and productivity was again enhanced. Electronic prescription writing was faster than any paper equivalent. Coding was frustrating. Coding is a process that normally is performed by the front office staff. Provider coding will enhance coding accuracy. Provider coding is a necessity to avoid rejected insurance claims and to prevent accusations of fraud under Medicare law. Diagnosis coding was difficult because ICD-9CM does not have practicing physicians in mind as its user. Procedural coding seemed easier, yet still more trouble than writing a five-digit number or circling a superbill entry. I slowed down coding. My neck began to hurt as I realized that I had the keyboard at the wrong height and the mouse was on the wrong side.

I felt lost at many times during the first day, even if only for a moment. Despite my computer skills, I could not remember where I was within the office visit. It was a horrible feeling of not only trying to determine what was wrong with the patient but also trying to document it appropriately without a scrap of paper. Although the first day was only to be for practice, I had to have the documentation for the legal medical record and I was no longer dictating.

In an electronic system, disposition, instructions, patient education, and referral are all different. The process is markedly different yet more complete. A learning curve is required.

We were late going to lunch as we tried to get the last patients through the system. The first morning we had had a 10% loss of efficiency, but I had expected much worse. At lunch the staff discussed what was happening to other employees. Soon they began to check in our afternoon patients as we missed most of our lunch. Throughout the afternoon, minor delays occurred as the original trained staff members began to show other employees how the system worked. The technical support staff graciously taught other staff how to use the system in brief lessons. Twice the anticipated number used the system by the first afternoon. Less hectic patient flow in the afternoon allowed for more comfort with the software.

Adequate on-site technical support prevented any hardware failures until the last hour when a computer failure prevented data entry. Aside from that computer hiccup, the day went surprisingly well. Nobody was abandoned in the waiting room unseen for hours. No patient was left in an exam room asleep. No patient departed without a prescription. Indeed, most were given a patient education handout. Patients were favorably impressed that they could see their medical record appearing before their eyes.

The day had gone much better than I had anticipated. My neck hurt as I arrived home. I self-diagnosed a job-related injury from twisting toward the screen on my ill-positioned stool. I denied that my neck pain was tension from the stress of taking a medical office paperless in less than a day. I knew how the Wright brothers felt a hundred years ago. I went to bed early contemplating the day knowing we would never go back again. We had left the world of the paper medical record forever.

The advantage of the system is clear. The paperwork is finished at the time the patient leaves the exam room. Patient education is possible. The software assures full documentation of the visit as it is happening. But the most amazing part of it all was that I spent 100% of my day sitting next to my patients. I never left them once!

Applying Your Knowledge

In the next exercise, you will apply what you have learned in this chapter to completely document Rosa Garcia's visit. In a second exercise, you will learn to print out your work to hand in to your instructor. You must complete both exercises in a single session, so if you are running out of class time this is a good stopping point.

During the course of these exercises you will create your first patient exam note. The goal of the exercises is to learn to use features of the software; therefore, the completed note is not intended to represent a complete medical exam.

Hands-On Exercise 21: Documenting a Visit for Headaches

Rosa Garcia visits her doctor's office complaining of headaches for the last 5 days.

Step 1

If you have not already done so, start the Student Edition software.

Locate the Medcin icon shown at the beginning of the chapter, as Figure 3-1. If you do not see it on the computer desktop, click on the Start button, and look in Programs or All Programs for the program named Medcin SE.

Step 2

When the Student Edition login screen is displayed, type into the field either your name or student ID.

> ### Note
>
> **Throughout the remainder of this book, red or blue circles will be printed in the text as a visual cue to instructions to click on a red or blue button to select a finding.**

When your name or ID is exactly as you want it to be, position the mouse pointer over the button labeled "OK," and click the mouse. The Student Edition software window will be displayed.

Step 3

Position the mouse pointer over the word Select in the menu at the top of the screen and click the mouse button once. A list of the Select menu options will appear.

Click the mouse on the word Patient to invoke the Patient Selection window shown in Figure 3-41.

Select the patient named **Rosa Garcia**.

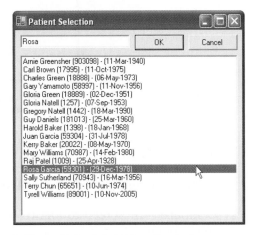

▶ Figure 3-41 Select Rosa Garcia from Patient Selection Window.

Step 4

Position the mouse pointer again over the word Select, and click the mouse button. Move the mouse pointer vertically down the list until the item New Encounter is highlighted. Click the mouse button.

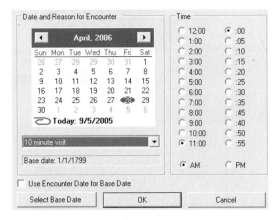

▶ Figure 3-42 New Encounter for a 10 Minute Visit, April 28, 2006 11:00 AM.

Using what you have learned in previous exercises, move the calendar to the date from the Select menu, click New Encounter. Use the date **April 28, 2006**, select the hour for **11:00**, the minutes for **:00**, and select **AM**. Then select the reason **10 minute visit** from the drop-down list.

Make certain you set the date, time, and encounter reason correctly. Compare your screen to Figure 3-42 before clicking on the OK button.

The left pane should display the Medcin Symptoms list and the right pane should display your student ID and Rosa Garcia's information. Before proceeding, confirm that the patient, date, time, and reason for visit (displayed in the title of the window) are all correct.

▶ **Figure 3-43 Chief Complaint Headaches More Than 5 Days.**

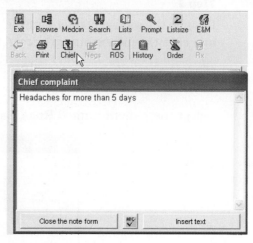

Step 5

Enter the Chief complaint by locating the button in the Toolbar labeled "Chief" and clicking on it.

The Chief complaint window will open; type: "Headaches for more than 5 days."

Compare your screen to Figure 3-43. If it is correct, click button labeled "Close the note form."

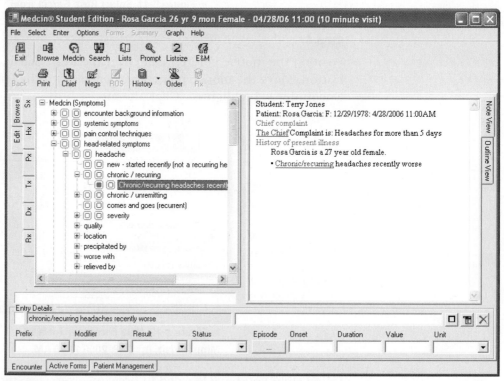

▶ **Figure 3-44 Sx Tab—Chronic Recurring Headaches Recently Worse.**

Step 6

Make sure that you have the Sx tab in the left pane selected. If you are uncertain, position the mouse pointer over the Sx tab and click the mouse once. Using the skills you have acquired in previous exercises, navigate the list of findings.

Locate and expand the tree of head-related symptoms.

Click on the small plus sign next to "head-related symptoms."

Click on the small plus sign next to "headache."

Click on the small plus sign next to "chronic/recurring."

Locate and click on the red button next to the following finding:

- (red button) episodes worse recently

The description of the finding will change to Chronic Recurring Headaches Recently Worse. Compare your screen to Figure 3-44.

▶ **Figure 3-45 Episodes 1 Per Day Lasting 2 to 4 Hours.**

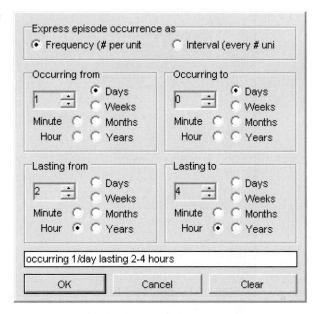

Step 7

Add information about the episodes of Ms. Garcia's headaches by clicking on the Episode button located at the bottom of your screen. (The button has an ellipsis on it.) The Episode window will be invoked.

Locate "Occurring from." Set it to 1 day by clicking on the up arrow button once and then clicking on the circle next to Days.

Locate "Lasting from." Set it to 2 hours by clicking on the up arrow button twice and then clicking on the circle next to Hours.

Locate "Lasting to." Set it to 4 hours by clicking on the up arrow button four times and then clicking on the circle next to Hours.

Compare your screen to the Episode window in Figure 3-45. If it is correct, click on the OK button.

▶ **Figure 3-46 Select Inade-quately Controlled from the Status Drop-Down List.**

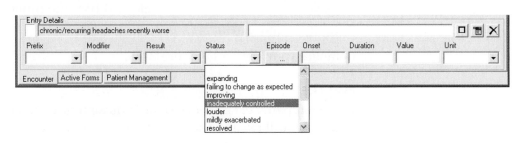

Step 8

Locate the Status field in the Entry Details section at the bottom of the screen. Click your mouse on the button with the down arrow in the status field. A drop-down list of status phrases (as shown in Figure 3-46) will appear.

Position your mouse pointer on the status "inadequately controlled" and click the mouse button.

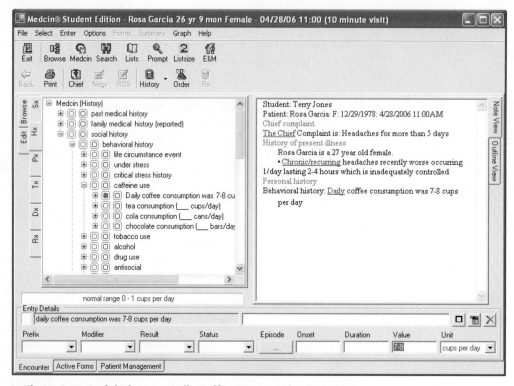

▶ Figure 3-47 Social History—Daily Coffee Consumption Was 7-8 Cups.

Step 9

Position the mouse pointer over the Hx tab and click the mouse once.

Locate and expand the tree of Social History.

Click on the small plus sign next to "social history."

Click on the small plus sign next to "behavioral history."

Click on the small plus sign next to "caffeine use."

Locate and click on the red button next to the following finding:

● (red button) "coffee consumption (cups/day)"

Step 10

Locate the Value and Unit fields in the Entry Details section at the bottom of the screen. Notice that the Unit field already contains the words "cups per day."

Click your mouse on the Value field and type the numerals **7-8**.

Press the Enter key on your keyboard.

Compare your screen to Figure 3-47.

Step 11

In the left pane, click on the small plus sign next to "Daily Coffee Consumption." This will expand the tree.

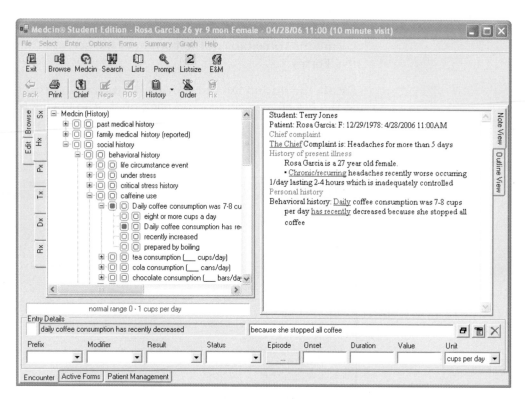

Locate and click on the red button next to the following finding:

- (red button) "recently decreased"

Step 12

Locate the free-text field in the first row of the Entry Details section, under the right pane.

Click your mouse in the free-text field. Type "**because she stopped all coffee**" in the field and then press the Enter key on your keyboard. Compare your screen with Figure 3-48.

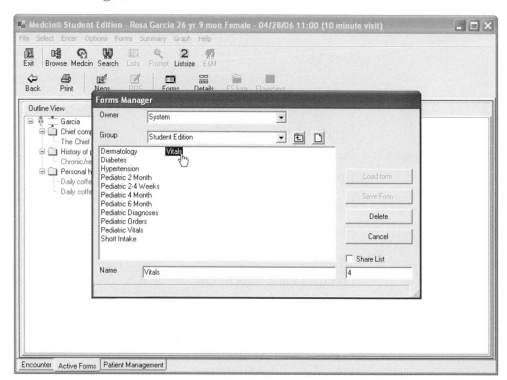

Step 13

Locate the three tabs at the bottom of the screen. Click on the tab labeled "Active Forms."

Locate the button labeled "Forms" in the second row of buttons on the Toolbar at the top of your screen and click on it. The Forms Manager will be invoked.

Locate and click on the form labeled Vitals.

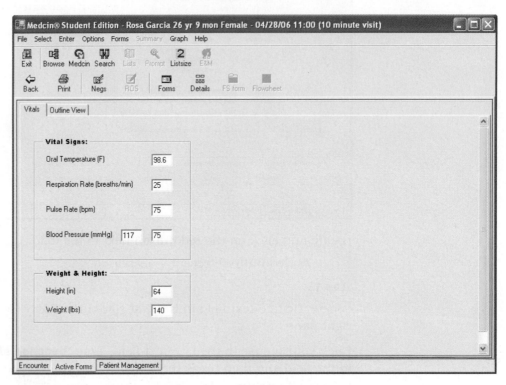

► Figure 3-50 Information for Rosa Garcia Entered in Vitals Form.

Step 14

Enter Ms. Garcia's Vital Signs into the corresponding fields as follows:

Temperature:	**98.6**
Respiration:	**25**
Pulse:	**75**
BP:	**117/75**
Height:	**64**
Weight:	**140**

When you have entered all of the vital signs, compare your screen to Figure 3-50 and then click your mouse on the Encounter tab at the bottom of the screen.

Step 15

Position the mouse pointer over the Px tab and click the mouse once. Notice that the vital signs information has been recorded in the exam note under the Physical Findings section.

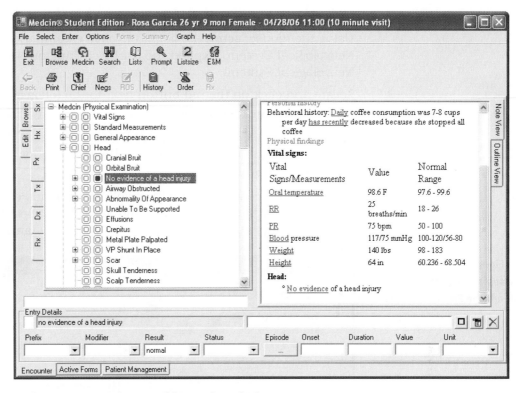

▶ **Figure 3-51 Px Tab—No Evidence of Head Injury.**

Click on the small plus sign next to "Head" to expand the list.

Locate and click on the blue button next to the following finding:

● (blue button) "evidence of injury"

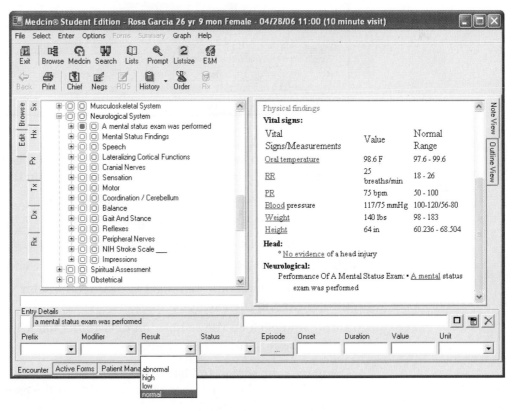

▶ **Figure 3-52 Px Tab—Mental Status Normal.**

Step 16

Using the mouse, scroll the list of physical examination findings until you see Neurological System. Expand the list by clicking on the small plus sign next to Neurological System.

Locate and click on the red button next to the following finding:

● (red button) "A mental status exam was performed"

Locate the Result field in the Entry Details section at the bottom of the screen. Click your mouse on the button with the down arrow in the Result field. A drop-down list will appear.

Position your mouse pointer on the result "normal" and click the mouse button. The field will display the word "normal," and the text in the exam note will change from "A mental status exam was performed" to "A mental status exam was normal."

▶ **Figure 3-53 Dx Tab—Assessment Withdrawal Headache From Caffeine .**

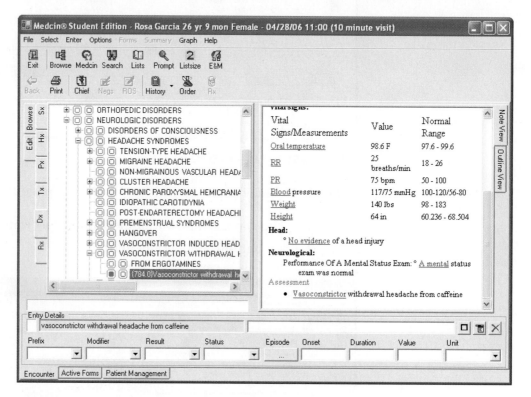

Step 17

Position your mouse pointer on the tab "Dx" and click the mouse. The Diagnosis, Syndromes, and Conditions list should be displayed in the left pane of the window.

Scroll the list until you see "Neurological Disorders."

Click on the small plus sign to expand the list.

Locate "Headache Syndromes" in the list.

Click on the small plus sign to expand Headache Syndromes.

Click on the small plus sign next to "Vasoconstrictor withdrawal headache" to further expand the list.

Locate and click on the red button next to the following finding:

● (red button) "From Caffeine"

Compare your screen to Figure 3-53. The finding "Vasoconstrictor withdrawal headache from caffeine" should be recorded in the exam note under a new heading: "Assessment."

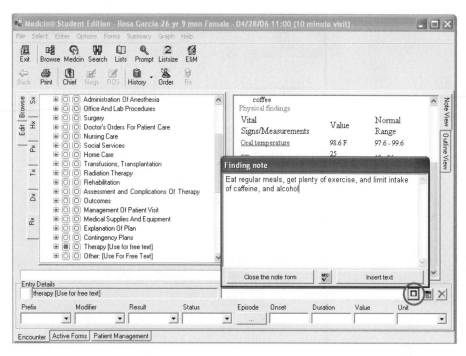

▶ **Figure 3-54 Rx Tab—Free-Text Therapy Note.**

Step 18

Position the mouse pointer on the Rx tab and click the mouse button. The Medcin Therapy list will be displayed.

Scroll the list until you see "Free Text," then and click on the red button next to the finding:

- (red button) "Free Text"

Locate and click on the Finding Note button (circled in red in the lower right corner of your screen). A Small Finding Note window will be invoked.

Type the following text into the Finding Note window: "Eat regular meals, get plenty of exercise, and limit intake of caffeine, and alcohol."

When you have finished, compare your screen to Figure 3-54. If it is correct, click your mouse on the button labeled "Close the note form." This will add your text to the exam note.

> **You have now successfully created your first complete exam note. However, do not stop or close the program until you complete the following exercise.**

Hands-On Exercise 22: Printing the Narrative Report

The Student Edition software does **not** save your entries to the patient's permanent medical record; therefore, you will **keep a record of your work by printing it**. In this exercise, you will learn to print the exam note.

You will be ask to give your finished printout to your instructor. **Do not quit or exit the program until you are sure the exam note has printed.** Once you exit, you will lose your work.

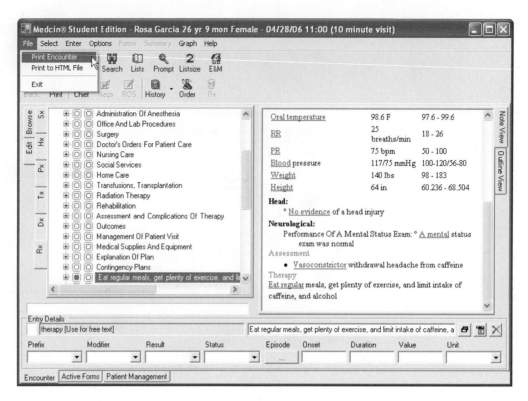

▶ Figure 3-55 File Menu Showing Print Options.

Step 1

There are two methods of printing your work, to a printer or to a file.

Position your mouse pointer over the menu item File at the top of the screen and click your mouse button. You will see the following two print options:

Print Encounter prints the Exam Note to a local or networked printer. This produces a paper copy you can hand in to your instructor.

Print to HTML File outputs the Exam Note to a file on your local computer. The file can be copied to a disk or e-mailed to your instructor.

Your instructor will tell you which method is appropriate for your class.

Step 2

Print Encounter

If the instructor wants you to print to a file, skip this—proceed to Step 3.

If the instructor wants you to print out a paper copy, move the mouse pointer down the list to highlight "Print Encounter" and click the mouse.

Depending on how your computer is set up, an additional print dialog from the operating system may appear. Figure 3-56 shows an example from Windows XP. Your computer may differ. But if you see a printer dialog similar to this, verify that the printer name is the printer you want to use and then click your mouse on the button labeled "Print."

If you need assistance printing, ask your instructor.

> **! Alert**
>
> **Some printers may close the dialog window before the printing has even started. Therefore, *do not exit the program until you have your printout in hand.* You could lose your work.**

► **Figure 3-56 Print Dialog for Windows XP.**

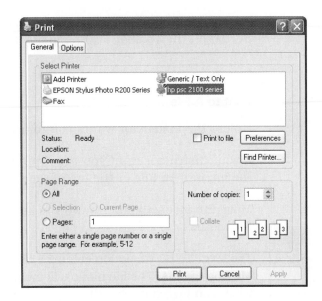

Compare your print out to Figure 3-57 and then give it to your instructor. You may print extra copies by repeating steps 1 and 2 before exiting the Student Edition software.

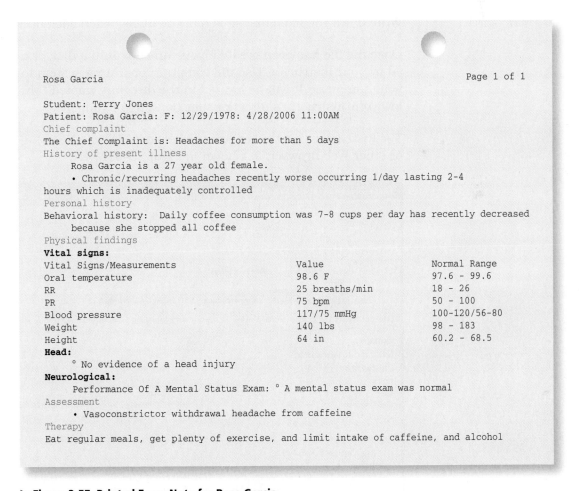

Rosa Garcia   Page 1 of 1

Student: Terry Jones
Patient: Rosa Garcia: F: 12/29/1978: 4/28/2006 11:00AM
Chief complaint
The Chief Complaint is: Headaches for more than 5 days
History of present illness
     Rosa Garcia is a 27 year old female.
     • Chronic/recurring headaches recently worse occurring 1/day lasting 2-4
hours which is inadequately controlled
Personal history
Behavioral history: Daily coffee consumption was 7-8 cups per day has recently decreased
     because she stopped all coffee
Physical findings
Vital signs:
Vital Signs/Measurements   Value   Normal Range
Oral temperature   98.6 F   97.6 - 99.6
RR   25 breaths/min   18 - 26
PR   75 bpm   50 - 100
Blood pressure   117/75 mmHg   100-120/56-80
Weight   140 lbs   98 - 183
Height   64 in   60.2 - 68.5
Head:
     ° No evidence of a head injury
Neurological:
     Performance Of A Mental Status Exam: ° A mental status exam was normal
Assessment
     • Vasoconstrictor withdrawal headache from caffeine
Therapy
Eat regular meals, get plenty of exercise, and limit intake of caffeine, and alcohol

► **Figure 3-57 Printed Exam Note for Rosa Garcia.**

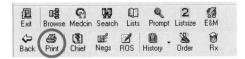

► **Figure 3-58 Print Button on Toolbar (circled in red).**

You also can print out copies of the exam note at anytime by clicking the Print button on the Toolbar at the top of your screen (shown in Figure 3-58).

Step 3

Print to A File

Unless the instructor wants you to print to a file, omit this step.

If your instructor want you to print to a file, position your mouse pointer over the menu item File at the top of the screen and click your mouse button.

Move the mouse pointer down the list to highlight "Print to HTML," and click the mouse.

The Print To HTML option creates a file on your computer in the directory named My Documents. The file name will include the student name or ID you entered when you logged in plus the date and time. The file name ends in "htm."

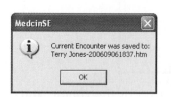

► **Figure 3-59 Print to HTML Confirmation.**

When the file has been successfully created, a Print To HTML confirmation similar to Figure 3-59 will be displayed.

Write down the file name shown in the dialog, then click on the OK button.

Once the file has been created, you can copy it to a disk or e-mail it, as directed by your instructor. Use the computer operating system to locate the file on your computer. It will be located in the directory named "My Documents." Follow your instructor's directions for handing in your file.

The instructor can view or print the student HTML file using Internet Explorer or other Web browser, as shown in Figure 3-60.

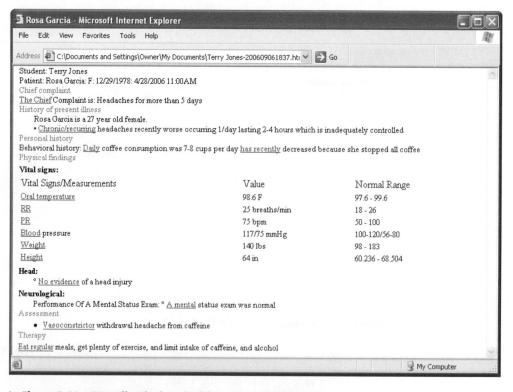

► **Figure 3-60 HTML File Displayed with Internet Explorer.**

Chapter Three Summary

EHR software allows clinicians to document the patient exam by selecting findings for symptoms, history, physical examination, tests, diagnoses, and therapy.

The Medcin Student Edition software has been specially created for this course. Therefore, it will be different in some aspects from EHR systems you will encounter when working in a medical office, but the concepts, skills, and familiarity with EHR systems you will acquire by practicing with the Student Edition will transfer directly into the workplace.

To more easily understand the Student Edition software, we divided the screen into four sections and discussed each of them.

1. The Menu bar and Toolbar are located at the top of the window.

The Menus are: File, Select, Enter, Options, Forms, Summary, Graph, and Help. Within them are lists of functions in the Student Edition software.

You select a menu item by positioning the mouse pointer over one of these words and click the mouse once; a list of functions will drop down below the word. Moving the mouse pointer vertically down the list will highlight each item. Clicking on the highlighted item will invoke that function. Clicking the mouse anywhere on the screen other than the list will close the list.

In the Student Edition, highlight means a blue rectangle appears over the item.

The Toolbar is also located at the top of your screen. It consists of two rows of buttons, each containing a small picture called an icon, and a brief label. The purpose of the Toolbar is to allow quick access to commonly used functions. Clicking on a button in the Toolbar invokes a function or feature. The Exit, Print, and Form Manager buttons on the Toolbar were used in this chapter.

2. The Medcin Nomenclature Pane is located in the left pane of the window. The left pane displays the lists of Medcin findings from which you choose when documenting a patient exam. On the left of the nomenclature pane there are 8 tabs. These look like tabs on file folders. Six of the tabs, labeled Sx (symptoms), Hx (history), Px (physical examination), Tx (tests), Dx (diagnosis, syndromes, and conditions), and Rx (therapy), are used to group the findings logically into six broad categories. The tab labeled Edit is used when editing a finding that has already been selected. The Browse tab was not covered in this chapter.

3. The Encounter View Pane is located in the right pane of the window. It has two tabs, labeled Note View and Outline View. When the clinician selects a finding from the Medcin nomenclature list in the left pane, the text for that finding will display in the right pane.

The Exam Note tab dynamically displays the findings accompanied by narrative text automatically generated by MEDCIN. Titles for the sections of the note also are added dynamically as findings are selected. Free-text also may be entered through the software and it will appear in the exam note pane as well.

The Outline View displays findings that have been selected as well as appropriate ICD-9CM or CPT-4 codes. The extra narrative text is omitted in the Outline View.

4. The Entry Details fields are located at the bottom portion of the screen. The Entry Details section consists of two rows of fields and three buttons that affect only the currently selected finding. Using the Entry Details features, the user can add detail or free-text to the finding or remove a finding from the exam note.

The first row has two fields and three buttons. The first field displays the finding description as it appears in the text. The field cannot be directly edited. The second field may be used to add short free-text to notes to the finding.

The three buttons are also located in the first row of fields. The first button invokes the Finding Note window, which makes it easier to enter longer free-text notes and includes a spell checker. The second button invokes a context menu and was not covered in this chapter. The third button deletes the current finding from the exam note (but not from the nomenclature).

The fields in the second row are Prefix, Modifier, Result, Status, an Episode button, Onset, Duration, Value, and Unit. The fields add informational text to the finding in the exam note, and in some cases modify its meaning. The advantage of these fields over free-text is that they allow the EHR to store the status, result, and so on, as fielded data that can be used later, which free-text entries do not.

Documenting the Visit

The first step in every encounter is to select the patient, then open an existing encounter or create a new encounter. In this chapter, you learned to select patients and create new encounters.

It is important when creating new encounters to use the exact date, time, and reason given in the exercise.

Selecting patients, encounters, adding chief complaint, finding notes, and selecting forms open small windows that close when the user is finished.

The left pane displays lists of Medcin findings in a tree structure in which small plus signs indicate more detailed findings are available. Clicking on the small plus sign expands the list further like branches on a tree. When a tree is expanded, the button changes to a small minus sign, which, if clicked, collapses the expanded list back to its previous size.

Findings are selected by clicking on buttons with red or blue circles in them located next to each finding. When a finding is selected, circles in the button become filled with red or blue and the finding is displayed in the exam note. The solid colors in the buttons help you quickly identify which findings have already been selected. Generally, the red button records that a patient has the condition described in the finding. Clicking the blue button usually records that a patient did not have the symptom or the condition described in the finding. The description of the finding also changes in the left pane when a finding is selected.

Visually Different Button Styles

Many EHR software packages are based on the Medcin Nomenclature. Each vendor has created a unique visual style, and although they share a common nomenclature, the EHR may look quite different. One difference is the look of the buttons. In many systems, a large plus sign and a large minus sign similar to those shown in Figure 3-61 are used to select findings instead of the red and blue buttons used in the Student Edition. However, as you become familiar with the Medcin Student Edition software, you should have no trouble transitioning to a similar Medcin-based EHR in a medical practice.

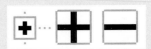

▶ Figure 3-61 Alternative Select Buttons Used to Select Findings in Some EHR Systems.

You can add or remove findings from the note in any order. Section titles are dynamically added or removed by the software based on the findings selected.

Using the Entry Detail fields at the bottom of the screen you can add text or a value to a finding, such as "quit smoking **3** months ago." Entry Detail fields also alter the meaning of a finding, for example, a prefix can change "smoking" to "history of smoking."

Some data will be easier to enter as a logical group. Medcin Forms allow a number of findings to be entered at once. Vital Signs is an example of a form that is used to enter data in almost every exam and medical practice.

Forms such as Chief Complaint also can be used as a means to add free-text that is automatically associated with a finding or a section of the exam note.

The bottom of the screen has three tabs: Encounter, Active Forms, and Patient Management. Except for Chief Complaint and Finding Note forms, most forms are located on the Active Forms tab. They are selected from the Forms Manager, which is a selection window invoked by a button on the Toolbar.

You can print the exam note at any time and as often as you like while practicing your exercises. However, the Student Edition of the Medcin software does **not** save your entries to the patient's permanent medical record; therefore, you will **keep a record of your work by printing it**. If your school permits, you may alternatively print it to an HTML file, which can be copied to a disk or e-mailed to your instructor.

Remember, do not quit or exit the program **until you are sure the exam note has printed**. Once you exit, you will lose your work.

Testing Your Knowledge of Chapter 3

You may run the Medcin Student Edition software and use your mouse on the screen to answer the following questions:

1. Which Menu did you use to Select the patient?

2. Which Menu did you use to start a New Encounter?

3. Where did you set the label "10 Minute Visit," which appeared in the title of the window?

The tabs on the left of the list of Medcin findings have medical abbreviations. Write the meaning of each of the following:

4. Sx _____

5. Hx _____

6. Px _____

7. Tx _____

8. Dx _____

9. Rx _____

10. How old was the patient?

11. How long had she been having headaches?

12. What was the clinical assessment (her diagnosis)?

13. How did you invoke the Vital Signs Window?

14. Why is it important to make sure you have your printout before exiting the Student Edition?

15. You should have produced a narrative document of a patient encounter, which you printed. If you have not already done so, hand it in to your instructor with this test. The printed exam note will count as a portion of your grade.

Data Entry at the Point of Care

Learning Outcomes

After completing this chapter, you should be able to:

◆ Use the Student Edition software to create exam notes for a variety of patients and conditions

◆ Search for a finding using the Search button

◆ Understand and use the Prompt feature

◆ Load and use Lists of Findings to speed up data entry

◆ Understand and use Forms

◆ Record orders for tests and therapies

◆ Record prescriptions

Increased Familiarity with the Software

In this chapter, you will practice documenting patient visits using the Student Edition software. One of the goals in this chapter is to increase your familiarity with the software and thereby increase your speed of data entry. Another is to explore methods of data entry that enable a clinician to document the visit while the patient is still present.

The exam notes you will produce will be similar to documents you would create in a medical office. Exercises in this chapter are intended to provide conceptual learning experiences with the software; however, they are not intended to represent full and complete medical exams.

In Chapter 3, you learned the basic layout of the screen and the concepts of adding, editing, and adding details to findings. Detailed instructions for scrolling and navigating the lists, which were provided in the previous chapter, should no longer be necessary. From this point forward, simplified instructions will guide you in areas where you are already familiar with the program.

Documenting a Brief Patient Visit

The next exercise will allow you to evaluate your knowledge of the software by using only the features you have learned in Chapter 3. If you have any difficulty with this exercise, you should review and repeat the exercises in Chapter 3 before continuing with this chapter.

Hands-On Exercise 23: Documenting a Visit for Common Cold

Patient Harold Baker feels like he has caught some sort of "bug." Like many patients who have a cold, he wants to see his doctor, and so the medical office has scheduled a brief 10-minute office visit for him. Using what you have learned so far, document Mr. Baker's brief exam.

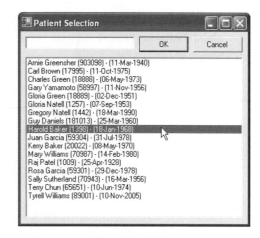

▶ **Figure 4-1 Selecting Harold Baker from the Patient Selection Window.**

Step 1

If you have not already done so, start the Student Edition software.

Click Select on the Menu bar, and then click Patient.

In the Patient Selection window, locate and click on **Harold Baker**.

Note that in the Patient Selection window patients are listed alphabetically by their first name. You also may type a portion of the first name in the field at the top of the window as you did in Chapter 3.

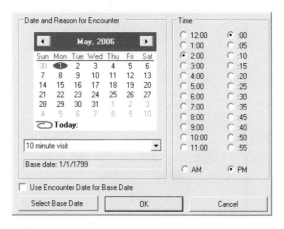

▶ **Figure 4-2 New Encounter for a 10 Minute Visit, May 1, 2006, 2:00 PM.**

Step 2

Click Select on the Menu bar, and then click New Encounter.

Select the date **May 1, 2006**, the time **2:00** PM, and the reason **10 minute visit**.

Make certain you set the date, time, and reason correctly. Compare your screen to Figure 4-2 before clicking on the OK button.

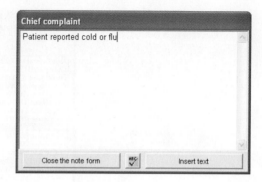

► **Figure 4-3 Chief Complaint Dialog for Patient Reported Cold or Flu.**

Step 3

Enter the Chief complaint by locating the button in the Toolbar labeled "Chief" and clicking on it.

In the dialog window which will open, type "Patient reported cold or flu."

Compare your screen to Figure 4-3 before clicking on the button labeled "Close the note form."

► **Figure 4-4 Symptom— Headache.**

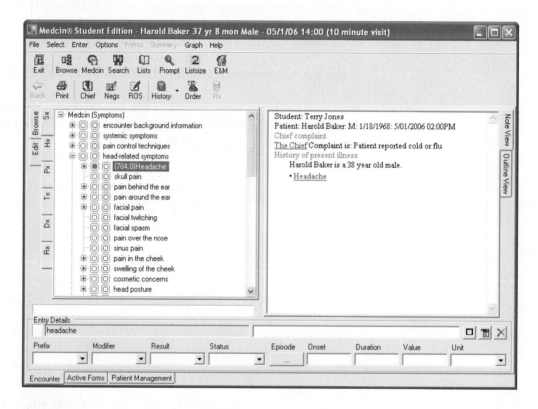

Step 4

The patient reports a headache, runny nose, and sneezing. Enter the patient's symptoms using the list of findings on the Sx tab.

Expand the tree of Medcin findings.

Locate and click on the small plus sign next to Head Symptoms.

Locate and click on the red button next to the following finding:

● (red button) Headache

Compare your screen to Figure 4-4.

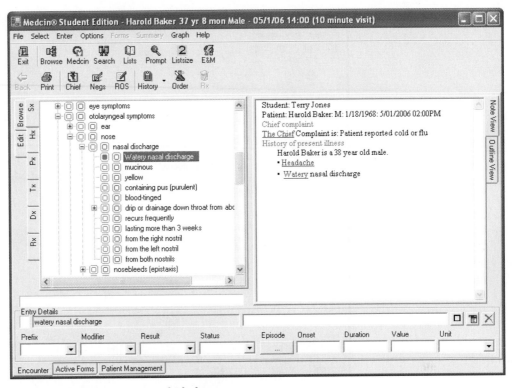

▶ **Figure 4-5 Symptom—Nasal Discharge.**

Step 5

Scroll the list of Sx findings downward to locate Otolaryngeal Symptoms.

Expand the tree of findings further.

Click on the small plus sign next to Otolaryngeal Symptoms.

Locate and click on the small plus sign next to Nose.

Locate and click on the small plus sign next to Nasal Discharge.

Locate and click on the red button for the following finding:

● (red button) Watery

Compare your screen to Figure 4-5.

Step 6

Scroll the list of Sx findings further downward to locate and click on the red button for the following finding:

● (red button) Sneezing

Compare your screen to Figure 4-6.

Step 7

The patient does not smoke. Enter this fact in the patient's History.

Click on the Hx tab.

Expand the tree of Medcin findings.

Locate and click on the small plus sign next to Social History.

Locate and click on the small plus sign next to Behavioral History.

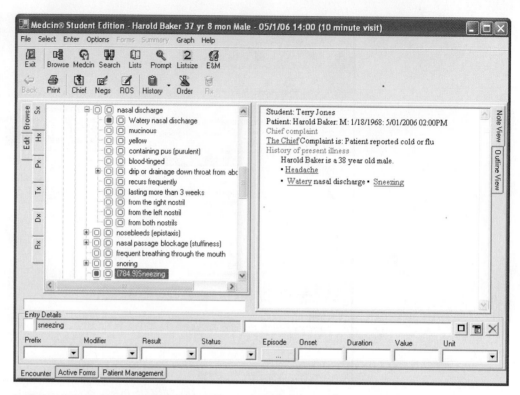

▶ **Figure 4-6 Symptom—Sneezing.**

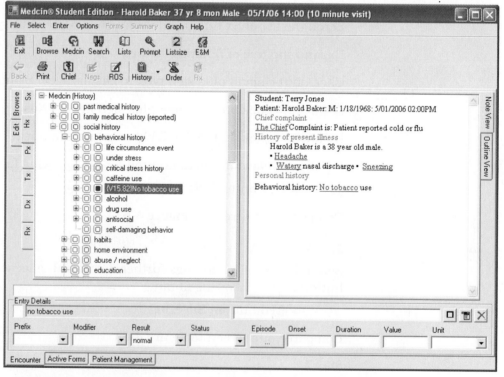

▶ **Figure 4-7 History—No Tobacco Use.**

Locate and click on the blue button next to the following finding:

> ● (blue button) Tobacco use

The description will change to "No Tobacco Use."

Compare your screen to Figure 4-7.

Step 8

Enter the patient's Vital Signs using the Vitals Form located in the Active Forms tab (as you did in Chapter 3).

Locate and click on the tab labeled Active Forms at the bottom of your screen (circled in Figure 4-8.)

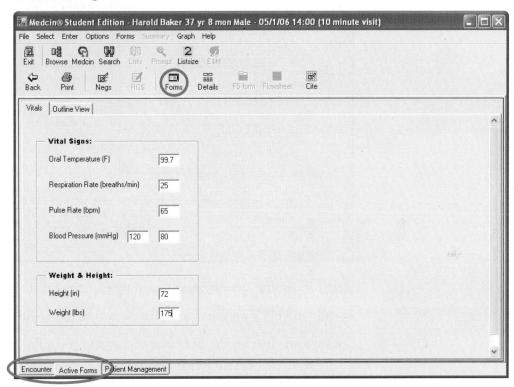

▶ **Figure 4-8 Vital Signs Form (with tabs and buttons circled in red).**

Locate and click on the button labeled "Forms" in the Toolbar at the top of your screen (also circled in Figure 4-8.) The Forms Manager window will be invoked.

Locate and click on the Form name "Vitals" in the list. The form shown in Figure 4-8 will be displayed.

Enter Mr. Baker's Vital Signs in the corresponding fields as follows:

Temperature:	**99.7**
Respiration:	**25**
Pulse:	**65**
BP:	**120/80**
Height:	**72**
Weight:	**175**

When you have entered all of the vital signs, compare your screen to Figure 4-8 and then click your mouse on the Encounter tab at the bottom of the screen.

Step 9

The clinician examines the patient's head, eyes, ears, nose, inside of mouth, and lungs.

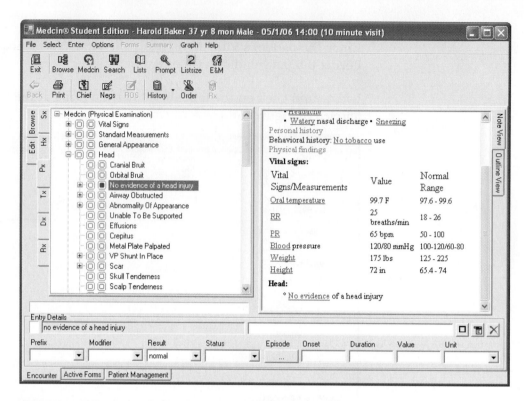

Begin recording the Physical Exam by clicking on the Px tab.

Locate and click on the small plus sign next to "Head."

Locate and click on the blue button next to the following finding:

● (blue button) Evidence of injury

The description will change to "No evidence of injury." Compare your screen to
Figure 4-9.

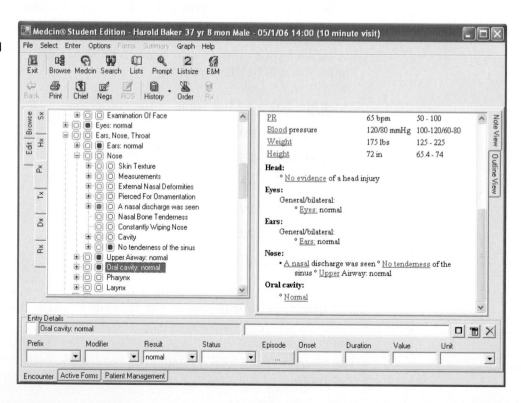

Step 10

Scroll the list of Physical findings downward to locate Eyes.

Locate and click on the blue button for the following finding:

- (blue button) Eyes

Expand the tree of findings further.

Locate and click on the small plus sign next to Ears, Nose, and Throat.

Locate and click on the small plus sign next to Nose.

Locate and click on the small plus sign next to Nasal Discharge.

Locate and click on the appropriate buttons for the following findings:

- (blue button) Ears
- (red button) Nasal Discharge
- (blue button) Sinus tenderness
- (blue button) Upper airway
- (blue button) Oral cavity

Compare your screen to Figure 4-10.

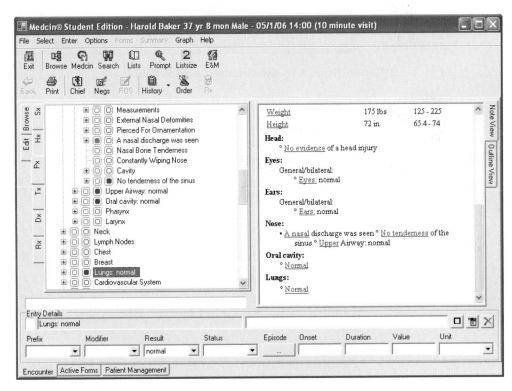

▶ Figure 4-11 Physical Exam—Lungs.

Step 11

Scroll the list of Physical findings further downward to locate Lungs.

Locate and click on the blue button for the following finding:

- (blue button) Lungs

Compare your screen to Figure 4-11.

The clinician concludes the patient has a common cold, and tells him to rest and drink plenty of fluids.

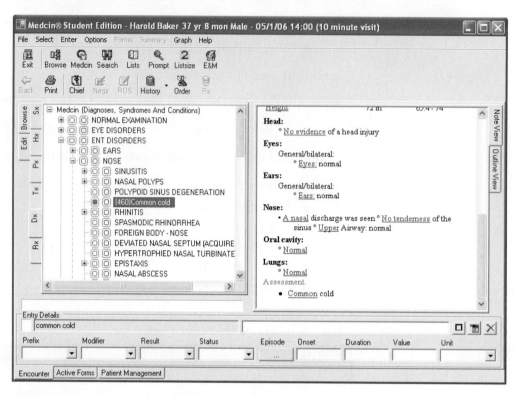

▶ Figure 4-12 Assessment—Common Cold.

Step 12

Record the Assessment by clicking on the Dx tab.

Expand the tree of findings.

Locate and click on the small plus sign next to ENT Disorders.

Locate and click on the small plus sign next to Nose.

Locate and click on the red button for the following finding:

   ● (red button) Common Cold

Compare your screen to Figure 4-12.

Step 13

Record the Plan by clicking on the Rx tab.

Expand the tree of findings.

Locate and click on the small plus sign next to Basic Management Procedures and Services.

Scroll the list downward until you locate "Nutrition and Hydration Services," then click on the small plus sign next to it.

Locate and click on the red button for the following finding:

   ● (red button) Fluids

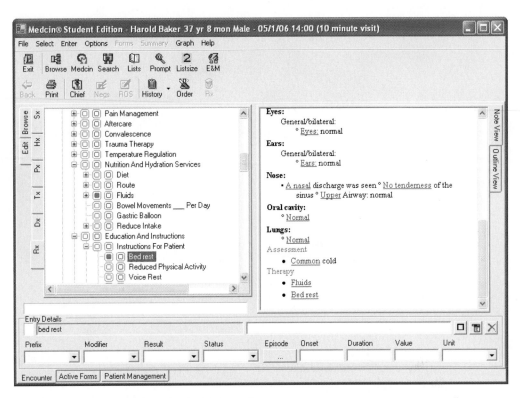

▶ **Figure 4-13 Therapy Plan—Patient Instructions.**

Expand the tree of findings further.

Locate and click on the small plus sign next to Education and Instructions.

Locate and click on the small plus sign next to Instructions to Patient.

Locate and click on the red button for the following finding:

● (red button) Bed rest

Compare your screen to Figure 4-13.

Step 14

Print your completed exam note.

Click File on the Menu bar, and then click Print Encounter or Print To HTML (as directed by your instructor).

Alert

Do not close or exit the Encounter until you have a printed copy in your hand. *You will lose your work if you exit before printing.*

If you are printing your work, you may click the Print button on the Toolbar at the top of your screen instead of selecting Print Encoounter from the Menu.

Compare your printout or file output to Figure 4-14. If it is correct, hand it in to your instructor. If there are any differences, review the previous steps in the exercise and find your error.

Once you have successfully completed this exercise, you should be comfortable with the general process of locating findings and expanding the tree to view additional findings. Future exercises in this book will instruct you to expand the tree where necessary without explicitly telling you to click the small plus sign.

```
Student: Terry Jones
Patient: Harold Baker: M: 1/18/1968: 5/01/2006 02:00PM
Chief complaint
The Chief Complaint is: Cold or flu
History of present illness
      Harold Baker is a 38 year old male.
      • Headache
      • Watery nasal discharge o Sneezing
Personal history
Behavioral history: No tobacco use
Physical findings
```

Vital signs:

Vital Signs/Measurements	Value	Normal Range
Oral temperature	99.7 F	97.6 - 99.6
RR	25 breaths/min	18 - 26
PR	65 bpm	50 - 100
Blood pressure	120/80 mmHg	100-120/60-80
Weight	175 lbs	125 - 225
Height	72 in	65.4 - 74

Head:
    ° No evidence of a head injury
Eyes:
General/bilateral:
    ° Eyes: normal
Ears:
General/bilateral:
    ° Ears: normal
Nose:
    • A nasal discharge was seen ° No tenderness of the sinus ° Upper Airway: normal
Oral cavity:
    ° Normal
Lungs:
    ° Normal
Assessment
    • Common cold
Therapy
      • Fluids
      • Bed rest

▶ **Figure 4-14 Printed Exam Note for Howard Baker.**

Why Speed of Entry Is Important in the EHR

In the previous chapter, it was stated that the goal of many EHR systems is to document the visit completely before the patient ever leaves the office. To document in real time, you must be able to quickly navigate and enter findings.

In real estate the cliché is that "the secret is location, location, location." This can be paraphrased in EHR as "the secret is speed, speed, speed."

Hardly anything is more frustrating than wanting to say something and not being able to remember the right word for it. Suppose you knew all the right words but you weren't allowed to use them unless you could find them and point to them. Such is the case with clinicians starting to use an EHR. They already know what they want to say, but they have to look it up and point to it with the mouse before they can record it. Add that to the average day in the clinic with a constant stream of patient visits intermingling acute illnesses with chronic disorders meaning terms that you found for the last patient are not the ones you will need for the next patient.

The schedule is full, the next patient is waiting, and the provider is ready to document the exam. To be successfully adopted in a medical practice, an EHR needs to present the finding the clinician needs when it is needed.

Methods to Increase Speed of Entry

The exercises so far have used relatively simple exams with findings that were fairly easy to locate. Patient visits to a medical office will involve different problems, more complex exams with less time to complete the exam note. Is there a faster way to find what you are looking for than just scrolling the navigation list and expanding the trees? Yes!

EHR vendors work constantly with EHR users to devise means to locate and present findings when they are most likely needed. The Student Edition software provides examples of a few of the ways EHR systems do this. In this chapter, you will learn about additional features that help a clinician enter data more quickly. These include using the Toolbar and features such as Search, Prompt, Lists, and Forms.

Encounter Tab Toolbar

Located at the top of your screen are two rows of icon buttons called a "Toolbar." You have previously used several of the buttons on the Toolbar. As you practice the remaining exercises in this book, you will learn about and use additional buttons on the Toolbar.

EHR systems frequently allow each provider to configure the Toolbar individually. This improves speed, by providing quick access to the features most needed by a particular clinician. The Toolbar in the Student Edition has been preset to match the exercises in the textbook.

You may have noticed that different buttons appear on the Toolbar when you switch to the Active Forms tab. Toolbar buttons also change when you access the Patient Management tab. These variations in the Toolbar on other tabs will be covered in subsequent chapters. For now, we will focus on the Toolbar as it appears when you use the Encounter tab (see Figure 4-15).

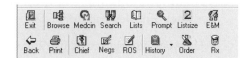

▶ **Figure 4-15 Toolbar as It Appears on the Encounter Tab.**

A quick reference guide to the buttons available on the Toolbar when you are on the Encounter tab is provided here. You will learn more about the buttons by using them in Hands-On Exercises. You can refer back to this guide any time you are unsure of the function of a button on the Toolbar.

Top Row:

Exit   Exits the Student Edition program and closes the window.

Browse   Displays the current finding's position in the Medcin nomenclature hierarchy using a separate tab.

Medcin   Displays the Medcin nomenclature in the data entry trees.

Search   Invokes the search dialogue window.

Lists   Invokes the Lists Manager window.

Prompt   Generates a list dynamically based on the currently selected finding.

List Size Increases or decreases the number of findings displayed from a list.

E&M   Calculates the Evaluation and Management (billing) code based on the findings recorded in the note.

Bottom Row:

Back   Reinvokes the previous entry mode selection.

Print   Prints the current Exam Note.

Chief   Invokes a finding note window specifically for Chief complaint.

Negs   Automatically selects the right button for all findings in the Sx or Px tab that are not already selected. In most cases, this is the blue button.

ROS   Review of Systems (On/Off). When On (button appears depressed), all symptoms selected are grouped in the Review of Systems category. When Off, symptoms selected are grouped in the History of Present Illness category.

History   Automatically sets the prefix of the current finding to "History of."

Order   Automatically sets the prefix of a current finding in the Tx or Rx tab to "Ordered."

Rx   Invokes the Prescription Writer window for medications in the Rx tab.

Using buttons on the Toolbar speeds up data entry by invoking windows when convenient and by reducing the number of items a clinician must click to complete a note.

Search and Prompt Features

As you learned in Chapter 2, medical nomenclatures such as SNOMED CT and Medcin have hundreds of thousands of findings. The challenges with large clinical vocabularies include:

◆ How can you locate a finding among hundreds of thousands?

◆ Does the nomenclature use the same term for the finding as you do?

◆ Where are other related findings?

The Search feature provides a quick way for the clinician to locate a desired finding in the nomenclature. Search produces a list of the findings almost instantly. Medcin addresses semantic differences in medical terms in several ways:

1. Search performs automatic word completion so if you search for knee but the finding is for knees it will still find it.

2. Medcin includes an extensive list of synonyms that are used in an alternate word search. For example, if you search for knee injury, the search results will also include findings for knee burns, knee trauma, and fractured patella, among others.

3. Search identifies related findings in other tabs so that when you search for a word or phrase in a particular tab, related findings are automatically available in the other tabs. This means that when you are using search when documenting a patient exam, as you proceed through the exam, the other tabs may already have related findings that you will use.

How Search Works

Search is not designed to find every instance that contains the words being searched because the search results would often have too many findings. Instead, search uses the Medcin hierarchy (the tree view you have expanded in previous exercises). It finds and shows the highest level match and does not list all the expanded findings below it.

For example, in Chapter 3 you did an exercise with Headache during which you expanded the tree to show many types of headache. If you searched for Headache, the search results would display the finding "Headache" with a small plus sign next to it. If you wanted to peruse the various types of headaches, you would click on the plus sign to expand the next level of the tree. If you were, however, searching for "migraine headache," the search results would have expanded the tree view for headache to show migraine, which is at a lower level.

Search always begins in the tab you are currently in when you start the search. If there are search results in another tab but none in the current tab, the software will automatically change tabs to the first one with results. The order of the tabs you see on the screen is the same order in which it will display the search results. For example, if you are on the Tx tab when you search and there are no results but there are results for the other tabs, it will automatically change the left pane to the Dx tab to display those results because that is the next tab in order.

Hands-On Exercise 24: Using Search

In this exercise, you will learn to use the Search and Prompt features as well as several new buttons on the toolbar. The exercise will not produce a very thorough exam note, but it will give you experience using the features.

The patient, Gary Yamamoto, has been referred to you with suspected Angina. The patient does not seem in any immediate danger, so you are going to schedule a complete work up later this week. In the meantime, you want to order some tests so that the results will be ready when the patient returns.

Rather than navigate the entire Medcin findings, you can start with a known symptom or disease and work forward. To quickly locate the desired findings, we will use the Search function.

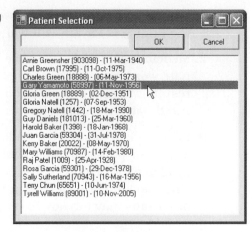

► **Figure 4-16 Selecting Gary Yamamoto from the Patient Selection Window.**

Step 1

If you have not already done so, start the Student Edition software.

Click Select on the Menu bar, and then click Patient.

In the Patient Selection window, locate and click on **Gary Yamamoto**.

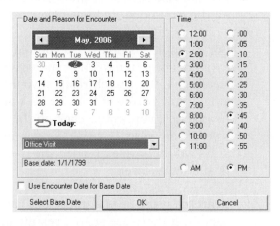

► **Figure 4-17 New Encounter for an Office Visit, May 2, 2006, 2:45 PM.**

Step 2

Click Select on the Menu bar, and then click New Encounter.

Select the date **May 2, 2006**, the time **2:45** PM, and the reason **Office Visit**.

Make certain you set the date, time, and reason correctly. Compare your screen to Figure 4-17 before clicking on the OK button.

► **Figure 4-18 Chief Complaint Dialog for Suspected Angina.**

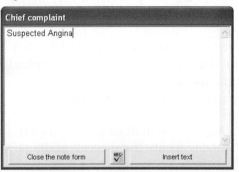

In the next two steps, the nurse enters the Chief complaint and vital signs.

Step 3

Enter the Chief complaint by locating the button in the Toolbar labeled "Chief" and clicking on it.

In the dialog window which will open, type "Suspected Angina."

Compare your screen to Figure 4-18 before clicking on the button labeled "Close the note form."

Step 4

Enter Mr. Yamamoto's Vital Signs using the Vitals Form located in the Active Forms tab (as you have done in the previous exercises).

Click on the Active Forms tab.

Locate and click on the button labeled Forms in the toolbar at the top of your screen.

(If you have difficulty locating the Active Forms tab or Forms button, refer to Figure 4-8 in the previous exercise.)

Select the form labeled Vitals from the list in the Form Manager window.

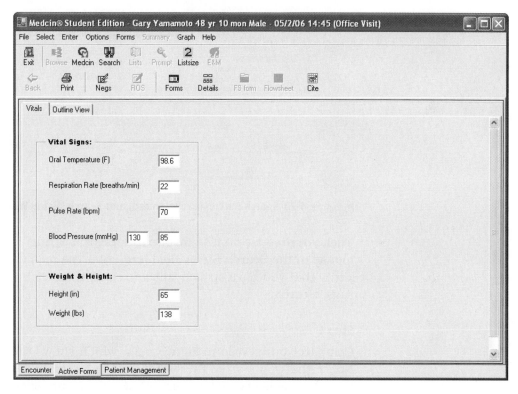

▶ **Figure 4-19 Vital Signs Form for Gary Yamamoto.**

Enter Gary Yamamoto's Vital Signs in the corresponding fields as follows:

Temperature: **98.6**

Respiration: **22**

Pulse: **70**

BP: **130/85**

Height: **65**

Weight: **138**

When you have finished, compare your screen to Figure 4-19. If it is correct, click on the tab labeled Encounter at the bottom of the window.

Step 5

Locate the Search button on the Toolbar near the top of the screen. The search icon resembles a small pair of binoculars. It is circled in red in Figure 4-20.

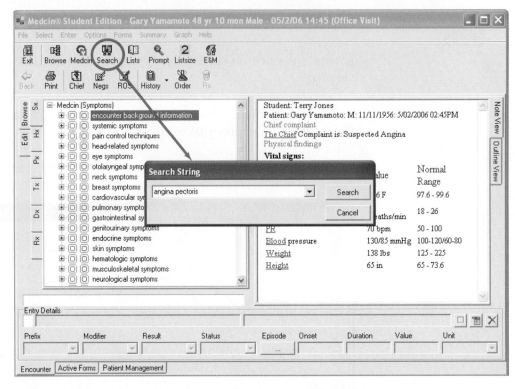

▶ **Figure 4-20 Search Button (circled in red) and Search Dialog Window.**

Click your mouse on it to invoke the "Search String" window. Position your mouse in the Search String field and enter the medical term "**angina pectoris**." Verify that you have spelled this correctly, then click the button in the box that says "Search."

Step 6

Compare your screen to Figure 4-21, which shows the search has succeeded. Notice that you started the search on the Sx tab but the screen is now on the Dx tab. This is because the search was for a very specific pair of words that did not exist in the other tabs.

As discussed earlier in this section, the Search result displays in the current tab if there are any findings that match the search string; otherwise, it displays in the first tab with findings that match. Had the search simply been for Angina, History of Angina would have been found and the Hx tab would have been displayed.

Note

No Results?

If your screen does not match Figure 4-21, or you received the message: "nothing found to match search," repeat Step 4 and verify that you have spelled the medical terms correctly. In this exercise you are doing a very specific match, and a spelling error will alter the search results.

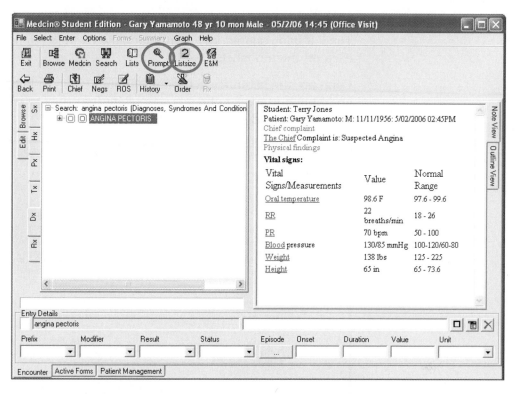

► Figure 4-21 Search Results (with Prompt and List buttons circled in red).

Step 7

Locate the button labeled "List Size" on the Toolbar near the top of the screen. The List Size icon is a teal square with a black numeral (from 1 to 3) in it. It is circled in red in Figure 4-21. As the name implies, the List Size controls the number of findings that will be displayed in a "prompt list."

Each time you click the mouse on the List Size button, it changes to the next number in sequence, from 1-3. When it reaches 3, it will start again at 1 the next time the button is clicked. You will visually see what this does in Step 9.

For this step, set the List Size to **1**. If the List Size is currently greater than 1, click your mouse over the icon repeatedly until it displays a **1**.

Step 8

Locate the Prompt button on the Toolbar near the top of the screen. The Prompt icon resembles a small magnifying glass. It is circled in red in Figure 4-21. The full name of the feature is "Prompt with current finding." This feature generates a list of findings that are clinically related to the finding currently highlighted. For this step, angina pectoris should be highlighted in blue on your screen.

Once the list is displayed, you can use it just like you have been using the full nomenclature in previous exercises. That is, you can record findings by clicking on the red or blue buttons next to the findings. You also can change tabs; however, the findings displayed in the other tabs will be limited to those that are clinically related to the finding that was highlighted when you clicked the Prompt button.

Click your mouse on the Prompt button at this time.

Step 9

The left pane should have automatically changed to the Sx tab; if it did not, click on the tab labeled Sx.

Compare the list in the left pane of your screen to Figure 4-22, ignoring the red and blue buttons for the moment. Note that the list of findings is much shorter than normally displays in the Sx tab.

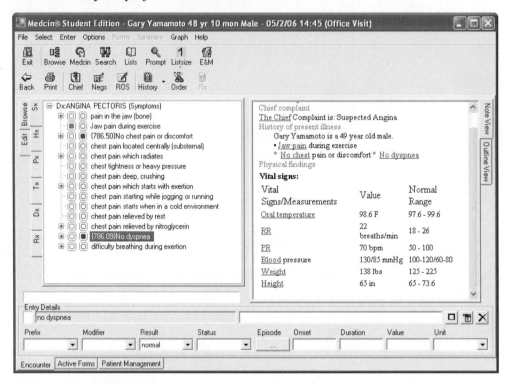

▶ **Figure 4-22 Sx Tab Displaying Findings Related to Angina (shown after findings selected).**

The first line in the left pane usually includes the name or source of the list. Heretofore, this was just the name of the tab, for example, Medcin (Symptoms); now, however, the first line reads "Dx: ANGINA PECTORIS (Symptoms)." This indicates that the list is limited to findings that are clinically related to the diagnosis *angina pectoris*.

Before you select findings for your exam note, this is a good opportunity to explore the function of the List Size button discussed in Step 7.

Click on the List Size button once. The icon should change to the numeral **2**; note that the number of findings has increased.

Click on the List Size button again and the icon should change to the numeral **3**; note that the number of findings has increased even more.

Click on the List Size button one more time and the icon should change back to a **1** and the list of findings should return to the shortest list.

Proceed with the exercise by locating and clicking on the following symptoms reported by the patient:

- (red button) Jaw pain while exercising
- (blue button) Chest pain or discomfort
- (blue button) Difficulty breathing (dyspnea)

Compare your screen to the selected red and blue buttons in Figure 4-22 before proceeding.

► **Figure 4-23 Hx Tab Displaying Findings Related to Angina.**

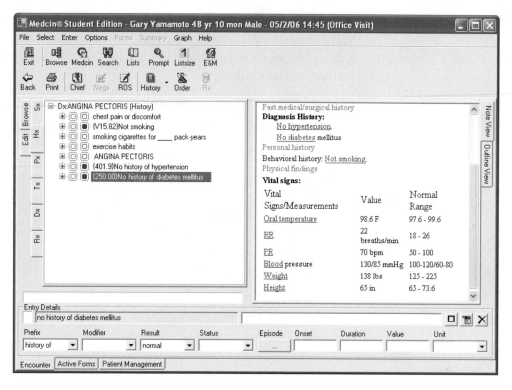

Step 10

The patient does not smoke, and denies any history of high blood pressure or diabetes. Click on the Hx tab and enter the patient's history information by locating and clicking on the following history findings:

- (blue button) Smoking
- (blue button) HYPERTENSION (Systemic)
- (blue button) DIABETES MELLITUS

Compare your screen to Figure 4-23 before proceeding.

► **Figure 4-24 Px Tab—Physical Exam Findings Related to Angina.**

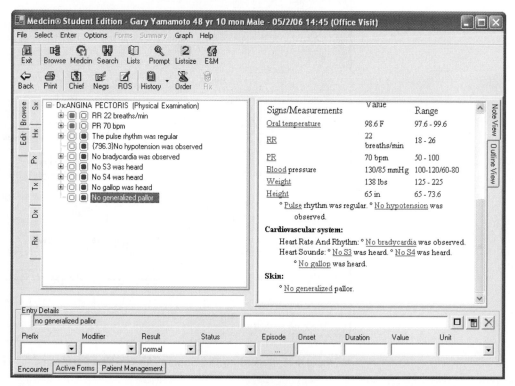

Step 11

Today's visit is preliminary and mainly to order and perform some tests before a complete exam scheduled later in the week. However, a brief physical is performed by the clinician.

Click on the List Size button until the list size is **2**.

Click on the Px tab. Notice that two findings are already selected; these are vital signs entered earlier.

Enter the physical exam information by locating and clicking on the following findings:

- (blue button) Pulse Rhythm Irregular
- (blue button) Hypotension
- (blue button) bradycardia
- (blue button) S3
- (blue button) S4
- (blue button) gallop
- (blue button) generalized pallor

Compare your screen to Figure 4-24 before proceeding.

Do not exit the program until you have completed the following exercise.

Hands-On Exercise 25: Ordering Diagnostic Tests

Continuing with Mr. Yamamoto's visit, this exercise will explore several methods of recording tests and orders.

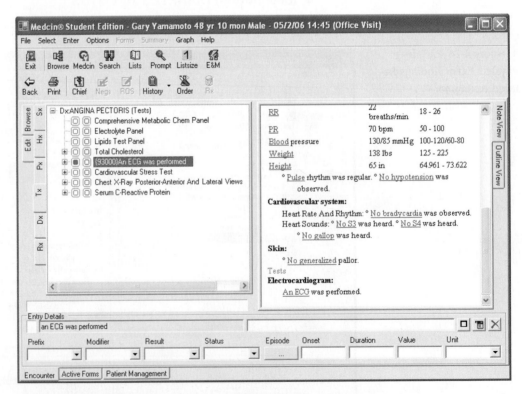

▶ **Figure 4-25 Recording The Finding "An ECG Was Performed."**

Step 12

Click on the List Size button until it displays the numeral **1**.

Click on the Tx tab which will display a list of tests that might be ordered for angina pectoris.

You can indicate that your office *performed* a test by clicking on the red button next to its name. Locate and click on the following finding:

● (red button) electrocardiogram

The exam note should now read "An ECG was performed," as shown in Figure 4-25.

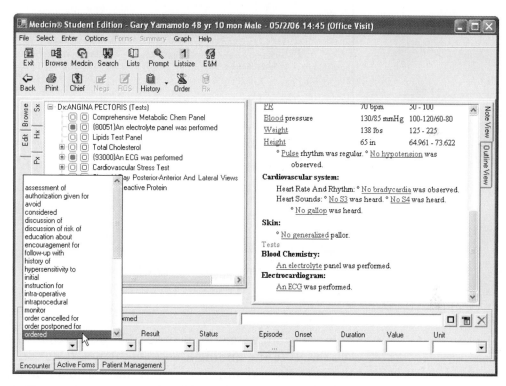

▶ **Figure 4-26 Drop-Down List of the Prefix Field Used for Electrolyte Panel.**

Step 13

Although some tests, such as electrocardiograms, are performed in the office, most lab tests and many radiology procedures are "ordered" by the physician, but the test is performed elsewhere.

In this exercise, you will order several lab tests. There are two ways to do this: by using the Entry Details Prefix field or by using the Orders button on the Toolbar. In this step, you are going to use a prefix.

Locate and click on the following test:

● (red button) electrolyte panel

Note that it appeared in the exam note under Tests "An Electrolyte Panel was performed." However, your office didn't really perform the Electrolyte test; the doctor just wanted to order it.

In Chapter 3, you practiced using the drop-down lists in the Entry Details fields. You are going to use that knowledge here. With the finding Electrolyte Panel still highlighted, click on the Prefix field in the bottom of the screen. A drop-down list will appear as shown in Figure 4-26. Locate and click on the word "Ordered" in the list of prefixes.

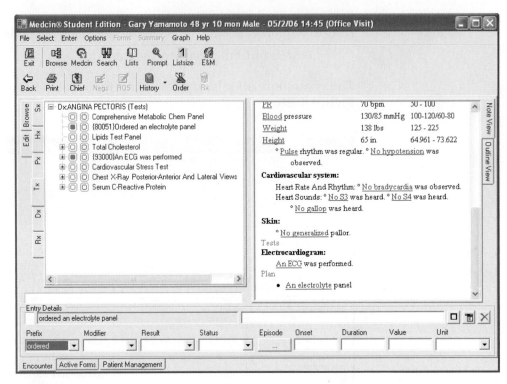

▶ **Figure 4-27 Electrolyte Panel "Ordered."**

Step 14

Compare your screen to Figure 4-27. Notice that when you added the prefix "Ordered" to the finding Electrolyte Panel, it not only changed the meaning in the exam note but also moved the test to a different category in the exam notes. Medcin assigns a test that was performed or has a result status to the category of test procedures but assigns a test that is ordered to the category "plan."

Step 15

Now that you are familiar with one method of ordering, you can see that it requires two steps. However, both of these actions can be accomplished in a single step by using the "Order" button on the Toolbar. To order a test using the order button, you only need to highlight the finding and click the "Order" button. You do not have to click either the red or blue button for the finding.

Locate and click on the description Lipids Test Panel to highlight it (as shown in Figure 4-28).

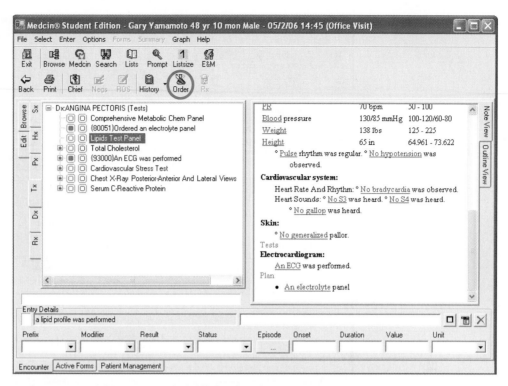

▶ **Figure 4-28 Lipids Test Panel Highlighted; Order Button (circled in red).**

Locate and click on the button labeled "Orders" in the Toolbar at the top of your screen. The Order icon resembles a lab beaker and test tube. It is circled in red in Figure 4-28.

Step 16

Using what your have learned in the previous step, order an additional test and an x-ray.

Highlight Total Cholesterol and click on the Order button in the Toolbar.

Highlight Chest X-Ray and click on the Order button in the Toolbar.

Compare your screen to Figure 4-29. From this example, you can see the advantage of using Toolbar buttons for orders. Similar buttons also are useful for History items and prescriptions, as you will learn in subsequent exercises.

Step 17

The clinician will determine the final assessment after the complete workup later this week. Therefore, the diagnosis at this time will be Possible Angina Pectoris.

Click on the Dx tab and record the assessment.

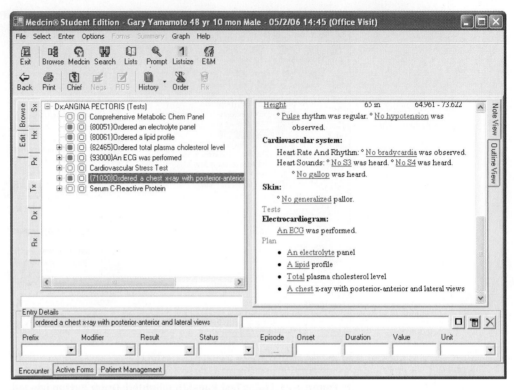

▶ Figure 4-29 Tests and X-Rays Ordered Using the Order Button.

Locate and click on the red button for the following finding:

- (red button) Angina Pectoris

Locate the Prefix field in the Entry Details section. Click the mouse on the button with the down arrow in the Prefix field.

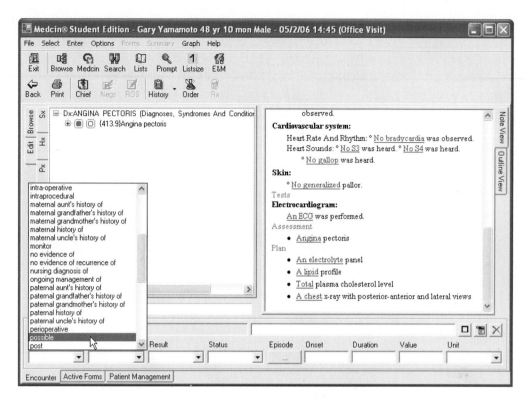

▶ **Figure 4-30 Dx Tab with Drop-Down List for Prefix—Possible Angina Pectoris.**

Scroll the drop-down list to locate and click on the word **Possible**, as shown in Figure 4-30.

This completes Mr. Yamamoto's preliminary visit. Print your completed exam note.

Step 18

Click File on the Menu bar, and then click Print Encounter or Print To HTML (as directed by your instructor).

If you are printing your work, you may click the Print button on the Toolbar at the top of your screen instead of selecting Print Encounter from the menu.

Compare your printout or file output to Figure 4-31. If it is correct, hand it in to your instructor. If there are any differences, review the previous steps in the exercise and find your error.

(!) **Alert**

Do not close or exit the Encounter until you have a printed copy in your hand. *You will lose your work if you exit before printing.*

```
Student: Terry Jones
Patient: Gary Yamamoto: M: 11/11/1956: 5/02/2006 02:45PM
Chief complaint
The Chief Complaint is: Suspected Angina.
History of present illness
      Gary Yamamoto is a 49 year old male.
      • Jaw pain during exercise.
      ° No chest pain or discomfort  °  No dyspnea
Past medical/surgical history
```

Diagnosis History:
```
      No hypertension.
      No diabetes mellitus
```
Personal history
Behavioral history: Not smoking.
Physical findings

Vital signs:

Vital Signs/Measurements	Value	Normal Range
Oral temperature	98.6 F	97.6 - 99.6
RR	22 breaths/min	18 - 26
PR	70 bpm	50 - 100
Blood pressure	130/85 mmHg	100-120/60-80
Weight	138 lbs	125 - 225
Height	65 in	65 - 73.6

```
         ° Pulse rhythm was regular.   ° No hypotension was observed.
```

Cardiovascular system:
```
      Heart Rate And Rhythm: ° No bradycardia was observed.
      Heart Sounds: ° No S3 was heard.   ° No S4 was heard.   ° No gallop was heard.
```

Skin:
```
      ° No generalized pallor.
```
Tests

Electrocardiogram:
```
      An ECG was performed.
```
Assessment
```
      • Possible angina pectoris
```
Plan
```
      • An electrolyte panel
      • A lipid profile
      • Total plasma cholesterol level
      • A chest x-ray with posterior-anterior and lateral views
```

▶ **Figure 4-31 Printed Exam Note with Angina Orders for Gary Yamamoto.**

Shortcuts That Increase Speed for Routine Exams

Search is fine for quickly locating findings related to anything that you don't see on a regular basis. However, most medical offices see a lot of patients with the same conditions. This is because of either the medical specialty or seasonal changes. For example, a pulmonary specialist sees primarily respiratory cases, nephrologists see patients with kidney problems, and during the cold and flu season family physicians see many patients with upper respiratory infections.

In each of these cases, physicians tend to perform the same type of exam, look for the same findings, order the same tests, and prescribe from a short-list of treatments recommended for the condition. Therefore, it is logical for the practice to create shorter, quicker methods of entering the data, by the type of exam or condition.

In the next two sections, we will explore two features of EHR systems that are used extensively in medical practices, Lists and Forms. This is not "canned medicine." These are templates to display findings that the doctor uses most frequently for different types of conditions or diseases so that the exam can be documented with minimal navigation or searching. Additionally, Lists and Forms can be shared or personalized to reflect the way in which each provider practices medicine.

The Concept of Lists

You may not have heard the term Lists used in the context of an EHR, but the concept should be very familiar to you because you have been scrolling and navigating the list of findings since Chapter 3. In the previous exercise, the Prompt function created a short-list of findings, relevant to the words you were searching for. You learned that you could select findings and create an exam from the Search/Prompt results the same as navigating the tree manually.

Now, imagine that you are a pediatrician who treats many children with ear-aches (*otitus media*) and that each time the patient's chief complaint was ear-ache the system could magically present the findings that you typically used to document the visit. That is the idea behind lists. Of course, lists don't magically appear. They are created by clinicians and their assistants for the many types of exams and conditions seen at their practice. However, the time spent making each list is saved again and again when subsequent patients are seen for the same or similar reasons.

The advantages of using lists are that they behave just like browsing the full Medcin Nomenclature except that only the desired subset is shown. The list can (and usually does) contain findings in every tab. This means that time savings are realized all the way through the exam. If only certain therapies or certain drugs are used for a particular condition, then when the clinician clicks the mouse on the Rx tab, only those items are shown. When using a list, if there is a finding that is needed but is not on the list, the provider can instantly switch to the full hierarchy of Medcin findings and then back to the list.

Lists are often limited to one particular condition such as *otitis media*, but this is not a rule; it is a convenience factor because shorter lists mean less scrolling. Lists are flexible and can contain as many findings as necessary to document a typical visit. With some types of exams, the assessment may turn out to be one of several different diagnoses. Therefore, a list with more findings reduces the possibility that the provider will need to switch to browsing the full Medcin tree.

A good example of this type of list is the one used for the next exercise. Adult Upper Respiratory Infections (URI) could include any of several possible infections such as *rhinitis*, *sinusitis*, or *bronchitis*. Therefore, it would be helpful for the list to include a larger list of relevant findings.

Over time, practices should create lists for any medical condition that is seen regularly. This will speed up entry of all routine exams and increase adoption of the EHR by clinicians in the practice. If clinicians differ in how they would document a particular exam, they should create personal copies of the list and tailor it to their style of medicine.

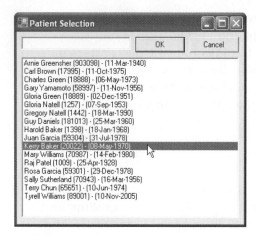

▶ **Figure 4-32 Selecting Kerry Baker from the Patient Selection Window.**

Hands-On Exercise 26: Using Adult URI List

URI is an acronym for Upper Respiratory Infection. During the cold and flu season, medical offices often see many patients with upper respiratory infections. Therefore, a list of findings for adults presenting with symptoms of URI can really speed up the documentation process.

Kerry Baker comes to the office complaining of sinus pain, stuffiness, and a runny nose. She says she has caught her husband's "bug." The medical practice has created a List of Medcin findings to use for this type of visit. They have named it Adult URI. In this exercise, you will learn to use the List feature as well as several additional buttons on the Toolbar.

Step 1

If you have not already done so, start the Student Edition software.

Click Select on the Menu bar, and then click Patient.

In the Patient Selection window, locate and click on **Kerry Baker**.

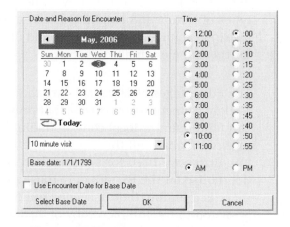

▶ **Figure 4-33 New Encounter for a 10 Minute Visit, May 3, 2006, 10:00 AM.**

Step 2

Click Select on the Menu bar, and then click New Encounter.

Select the date **May 3, 2006**, the time **10:00 AM**, and the reason **10 Minute Visit**.

Make certain that you set the date and reason correctly. Compare your screen to Figure 4-33 before clicking on the OK button.

Step 3

Enter the Chief complaint by locating the button in the Toolbar labeled "Chief" and clicking on it.

In the dialog window that will open, type "Patient reported cold or flu."

Compare your screen to Figure 4-34 before clicking on the button labeled "Close the note form."

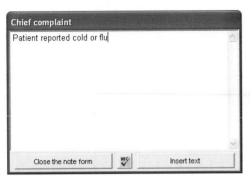

▶ **Figure 4-34 Chief Complaint Dialog for Patient Reported Cold or Flu.**

Step 4

In this exercise, the nurse will begin the visit by taking Kerry's Vital Signs.

Use the form labeled "Vitals," which you will select from the Forms Manager, invoked on the Active Forms tab (as you have done in previous exercises).

Enter Kerry's Vital Signs in the corresponding fields on the Form as follows:

Temperature:	**99**
Respiration:	**23**
Pulse:	**78**
BP:	**120/80**
Height:	**60**
Weight:	**100**

When you have finished, compare your screen to Figure 4-35 and, when it is correct, click on the Encounter tab at the bottom of the screen.

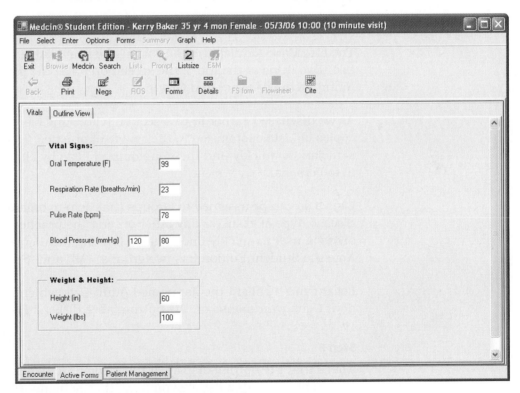

▶ **Figure 4-35 Vital Signs Form for Kerry Baker.**

Step 5

As the patient reported cold or flu symptoms, we will use a List created for this type of exam.

Locate and click on the Lists button in the Toolbar at the top of your screen (circled in red in Figure 4-36). The icon resembles an open book. The List Manager window will be invoked.

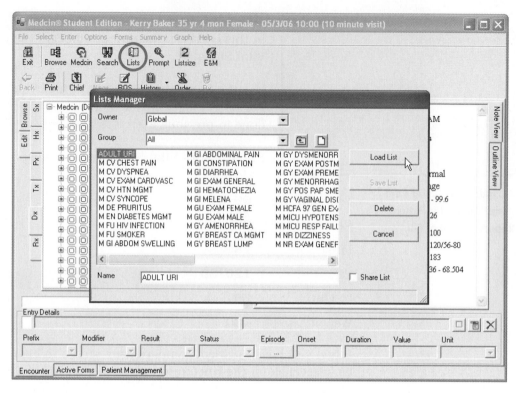

► **Figure 4-36 Select Adult URI from Lists Manager Window (invoked by Lists button circled in red).**

The List Manager displays the various Lists available to providers in the practice. Two fields at the top of the screen organize the display of List names, filtering them by Owner and Group.

As we discussed earlier in this section, clinicians also can create personal copies of Lists customized to their style of practice. The Owner field allows the clinician. to quickly find their customized Lists by changing the field from Global to Personal.

Lists also can be assigned to Groups that help to organize them by body system, disease, type of exam, or any other criteria the practice desires. The Group field allows a user to quickly find a list by limiting the display to a desired group. Note the Student Edition has two groups, "All" and "Student Edition."

Locate and highlight the list named Adult URI, which is the first list in the window. Click your mouse on the button labeled "Load List."

Step 6

Notice that the normal display of the Medcin Nomenclature in the left pane has been replaced with a list of symptoms that patients with upper respiratory infections are likely to report. Notice that the title of the first line "Templates (Symptoms)" indicates that the finding are limited by a List (referred to in the left pane as a Template).

Locate and click on the following symptom findings:
- (red button) Sinus pain
- (red button) Nasal discharge
- (red button) Nasal blockage (from stuffiness)

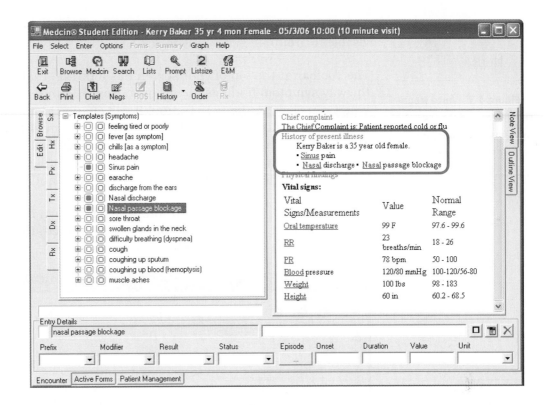

Compare your screen to Figure 4-37. Before proceeding, notice that Symptoms reported by the patient have been documented in "History of Present Illness" or "HPI" (circled in red).

Step 7

Review of Systems is a way of organizing an exam by body systems starting from the head down. You may be familiar with the body systems from other medical classes. The body systems in a standard ROS are: Constitutional symptoms, HEENT (Head, Eyes, Ears, Nose, Mouth, Throat), Cardiovascular, Respiratory, Gastrointestinal, Genitourinary, Musculoskeletal, Integumentary (skin and/or breast), Neurological, Psychiatric, Endocrine, Hematologic/Lymphatic, and Allergic/Immunologic.

Typically, a provider will document the symptoms directly related to the Chief complaint in the HPI. The remainder of the symptoms review is to rule out other causes. It is typically documented in a "Review of Systems" or "ROS."

For example:

A patient comes in with a headache. Typically the characteristics of the headache (location, quality, duration, etc.) and any other symptoms occurring with the headache (such as fever) would be documented in the History of Present Illness.

The clinician would then perform a symptomatic review of other systems such as stiff neck, facial pain, abdominal pain, any numbness or tingling, and so on. Most of these will be negative. Because they weren't reported by the patient and are not directly correlated to or the result of a headache, they would typically be documented in the ROS.

In Chapter 5, you will learn about the CMS coding guidelines used to determine the correct Evaluation and Management code for billing. Because the

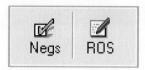

▶ **Figure 4-38 Auto Negative (Neg) and Review of Systems (ROS) Buttons (enlarged).**

CMS guidelines have specific rules for counting ROS body systems, it is *not* advisable to group all symptoms in the HPI.

The Toolbar at the top of your screen has a button that can be used to change the way symptom findings are grouped from HPI into a Review of Systems. When you click on the ROS button, it will change in appearance to look as though the button is pressed in (as shown in Figure 4-39 below, circled in red). This indicates that the ROS grouping is on. If you click on the button again, it will change back to its original appearance. This indicates that the ROS grouping is *not* on. The ROS button toggles between on and off.

Locate and click on the ROS button, which is shown in Figure 4-38. When you click on findings when the ROS button is depressed, the findings selected will be placed in the Review of Systems group.

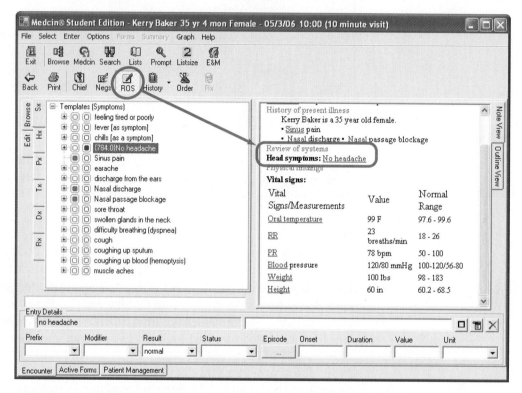

▶ **Figure 4-39 Symptom: No Headache in Review of Systems Group (circled in red).**

Step 8

Verify the ROS button is depressed, then locate and click on the following finding:

- (blue button) Headache

Compare your screen to Figure 4-39. Notice that the finding "No Headache" was placed in a new group "Review of Systems" that was created in the note (shown circled in red).

Step 9

Frequently, most of the symptoms in the ROS will be negative, as they were not reported by the patient in the HPI. Using a List such as Adult URI, you could quickly go down the list clicking a blue button on each of the remaining findings. However, that would still be a lot of mouse clicks.

There is another button on the Toolbar to speed up the documentation, which is called Auto Negatives. When the clinician has clicked a red or blue button for all the relevant positive findings, the remainder of the list can be set to the negative with one click on the "Negs" button on the Toolbar (shown enlarged in Figure 4-38).

The purpose of Auto Negatives is not to shortcut the exam process but to speed up the documentation of the exam. Clinicians find they can review systems much more quickly than they can document each finding. The Auto Negatives button allows them to complete this portion of the exam and then document it in fewer clicks.

The Auto Negative feature selects the button in the right column (usually a blue button) for all displayed findings that are not already set. The user can change any finding after the process is finished. Because all the findings displayed in the current tab are automatically selected, the Auto Negative feature works best with Lists or Forms because the List is already limited to findings the clinician would normally use in a particular type of exam.

Locate and click on the button labeled "Negs" in the Toolbar at the top of your screen. The icon resembles a box with a teal check mark. The Negs button is circled in red in Figure 4-40.

All symptoms that have not previously been selected have automatically had their blue buttons selected. Notice how quickly the documentation process was completed.

Compare the exam notes on your screen with Figure 4-40. (You may need to scroll the right pane upward to see the full effect.) Notice that the three findings with red buttons were not altered.

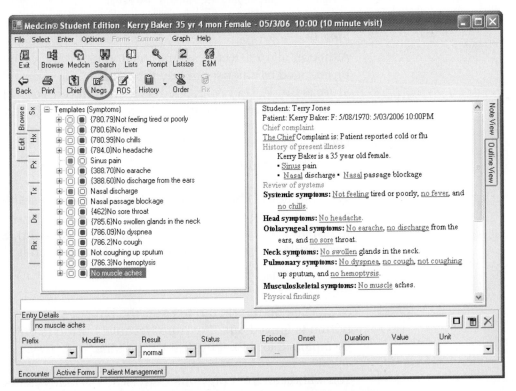

▶ **Figure 4-40 Auto Negative Button Quickly Completes Multiple Findings.**

The Auto Negative function will record the findings according to the state of the ROS button. Because the ROS button was depressed, the additional symptoms were recorded in the Review of Symptoms group, not the HPI group.

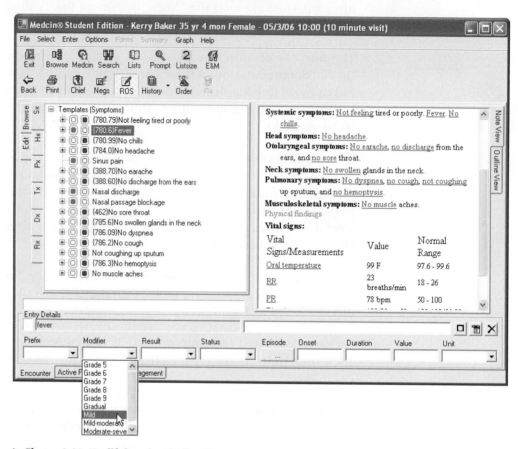

▶ Figure 4-41 Modifying the Finding "No Fever."

Step 10

Although all unselected symptoms findings were set by Auto Negative, they can be changed by the user at any time during the exam. Note that Kerry's temperature is 99° F. Therefore, she has a slight fever. You will change the finding "No Fever" from blue to red and add a modifier in the Entry Details field.

Locate and click on the following finding:

● (red button) No Fever

The finding will change to Fever. With the finding still highlighted, click your mouse on the button with the down arrow in the Entry Details field "Modifier" to display a drop-down list (as shown in Figure 4-41). Scroll the list of modifiers until you locate the word "Mild," then click on it.

Step 11

Next, click on the Hx tab to enter the patient's history. Note that the "Negs" button is grayed out. The Auto Negative button is only available on the Sx (Symptoms) and Px (Physical Exam) tabs.

You will recall from previous exercises how many items are typically in the Hx tab, but, because you are using a list, only those items related to Adult URI are

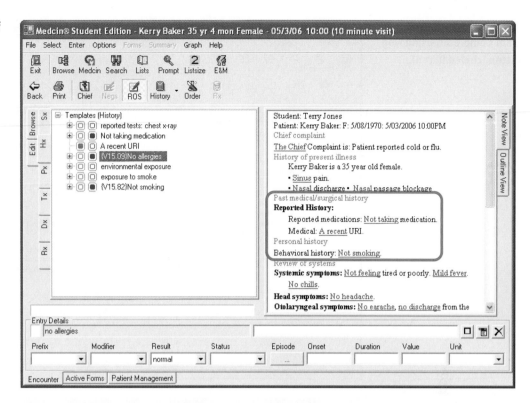

displayed. This makes navigation of the list quicker because the list is shorter. Locate and click on the following History findings.

- (blue button) Taking Medications
- (red button) Recent upper respiratory infection (URI)
- (blue button) Allergies
- (blue button) Smoking

Compare your screen to the Reported History circled in red in Figure 4-42. Note that Allergy findings are in their own group below Physical Exam. Now scroll your screen upward. Note that even though the findings were listed together in the left pane, they were actually from three different history groups (Past Medical History, Social History and Allergies).

Step 12

Click on the Px tab to document the physical exam. Note that the "Negs" button in the Toolbar is available when you are on this tab.

Locate and click on the following Physical Exam findings.

- (blue button) Both tympanic membranes were examined
- (red button) Nasal discharge purulent
- (red button) Sinus tenderness

Now locate the button labeled "Negs" in the Toolbar and click it once.

Compare your screen to Figure 4-43. Notice that the first and third findings (ears and nasal discharge) were not set. This because the Auto Negative feature correctly determined that the tympanic membrane finding was an examination of the ears, and the purulent discharge finding was a refinement of the nasal discharge finding. Note also that although the ROS button may still be depressed on your Toolbar, ROS has no effect in the Px tab.

▶ **Figure 4-43 Physical Exam Completed Using Neg Button (circled in red).**

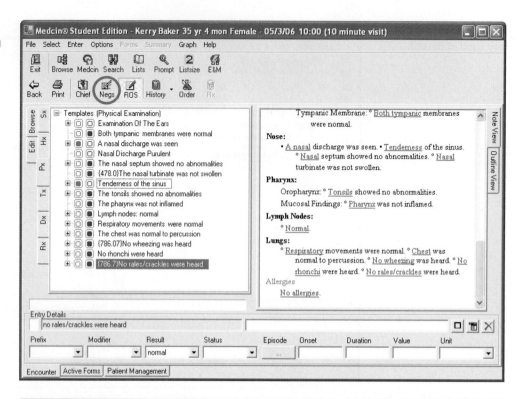

▶ **Figure 4-44 Assessment—Acute Sinusitis.**

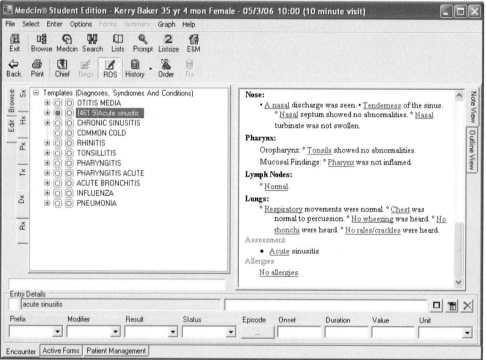

Step 13

The clinician has determined that the patient has Acute Sinusitis. Click on the Dx tab and notice that the Adult URI list contains only diagnoses that the practice has decided are likely to present for this type of condition.

Locate and click on the following finding:

● (red button) Sinusitis Acute

Compare your screen to Figure 4-44.

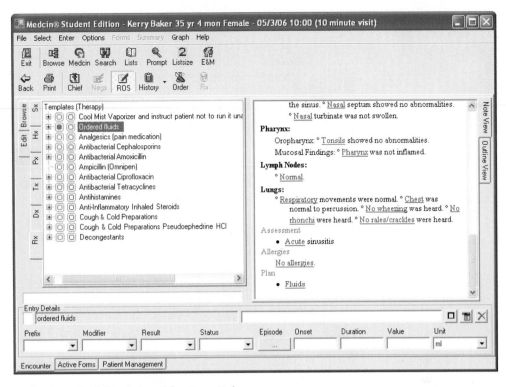

▶ Figure 4-45 Fluids Ordered for Kerry Baker.

Step 14

Click on the Rx tab and again appreciate the fact that the tab contains only types of treatments that the practice is likely to prescribe for an Adult upper respiratory infection. The clinician is going to order fluids and an antibiotic.

Locate and click on the following finding:

- (red button) Fluids

Compare your screen to Figure 4-45.

Do not exit the program until you have completed the following exercise.

Hands-On Exercise 27: Writing Prescriptions in an EHR

Step 15

Locate the Prescription button in the Toolbar at the top of your screen. The icon resembles a small prescription bottle, but as the finding "Ordered Fluids" is still highlighted, the button will appear grayed out. The button is shown circled in red in Figure 4-46.

Locate and highlight the finding "Antibacterial Amoxicillin." The button labeled Rx on the Toolbar will become available when you highlight the finding. The prescription (Rx) button is enabled only when you are on the Rx tab and only if the highlighted finding is a medication.

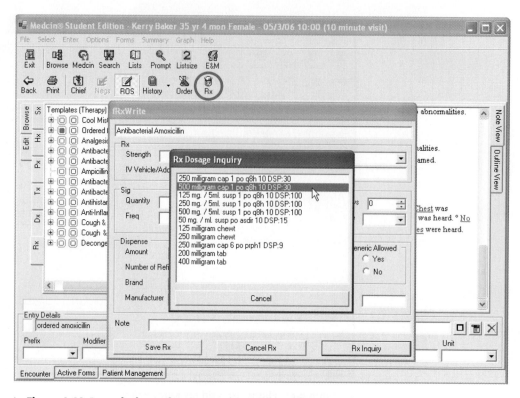

▶ **Figure 4-46 Prescription Writer Button (circled in red) with Dosage Window.**

With the finding "Antibacterial Amoxicillin" highlighted, click on the Prescription button in the Toolbar. A simple Prescription writer window will be invoked, as shown in Figure 4-46.

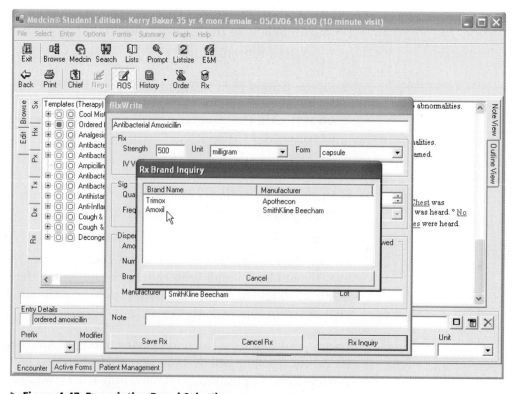

▶ **Figure 4-47 Prescription Brand Selection.**

Step 16

When you clicked on the prescription (Rx) button and invoked the prescription writing window, the drug was automatically selected from the finding. A list of available dosages is automatically displayed. This is the "Sig" information that the pharmacist will include on the label. It consists of the quantity prescribed, the number of times per day, capsules to take each time, number of days to take the drug, the total quantity prescribed, the number of refills allowed, and any free-text instructions to the patient. The list of available Sig choices makes writing the prescription very fast. It is found in virtually all commercial EHR prescription systems.

Locate and click your mouse on the Sig: "**500 milligram cap 1 po q8h 10 DSP:30**," shown highlighted in Figure 4-46.

The next window displaying available brands (as shown in Figure 4-47) will be displayed automatically.

Step 17

Locate and click on "Amoxil SmithKline Beecham," as shown in Figure 4-47.

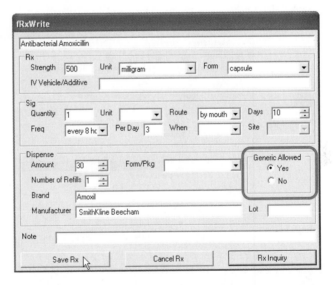

▶ **Figure 4-48 Prescription for Amoxicillin (generic circled in red).**

Step 18

Compare your screen to Figure 4-48. Locate the "Generic Allowed" fields. The "Yes" and "No" indicate if the pharmacist is allowed to substitute a generic drug for a prescribed brand. Click in the small circle next to **Yes**. The small circle is then filled in.

If you need to make any changes or corrections in the prescription, click on the button labeled "Rx Inquiry" to invoke the Dosage and Brand windows again.

When everything in your prescription screen matches Figure 4-48, click on the Save Rx button.

Electronic Prescription Writers

An EHR Prescription writer is more than just a replacement for a paper prescription pad. Commercial EHR systems offer sophisticated systems that make extensive use of the patient's current and previous medications, allergy data as well as insurance formulary, and extensive drug databases to perform automatic Drug Utilization Review, as well as formulary compliance checking during the prescription writing process. Prescriptions written in these systems can be transmitted electronically directly to the patient's preferred pharmacy. Additional benefits of electronic prescription writing will be covered in Chapter 7.

The Student Edition does not contain a true electronic prescription writer. The prescription window in this exercise is only a simulation intended to give you the feel for writing a prescription on a computer. You cannot use it to write or send actual prescriptions to a pharmacy, as this would be inappropriate in a student edition.

The prescription information will be written into your patient Exam Note as shown in Figure 4-49.

In this exercise you learned to use the List feature as well as the ROS and Auto Negative buttons. You also learned to use the Modifier field and the prescription writer.

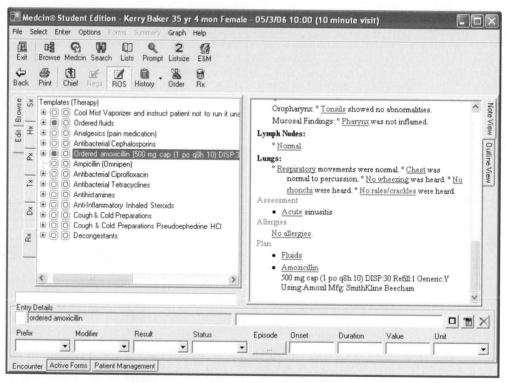

▶ **Figure 4-49 Completed Adult URI Exam for Kerry Baker.**

Step 19

Click File on the Menu bar, and then click Print Encounter or Print To HTML (as directed by your instructor).

If you are printing your work, you may click the Print button on the Toolbar at the top of your screen instead of selecting Print Encounter from the Menu.

Compare your printout or file output to Figure 4-50. If it is correct, hand it in to your instructor. If there are any differences, review the previous steps in the exercise and find your error.

Kerry Baker

Student: Terry Jones
Patient: Kerry Baker: F: 5/08/1970: 5/03/2006 10:00AM
Chief complaint
The Chief Complaint is: Patient reported cold or flu.
History of present illness
     Kerry Baker is a 35 year old female.
     • Sinus pain.
     • Nasal discharge o Nasal passage blockage
Past medical/surgical history
Reported History:
     Reported medications: Not taking medication.
     Medical: A recent URI.
Personal history
Behavioral history: Not smoking.
Review of systems
Systemic symptoms: Not feeling tired or poorly. Mild fever. No chills.
Head symptoms: No headache.
Otolaryngeal symptoms: No earache, no discharge from the ears, and no sore throat.
Neck symptoms: No swollen glands in the neck.
Pulmonary symptoms: No dyspnea, no cough, not coughing up sputum, and no hemoptysis.
Musculoskeletal symptoms: No muscle aches.
Physical findings
Vital signs:

Vital Signs/Measurements	Value	Normal Range
Oral temperature	99 F	97.6 - 99.6
RR	23 breaths/min	18 - 26
PR	78 bpm	50 - 100
Blood pressure	120/80 mmHg	100-120/56-80
Weight	100 lbs	98 - 183
Height	60 in	60.2 - 68.5

Ears:
General/bilateral:
Tympanic Membrane: ° Both tympanic membranes were normal.
Nose:
     • A purulent nasal discharge was seen. • Tenderness of the sinus. ° Nasal septum
          showed no abnormalities. ° Nasal turbinate was not swollen.
Pharynx:
     Oropharynx: ° Tonsils showed no abnormalities.
     Mucosal Findings: ° Pharynx was not inflamed.
Lymph Nodes:
     ° Normal.
Lungs:
     ° Respiratory movements were normal. ° Chest was normal to percussion.
     ° No wheezing was heard. ° No rhonchi were heard. ° No rales/crackles were heard.
Assessment
     • Acute sinusitis
Allergies
     No allergies.
Plan
     • Fluids
     • Amoxicillin
     500 mg cap (1 po q8h 10) DISP:30 Refill:1 Generic:Y Using:Amoxil
     Mfg: SmithKline Beecham

▶ **Figure 4-50 Printed Exam Note (with Prescription) for Kerry Baker.**

Hands-On Exercise 28:
Timed Experiment for Extra Credit (optional)

Now that you have learned that the Lists and Auto Negative feature can help you enter EHR data more quickly, prove it to yourself with the following experiment.

Step 1

Look at the clock and write down the current time.

Step 2

Select the same patient, **Kerry Baker**, and create a New Encounter for the same date, but use a different appointment time.

Use the date **May 3, 2006**, the time **10:15 AM**, and the reason **10 Minute Visit**.

Steps 3–18

Turn back to the previous exercises (Hands-On Exercises 26 and 27) and repeats steps 3–18 exactly. Work carefully but as quickly as you can.

Step 19

Look at the clock and write down the time you finished.

Click File on the Menu bar, and then click Print Encounter or click the button labeled "Print" on the Toolbar. Write your start and stop time on your printout and hand it in to your instructor.

Were you surprised how quickly you completed the complete Exam Note?

> **Note**
>
> The time printed next to the patient's name on your printed exam note must be 10:15 AM to receive extra credit.

The Concept of Forms

In this chapter, you experienced the use of lists dynamically created by the search and prompt features and the value in using predesigned lists for specific types of exams such as Adult URI. The other type of template that can speed up data entry is called a Form. You already have worked briefly with Forms, because the Vital Signs screen is actually a form.

The concept of Forms is to display a desired group of findings in a presentation that allows for quick entry of not only positive and negative findings but of any Entry Details fields such as value or results as easily. The Vitals Signs form is a good example. You could enter Vitals on the Encounter Px tab by locating and clicking on individual findings on the Px tab, then repositioning your mouse at the bottom of the screen, then entering the value and unit of measurement for each vital sign. This would obviously be a time-consuming way to do it. As you have already experienced, vitals are much easier to enter using the Vitals form on which all the necessary findings are arranged with the value fields ready for data entry and the unit of measurement fields preset.

The Vitals form is only a very small example of what can be done with forms. Complete multipage forms can be created that make it fast and easy to document standard types of exams.

Comparison of Lists and Forms

Forms provide a feature that lists cannot; they are static. The value of lists is that they are dynamic and expand as necessary. The inverse effect of this is that sometimes findings do not appear on the screen, because they are in the nonexpanded

Family Practice Medical Center
Anytown, USA

What is the reason you are here today?

Date: _____
Patient Name: _____
Date of Birth: _____
☐ Male   ☐ Female

Race: _____

_____

Please check any of the following conditions which you have had

General
☐ Serious Infections
  (e.g. pneumonia)
☐ Diabetes Mellitus
☐ Rheumatic fever
☐ HIV Infection
☐ Cancer

Cardiovascular
☐ High Blood Pressure
☐ Congestive Heart failure
☐ Heart Murmur
☐ Heart Valve Disease
☐ Angina
☐ Heart Attack
☐ High Cholesterol
☐ Abnormal Heart Rhythm
☐ Blood Clot in Veins
☐ Blocked Arteries in Neck
☐ Blocked Arteries in Legs

HEENT
☐ Glaucoma
☐ Allergies "hay fever"
☐ Frequent Ear Infections
☐ Frequent Sinus Infections

Respiratory
☐ Asthma
☐ Emphysema
☐ Blood Colt in Lungs
☐ Sleep Apnea

**Musculoskeletal /
Extremities**
☐ Osteoporosis
☐ Rheumatoid Arthritis
☐ Degenerative Joint Disease
☐ Fibrmyalgia
☐ Neck Pain (herniated disk)
☐ Back Pain (herniated disc)

GI/GU
☐ Stomach Ulcers
☐ Ulcerative Colitis
☐ Crohns Disease
☐ Bleeding from Intestines
☐ Diverticulitis
☐ Colon Polyps
☐ Irritable Bowel Disease
☐ Hepatitis
☐ Cirrhosis of the liver
☐ Liver Failure
☐ Pancreatitis
☐ Gallstones
☐ Kidney Stones
☐ Kidney Failure
☐ Prostate Disease
☐ Endometriosis
☐ Sex Transmitted Infection

Lymphatic / Hematologic
☐ Thyroid Goiter
☐ Over Active Thyroid
☐ Under Active Thyroid
☐ Transfusions
☐ Anemia

Skin / Breast
☐ Acne
☐ Eczema
☐ Psoriasis
☐ Fibrocystic Breast Disease

Neurological / Psychiatric
☐ Chronic Vertigo (Meniere's)
☐ Peripheral Nerve Disease
☐ Migraine Headaches
☐ Stroke
☐ Multiple Sclerosis
☐ Depression
☐ Anxiety

Please check any of the following major illnesses in your family members:
☐ Tuberculosis
☐ Emphysema
☐ Heart Disease
☐ High Blood Pressure
☐ Osteoporosis

☐ Diabetes Mellitus
☐ Thyroid Disease
☐ Anemia
☐ Hemophilia
☐ Other _____

☐ Kidney Disease
☐ Epilepsy
☐ Neurological Disorder
☐ Liver Disease
☐ Other _____

☐ Breast Cancer
☐ Ovarian Cancer
☐ Colon Cancer
☐ Prostate Cancer
☐ Other _____

If you have had surgery please indicate the year:

Year	Surgery	Year	Surgery	Year	Surgery	Year	Surgery
____	Angioplasty	____	Colonoscopy	____	Neurosurgery	____	Tubal ligation
____	Appendectomy	____	Coronary Bypass	____	Sinus Surgery	____	C-Section
____	Back or Neck Surgery	____	Ear Surgery	____	Stomach Surgery	____	Hysterectomy
____	Bladder Surgery	____	Gallbladder	____	Thyroid Surgery	____	Ovary Removed
____	Carotid Artery Surgery	____	Hip Surgery	____	Tonsillectomy	____	Breast Surgery
____	Carpal Tunnel Surgery	____	Inguinal Hernia	____	Trauma Related Surgery	____	Thyroid Surgery
____	Chest/lung Surgery	____	Knee Surgery	____	Vascular Surgery	____	Other

Please indicate when you had the following preventative services:

Date	Immunizations	Date	Tests	Date	Tests / Exams	Date	Tests / Exams
____	Flu Vaccine	____	Chest X-ray	____	Colon Cancer Stool Test	____	Breast Exam
____	Hepatitis Vaccine	____	EKG	____	Flexible Sigmoidoscopy,	____	Mammogram
____	Pneumonia Vaccine	____	Echocardiogram	____	Rectal Exam	____	Pap Smear
____	Tetanus Booster	____	Stress Test	____	Barium Enema	____	Bone Density Test
____	Other	____	Cardiac Angiogram	____	Prostate Cancer Blood Test	____	Date of last Physical Exam

Personal Habits

Tobacco	Alcohol	Caffeine	Illicit Drugs
☐ Never	☐ Never	☐ Never	☐ Never
☐ Previous user	☐ Previous user	☐ Previous user	☐ Previous user
☐ Current user	☐ Current user	☐ Current user	☐ Current user
# packs per day _____	# drinks per day _____	# cups per day _____	

▶ **Figure 4-51 Sample Intake Form from a Paper Chart.**

portion of the tree, or the user must scroll the screen to find them. With Forms, however, findings have a fixed position on the screen and will remain in that location every time the form is used.

Lists arrange findings in the appropriate tab (Sx, Hx, Px, Tx, Dx, and Rx); however, this means the clinicians must change tabs as they work through the exam. This is not a limitation with forms. The form designer is free to put any finding anywhere on the form. This allows each form to be designed to allow the quickest entry of data for a particular type of exam. For example, if a nurse routinely enters the Chief complaint and records the patient's symptoms at the same time she takes the vital signs, these could all be placed on one page of the form, even though the findings will appear in three different sections of the note.

Forms offer many additional features to the designer. These include check boxes, drop-down lists, and most of the fields in the Entry Details section. Free-text boxes in a form can be preassigned to a finding; therefore, they do not require the user to locate a free-text finding to record comments.

Just as Lists can contain additional findings that broaden the type of exams for which the list is used, the same is true of Forms. Forms can contain findings that are required and those that are optional. Every question on a Form does not have to be answered for every visit. Clinicians often use clinical judgment when deciding what to document.

Standard Initial Visit Intake for Adult

The intake form used in the following exercise provides an example of different looks and features that are possible with forms. These include the unique ability to record two types of history at once, Auto-negative, and other features you will explore during the exercise.

Figure 4-51 is an example of a form that might be found in an office that used paper medical records. You have probably seen a similar form at your own doctor's office. As you complete the following exercise, notice the similarities to the design of the EHR form. Electronic Forms are one of the easiest ways to use an EHR.

Hands-On Exercise 29: Using Forms

In this exercise, you will use an EHR form to record symptoms, history, and a physical exam. In this case, the EHR form has been abridged to shorten the time it takes a student to complete the exercise; a full version of the form as it is used in a medical office would have much more detail. A short intake form might be used by a nurse or medical assistant for prescreening. The clinician would then complete the exam, following up on any abnormal findings.

Step 1

If you have not already done so, start the Student Edition software.

Click Select on the Menu bar, and then click Patient.

In the Patient Selection window, locate and click on **Terry Chun**.

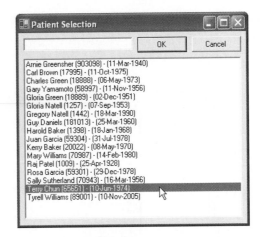

▶ Figure 4-52 Selecting Terry Chun from the Patient Selection Window.

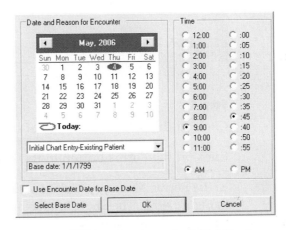

▶ Figure 4-53 New Encounter for Initial Chart Entry, May 4, 2006, 9:45 AM.

Step 2

Click Select on the Menu bar, and then click New Encounter.

Select the date **May 4, 2006**, the time **9:45 AM**, and the reason **Initial Chart Entry-Existing Patient**.

Make certain you set the date, time, and reason correctly. Compare your screen to Figure 4-53 before clicking on the OK button.

Step 3

Enter the Chief complaint by locating the button in the Toolbar labeled "Chief" and clicking on it.

In the dialog window which will open, type "New Patient Chart."

Compare your screen to Figure 4-54 before clicking on the button labeled "Close the vote form".

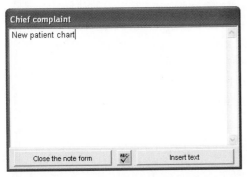

▶ Figure 4-54 Chief Complaint Dialog for New Patient Chart.

▶ Figure 4-55 Select Short
Intake in Forms Manager
Window.

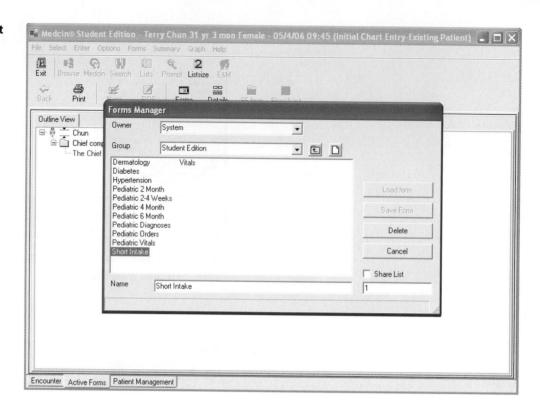

Step 4

Click on the Active Forms tab at the bottom of your screen.

Click on the Forms button in the Toolbar at the top of the screen.

In the Forms Manager window, select the Form labeled "Short Intake," as shown in Figure 4-55. The Short Intake form shown in Figure 4-56 will be displayed.

▶ Figure 4-56 Short Intake
Form—Review of Symp-
toms Tab.

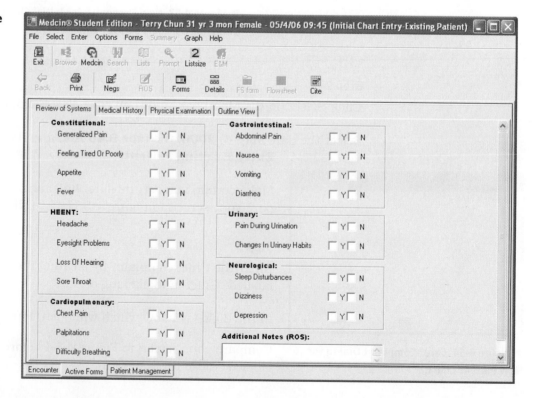

Step 5

Compare your screen to Figure 4-56. Take a few minutes to study the Form on your screen.

Note that at the top of the form there are tabs, labeled Review of Systems, Medical History, and Physical Examination. This form has three pages on which you may enter data. In subsequent steps, you will use each of these pages to explore the features of this form.

Probably the first thing you noticed are columns of check boxes with Y and N next to them. This is very similar to a paper form and very intuitive. With almost no training, people understand Y means Yes and N represents No.

Check boxes work very simply, here is how:

✓ If you click your mouse on an empty box, a check mark appears. The finding will be recorded in the patient's record.

✓ If you change your mind and click in the opposite box, the check mark moves to the box you just clicked.

✓ If you didn't want either box checked, click on whichever box already has the check mark and you will be asked to confirm that you want the finding removed (as shown in Figure 4-57).

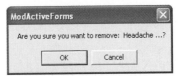

▶ **Figure 4-57 Confirmation That You Want to Remove a Finding.**

Step 6

On the Review of Symptoms tab, if you put a check in the Y box, it means that the patient has that symptom. If you put check in the N box, this means that the patient does not have that symptom.

Practice using the check boxes with the finding Headache, which is located in the section of the form labeled "HEENT." Remember, HEENT stands for *head, eyes, ears, nose and throat.*

Locate the finding Headache and click in the check box next to the letter **Y**.

Now click the mouse in the check box next to the letter **N**. Did the check mark move?

Although you cannot see the exam note at this moment, you just changed the note from the "headache" to "No headache."

Click the mouse again in the same box that already has the check mark in it; this should be next to the letter N. The confirmation message shown in Figure 4-57 should appear. Click on the OK button. Both check boxes should now be empty.

Remember, even though the form looks different than the Encounter tab, you really are adding and removing findings on the patient note when you work with the form.

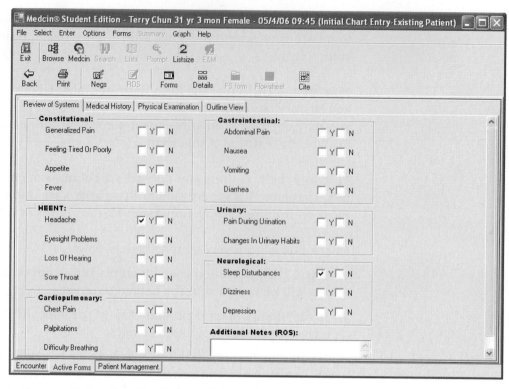

▶ **Figure 4-58 Recording Headache and Sleep Disturbances.**

Step 7

The patient reports that she has headaches and some nights has trouble sleeping.

Locate the finding Headache and click in the check box next to the letter **Y**.

Locate the finding Sleep Disturbances and click in the check box next to the letter **Y**.

Compare your screen to Figure 4-58.

Step 8

A feature that is included in many EHR forms is the ability to see where in the nomenclature hierarchy the current finding exists. This feature is not necessarily designed into all forms, but it has been included on the Short Intake form for the Student Edition.

Left and Right Mouse Buttons

A computer mouse typically has at least two buttons, usually referred to as the "left click" and "right click" buttons. In this step you will use the right click button. If your mouse has only one button, use the Alternate Instructions For Left Mouse Button provided here.

Position the mouse pointer over the word "headache" (not over the Y/N check boxes.) The finding will become highlighted in white and the mouse pointer will change shape to include a question mark. When your mouse pointer looks like the one circled in red in Figure 4-59, click the **right click** button on your mouse. A small pane of Medcin findings will open in the middle of the form.

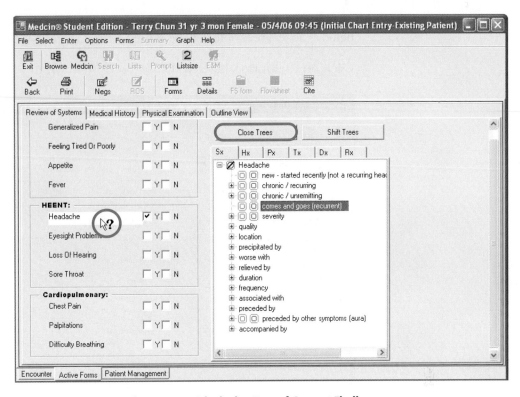

▶ **Figure 4-59 Nomenclature Pane Displaying Tree of Current Finding.**

The nomenclature pane shows the highlighted finding in context of the Medcin Tree Structure. When the nomenclature pane is displayed, you can expand the tree structure as well as select additional or different findings.

One reason for invoking the Medcin tree is to locate a more specific finding. In the previous step you recorded the finding "Headache," but the patient informs you that the headaches come and go.

Locate and click on the following finding in the Medcin tree currently displayed on your screen:

● (red button) Comes and goes (recurrent)

Two buttons at the top of the pane allow you to close or reposition it. The button labeled "Shift Trees" moves the browser pane left or right so you can see a

---

Note ▶

Alternate Instructions for Left Mouse Button

An alternative to using the right mouse button to open the nomenclature pane in a form is to click the left button of your mouse on the finding name "Headache" (not over the Y/N check boxes).

Headache ☑ Y ☐ N

▶ **Figure 4-60 Check Boxes Outlined with a Rectangle.**

When you see the check boxes outlined with a rectangle (as shown in Figure 4-60), then move your mouse pointer to the Toolbar and locate and click on the button labeled "Browse." A small pane of Medcin findings will open in the middle of the form and should be positioned in the Tree on the finding "Headache." Continue with the remainder of Step 8.

part of the form that might otherwise be covered by the pane. The button labeled "Close Trees" closes the pane to restore your view of the entire form.

Click on the button labeled "Close Trees" (shown in Figure 4-59 circled in red).

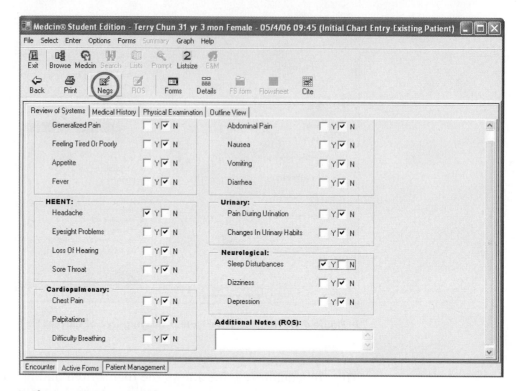

▶ **Figure 4-61 Auto Negative in a Form.**

Step 9

The Auto Negative button, which you learned to use in Exercise 26, also can be enabled in forms. This feature allows you to complete form pages quickly whenever most of the answers are "No" or "Normal."

Locate the "Negs" button in the Toolbar at the top of your form. Click your mouse on the Negs button (circled in red in Figure 4-61).

Compare your screen to Figure 4-61. Note what happened. Note that Auto Negative does not alter findings that are already recorded, as in this example, "Headache" and "Sleep Disturbances."

Step 10

Forms also can allow entry of free-text notes right on the form. This saves the clinician the time it takes to add notes to entry details, or open free-text findings. In this step, add a clinical impression to the ROS findings.

In the box at the bottom of your screen labeled "Additional Notes ROS," type the following text: **Patient denies depression but seems very sad**.

Compare your screen to Figure 4-62 before proceeding.

Step 11

During the course of this exercise, you have been recording findings in the exam note with every click of your mouse on the form, but you cannot see them as you can on the Encounter tab.

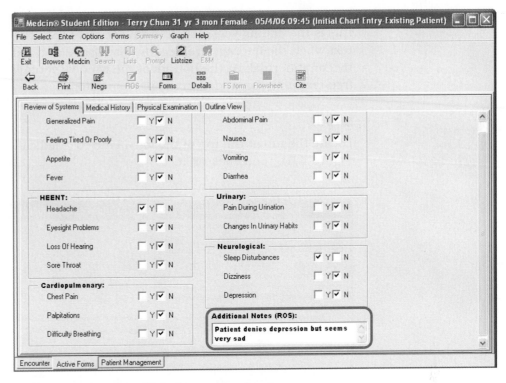

► **Figure 4-62 Free-Text Clinical Impressions in a Form.**

In Forms, the Outline View allows you to take a quick look at the findings you have selected for the exam note. Before entering data in the rest of the form, take a moment to see what has been entered so far.

Locate the tab labeled "Outline View" at the top of your form. Click on the Outline tab (circled in red in Figure 4-63).

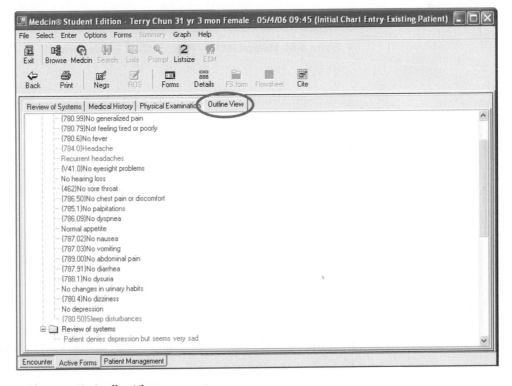

► **Figure 4-63 Outline View.**

Compare your screen to Figure 4-63. Notice the headaches are also recurrent; this is the finding you entered from the tree view. The Outline View uses blue text when the findings are negative or normal and red text when they are positive or abnormal. At the bottom of the window you also can see in red text the free-text note you added in the previous step.

Step 12

Locate the tab at the top of the form labeled "Medical History" (circled in red in Figure 4-64), and click on it.

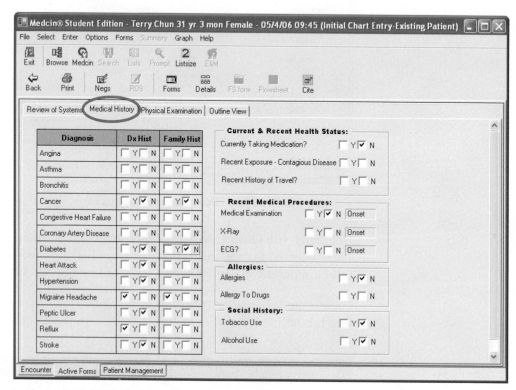

▶ **Figure 4-64 Medical History Page of Short Intake Form.**

This page illustrates another advantage of forms. Normally, when you do an intake history on a patient, you go through many items twice: "Have you ever had a heart attack? Has anyone in your family ever had a heart attack?" On this page, the form has been designed to save the clinician time, by making it easy to record answers to either personal, family history, or both in two columns. Compare the information on this tab of the EHR form with the paper form in Figure 4-51.

Step 13

Sometimes patients do not know the medical history of other family members; therefore, you will only record findings the patient is sure about. As the medical assistant asks Ms. Chun the history questions, the patient will only know the answer to some of them.

Enter the Dx History and Family History only for the following items:

Diagnosis	Dx Hist	Family Hist
Cancer	✓ N	✓ N
Diabetes	✓ N	✓ N
Heart Attack	✓ N	
Hypertension	✓ N	
Migraine	✓ Y	✓ Y
Peptic Ulcer	✓ N	
Reflux	✓ Y	
Stroke	✓ N	

Complete the rest of her Medical History in the right side of the form by locating and clicking on the check boxes as follows:

Currently Taking Medication	✓ N
Recent Medical Examination	✓ N
Allergies	✓ N
Tobacco	✓ N
Alcohol	✓ Y

Carefully compare your screen to Figure 4-64 before proceeding.

Step 14

Locate the tab at the top of the form labeled "Physical Examination" (circled in red in Figure 4-65), and click on it.

The first thing you will notice about this page is that it includes the Vital Signs (in the upper left corner of the page). Recording vital signs as part of the intake physical saves the time it would take to load the vitals form separately. This page illustrates how forms can combine many different elements to make data entry more convenient.

Enter the following Vital Signs for Terry Chun:

Temperature: **97**

Respiration: **22**

Pulse: **65**

BP: **118/81**

Weight: **133**

Step 15

During the exam, the clinician observes Sinus Tenderness. Locate the finding Sinus Tenderness and click the check box for **Y**.

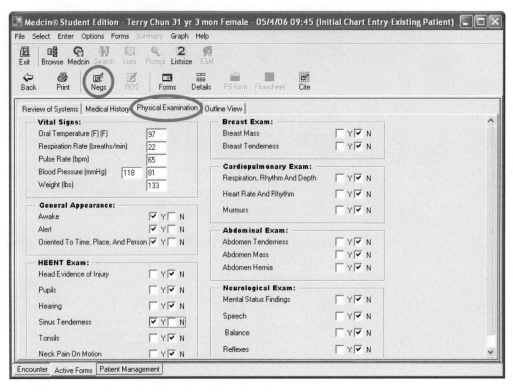

► **Figure 4-65 Physical Exam Page of Short Intake Form.**

Everything else is normal. Click on the button labeled "Negs" on the Toolbar at the top of your screen (circled in red in Figure 4-65).

Remember you can use the button to quickly document "normals" on Symptoms and Physical Exam findings.

Compare your screen to Figure 4-65.

Did you see that the findings in the General Appearance group were checked Y instead of N by the Auto Negative feature? That is because for some findings such as these, the normal state is to be *awake*, *alert*, and *oriented*. If these were checked No, the condition would be abnormal. The Auto Negative feature is really an Auto Normal feature.

Step 16

Click on the Encounter tab at the bottom of your screen, to view the full text of the exam note that was completed from within the form.

Click on the Dx tab in the left pane and enter an assessment.

Locate and click the red button for the following finding:

● (red button) Normal examination

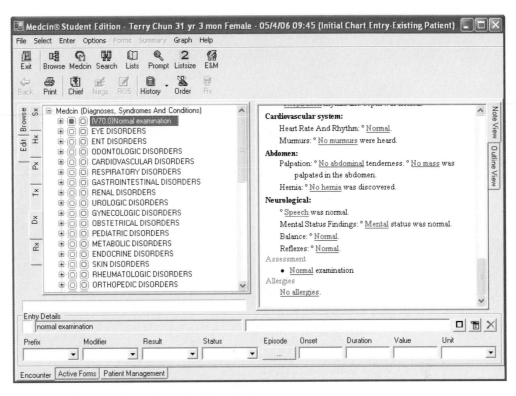

▶ **Figure 4-66 Exam Note Entered Using a Form.**

Compare your screen to Figure 4-66. Scroll the right pane so that you can view the entire contents of the note.

Forms are not limited to the pages used in this exercise. Forms also allow you to organize questions in the order you would ask them, regardless of where the findings may be grouped in the Medcin Nomenclature hierarchy.

Forms can be designed to include pages for any of the findings expected to be needed for a particular type of visit. For example, a therapy page is an excellent means of having quick access to standard treatments for specific conditions.

Medical offices that have a large number of forms customized to their style of practice succeed very well in implementing an EHR. Form Design tools are a part of almost every EHR system on the market. Forms take longer for the designer to create than Lists, but, if well constructed, make it significantly easier to record patient exams as they happen. (See the Real-Life Story by Dr. Lukowski later in this chapter.)

Step 17

This exercise was intended to demonstrate how forms can be used to speed through pages of routine questions, and provide the convenience of free-text or Entry Details fields as part of the form. Although the exercise does not create a medically complete intake history and a physical, you have successfully completed the goals of this exercise.

```
Student: Terry Jones
Patient: Terry Chun: F: 6/10/1974: 5/04/2006 09:45AM
```

Chief complaint

```
The Chief Complaint is: New Patient Chart.
```

History of present illness

```
     Terry Chun is a 31 year old female.
     • Headache recurrent.
     ° No depression  o Sleep disturbances
     ° No generalized pain ° , Not feeling tired or poorly ° , and No fever
     ° No eyesight problems  °  No hearing loss °  and No sore throat  °  No chest pain or
        discomfort °  and No palpitations °  No dyspnea °  Normal appetite ° , No nausea
        ° , No vomiting ° , No abdominal pain ° , and No diarrhea  °  No dysuria °  and
        No changes in urinary habits   °  No dizziness
```

Past medical/surgical history

Reported History:

```
     Reported medications: Not taking medication.
```

Diagnosis History:

```
     No acute myocardial infarction.
     No hypertension.
     No esophageal reflux
     No peptic ulcer.
     No diabetes mellitus.
     Migraine headache.
     No stroke syndrome.
     No cancer
```

Personal history

```
Behavioral history:  No tobacco use.
Alcohol: Alcohol use.
Habits: No recent medical examination.
```

Family history

```
     No diabetes mellitus
     Migraine headache
     No cancer.
```

Review of systems

```
Patient denies depression but seems very sad.
```

Continued on the following page…

▶ **Figure 4-67a Printout of Exam Note for Terry Chun Created Using a Form (Page 1 of 2).**

At this point, print out your Patient Exam note, compare it to Figure 4–67, and turn it into your instructor.

Click File on the Menu bar, and then click Print Encounter or Print To HTML (as directed by your instructor).

If you are printing your work you may alternatively click the Print button on the Toolbar at the top of your screen.

Compare your printout or file output to Figure 4-67. If it is correct, hand it in to your instructor. If there are any differences, review the previous steps in the exercise and find your error.

(Note your computer will print out two pages; however, the page breaks may not be in the same place as Figure 4-67. The page breaks vary by the type of printer and will not affect your grade.)

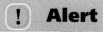

! Alert

Do not close or exit the Encounter until you have a printed copy in your hand. *You will lose your work if you exit before printing.*

Physical findings

Vital signs:

Vital Signs/Measurements	Value	Normal Range
Oral temperature	97 F	97.6 - 99.6
RR	22 breaths/min	18 - 26
PR	65 bpm	50 - 100
Blood pressure	118/81 mmHg	100-120/56-80
Weight	133 lbs	98 - 183

General appearance:
    ° Awake. ° Alert. ° Oriented to time, place, and person.

Head:
    ° No evidence of a head injury.

Eyes:
    General/bilateral:
      Pupils: ° Normal.

Ears:
    General/bilateral:
      Hearing: ° Normal.

Nose:
    • Tenderness of the sinus.

Pharynx:
    Oropharynx: ° Tonsils showed no abnormalities.

Neck:
    ° Pain was not elicited by motion.

Breasts:
    General/bilateral:
      ° No breast mass was found. ° No tenderness of the breast.

Lungs:
    ° Respiration rhythm and depth was normal.

Cardiovascular system:
    Heart Rate And Rhythm: ° Normal.
    Murmurs: ° No murmurs were heard.

Abdomen:
    Palpation: ° No abdominal tenderness. ° No mass was palpated in the abdomen.
    Hernia: ° No hernia was discovered.

Neurological:
    ° Speech was normal.
    Mental Status Findings: ° Mental status was normal.
    Balance: ° Normal.
    Reflexes: ° Normal.

Assessment
    • Normal examination

Allergies
    No allergies.

▶ **Figure 4-67b Printout of Exam Note for Terry Chun Created Using a Form (Page 2 of 2).**

By Michael Lukowski, M.D.

Michael Lukowski is a specialist in obstetrics and gynecology. He has been practicing more than 20 years. He uses an EHR in his practice, enters his own data, and has designed his own EHR forms.

I started using forms right away. When the trainer told me about forms, I thought "this is the way to go." It slows you down if you have to search a lot. Forms gave me a discrete window into the database so that I could pick out things that I use day in and day out.

I try to put as much of my exam in as data points (findings) rather than just free-text. I use free-text only as a comment to a finding. To me the whole idea of this is to have retrievable information that I can analyze over time. So I always try to use the (nomenclature) database as my main way to construct a note and then add free-text to that if I have to. I find that I use less and less free-text because I can pick out findings that say pretty much what I need to say.

Workflow

Using forms I do what I have always done. My nurse puts in the vital signs; we do some simple lab tests like a hematocrit. The patient is sitting in the exam room when I go in. I sit down and talk with her. As we are talking, I am filling in her history using a tablet computer, just like I used to do with a paper chart. When I am done with that part of the exam, I call my nurse in and do the physical exam.

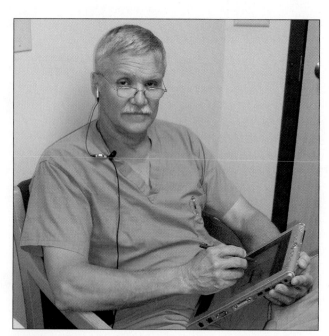

Photo by Richard Gartee.

Dr. Lukowski Enters Data in the Exam Room on a TabletPC Using a Form He Designed.

When the physical exam is finished, I leave and come back to my office. While the patient gets dressed, I finish filling out the rest of the encounter. The patient comes to my office once she is dressed and we talk a little bit more; I finalize her note and write any prescription. If the patient has a pharmacy that receives electronic prescriptions, I transmit them directly to the pharmacy. If the pharmacy does not, I print it on paper and the staff brings it to me to sign.

Forms

I use four forms: Gyn, Post-partum, Pre-op, and then one that contains all the procedures I do, which is still a work in progress, but it covers a lot.

I have a number of tabs within each form. For instance, the Gyn form starts with the intake page. My assistant fills in the menstrual history, pap smear, mammograms, methods of birth control, and so on.

I move through the rest of the tabs except at the right end of the form, I use three different tabs for assessment so that I can have all the diagnoses I normally use available without searching.

Figure 4-68 shows one of the forms I use every day. The Tabs are: Intake info, VS and Off Labs, Pain Hx, V & V, GI and UTI Sx, Meno & PMS, Fertility Eval, BC Counseling, Soc Hx, Med Hx, and three tabs for assessment.

The tabs are not necessarily in the order I use them but, rather, the order I made the form in—but I know where everything is. If I do want to browse, I have a search box right at the top of my form. I can type in a term I want and hit my search button.

I started learning to use the E&M (evaluation and management calculator) function to post my charges, but I wanted to spend more time on my forms development. So I haven't followed up on it. My front desk people are very astute and continue to do the coding.

This system, I'm in love with it. It takes either the same time or less time than it used to on paper and I get a note that is 10 times better.

▶ **Figure 4-68 Intake Tab of Gynecology Form Designed and Used by Dr. Lukowski.**

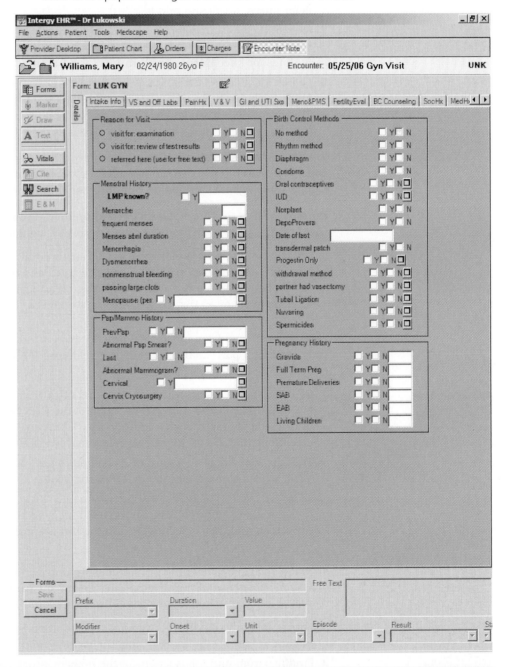

Chapter Four Summary

Completely documenting a visit before the patient ever leaves the office is the easiest way to use an EHR and provides the most rewarding benefits from the system. To document in real time you must be able to quickly navigate and enter findings. To help you do this, the EHR needs to present the finding the clinician needs, as it is needed.

EHR systems use features such as Search, Prompt, Lists, and Forms to preload the findings that are likely to be needed for each type of patient.

Search provides a quick way to locate a desired finding in the nomenclature. Medcin addresses semantic differences in medical terms in three ways:

1. Search performs automatic word completion, so if you search for knee but the finding is for knees, it will still find it.

2. Medcin includes an extensive list of synonyms that are used in an alternate word search. For example, if you search for knee injury, the search results will also include findings for knee burns, knee trauma, and fractured patella, among others.

3. Search identifies related findings in other tabs so that when you search for a word or phrase in a particular tab, related findings are automatically available in the other tabs. This means that when you are using search while documenting a patient exam, as you continue through the exam, the other tabs may already have findings that you will use.

Search is not designed to find every instance that contains the words being searched because the search results would often have too many findings. Instead, search finds and displays the highest level match but does not list all the expanded findings below it.

Prompt is short for "prompt with current finding." Prompt generates a list of findings that are clinically related to the finding currently highlighted.

The prompt list that is displayed is shorter than the full nomenclature, containing only relevant findings, making it easier to read and navigate. The list generated by the prompt feature populates all the tabs, creating shorter lists of any relevant findings in each tab (Sx, Hx, Px, Tx, Dx, and Rx).

Lists allow the clinician or medical practice to create a subset of the nomenclature typically used for a particular condition or type of exam. A List usually contains findings in every tab.

Because shorter lists mean less scrolling, Lists are a sure way to speed up data entry of routine exams and increase adoption of the EHR by clinicians in the practice. Over time, medical practices should build up a library of Lists covering the medical conditions that are frequently seen at their practice.

To keep them short, Lists are often limited to one particular condition, but this is not a rule; it is a convenience factor. Lists are flexible and can contain as many findings as necessary to document a typical visit.

A List is accessed by clicking on the button labeled Lists in the Toolbar at the top of the screen and then selecting it from the List Manager window.

Forms display a desired group of findings in a presentation that allows for quick entry of not only positive and negative findings but of any Entry Details fields such as value or results as well. Forms also provide other features that lists cannot, for example:

1. Forms are static; findings have a fixed position on Forms, and will consistently remain in that position, every time the form is used.

2. Findings from multiple sections of the nomenclature can be mixed on the same page of the form in any way that will enable the quickest data entry.

3. Forms may include check boxes, drop-down lists, the fields in the Entry Details section, the onset date, and free-text boxes to record comments.

4. Forms can control which findings are required and which are optional; every question on a Form does not have to be answered for every visit.

   The Outline View allows you to see the findings that have been selected without leaving the Active Forms tab.

   A Form is accessed by clicking on the Active Forms tab at the bottom of the screen then selecting it from the Forms Manager window.

The Medcin Toolbar The purpose of the Toolbar is to allow quick access to commonly used functions. The Toolbar has two rows of icon buttons that help you in three different ways:

1. Some buttons eliminate the need to access the menu for frequently used items.

2. Other buttons control the behavior or look of the panes in the Medcin window.

3. Several buttons set the prefix on a finding so you don't have to go to the Entry Details fields to do it.

In previous chapters, you used several of the buttons on the Toolbar. In this chapter, you learned to use the following new buttons:

Search	Invokes the word search allowing you to quickly locate all findings with matching words or synonyms.
Prompt	Generates a list of findings that are clinically related to the finding currently highlighted.
List	Invokes the List Manager window from which you may select and load a List.
List Size	Increases or decreases the number of findings in the displayed list. List sizes are 1–3.
Negs	Auto Negative button will automatically set all the findings (that are not already set) to "normal" when you are on the Sx or Px tab.
ROS	On/Off button; when On (depressed), history findings are recorded in the Review of Systems section; when Off, history findings are recorded in the History of Present Illness section.
Order	Prefaces the highlighted finding with the prefix "Ordered" and records the finding in the Plan section. The button is enabled only when a finding is "orderable" but not a medication.
Rx	Invokes the prescription writer. The button is enabled only if the highlighted finding is a medication.
Browse	Displays the current finding's position in the Medcin nomenclature hierarchy. This button was used in this chapter only if you did not have a right click button on your mouse.

After completing this chapter, you should be comfortable with the general process of locating findings and expanding the tree to view additional findings, using Lists, Forms Search, and Prompt features to create Patient Exam Notes. In this chapter, you completed four required exercises and one optional exercise. If you are having difficulty with any area, it is suggested that you repeat those exercises before proceeding.

Testing Your Knowledge of Chapter 4

You may run the Medcin Student Edition software and use your mouse on the screen to answer the following questions:

1. How do you select a List?

2. How do you select Forms?

3. List three features Forms have that Lists do not.

4. Describe what the Prompt button on the toolbar does.

Write the meaning of each of the following medical abbreviations (as they were used in this chapter):

5. ROS _____

6. HPI _____

7. HEENT _____

8. URI _____

9. Sig _____

10. How do you indicate a "possible" diagnosis?

11. Auto-Negative (the Negs button) functions on what two tabs?

12. Describe how to record a test that was ordered and describe how to record a test that was performed.

13. What Entry Details field is used with a finding to indicate the patient's fever was "mild"?

14. How do you change the numbers on the List Size button and what do the numbers do?

15. You should have produced four narrative documents of patient encounters, which you printed. If you have not already done so, hand these in to your instructor with this test. The printed encounter notes will count as a portion of your grade.

5

Electronic Coding from Medical Records

Learning Outcomes

After completing this chapter, you should be able to:

- Explain why billing codes are important in an EHR system
- Show how Evaluation and Management (E&M) codes are determined
- Name and describe key components of E&M codes
- Read and understand the tables used in CMS guidelines
- Explain how the level of key components determines the level of the E&M code
- Use E&M calculator software
- Correctly use and document the Time factor to change the level of an E&M code
- Use a diagnosis to find protocols
- Order tests to confirm or rule out a diagnosis

Acronyms are used extensively in both medicine and computers. Listed below are those that are used in this chapter.

CC	Chief complaint
CBC	Complete Blood Count (lab test)
CMS	Centers For Medicare and Medicaid Services
CPT-4	Current Procedural Terminology, 4th Revision
E&M	Evaluation and Management codes
EMR	Electronic Medical Record
ENT	Ears, Nose, and Throat
HCFA	Health Care Financing Administration (CMS predecessor)
HCPCS	Healthcare Common Procedure Coding System
HPI	History of Present Illness
ICD-9CM	International Classification of Disease, 9th Revision with Clinical Modifiers
MDM	Medical Decision Making (a key component)
OIG	Office of Inspector General (Department of Health and Human Services)
PFSH	Past History, Family History, and Social History
NEC	Not Elsewhere Classified (diagnosis codes)
NOS	Not Otherwise Specified (diagnosis codes)
ROS	Review of Systems
URI	Upper Respiratory Infection

CPT-4 and ICD-9CM Codes for Billing

Health care providers need to be paid for their work. The vast majority of those payments are the result of filing insurance claims, which require CPT-4 and ICD-9CM codes. Those codes are derived from the medical records made during the course of the patient exam or treatment. In a paper or manual system, billing experts called "medical coders" or "coding specialists" on the doctor's staff review the exam notes and create the coding. In a modern EHR, the software can evaluate the exam note and suggest the correct billing codes.

In Chapter 2, you learned about various national standard code sets, including CPT-4 and ICD-9CM. In this chapter, you will explore the relationship of those two code sets with an EHR.

A complete medical coding course cannot be taught in one chapter and that is not the intent of this chapter. The purpose of this section is to provide a basic understanding of government mandated guidelines for medical coding. Hands-On Exercises will compare the published guidelines with actual findings in the EHR using software that analyzes a patient encounter.

Understanding Evaluation and Management Codes

Most private and all public health plans follow standards set by CMS. The importance of documented exam notes is derived from a principle put forth by the CMS predecessor HCFA: *"If it isn't documented, it wasn't done."* This phrase meant that a clinician was required to keep a record of the patient exam. If an audit by Medicare or an insurance plan found the documented note did not support the charges on the claim, it would be assumed that the procedures were never performed.

Nowhere was this more important than in the most common procedure codes, the Evaluation and Management (E&M) codes. These CPT-4 codes are used to bill for nearly every kind of patient encounter, such as physician office visits, in-patient hospital exams, nursing home visits, consults, emergency room doctors, and scores of other services. E&M codes are used by virtually all specialties.

You will recall from Chapter 2 that the AMA originally created CPT codes for medical and surgical procedures. E&M codes were added later to provide billing codes for the (nonsurgical) time providers spent examining their patients and managing their health. The previous edition of CPT had four levels of E&M codes for each type of visit. The levels were intended to reflect the complexity of the exam but were often assigned by how much of the physician's time was required.

The four levels of codes for E&M services represent the least complicated exam (level 1) to the most complex exam (level 4). The level is important because a provider's "allowed payment" amount is proportionate to the level of the exam (level 1 paying the least, level 4 paying the most).

In 1994, while revamping Medicare rules to combat fraud and abuse, HCFA developed some strict guidelines for determining how the level of exam justified the level of E&M code. The time spent with the patient was no longer the controlling factor, and gone were the days when a physician might perform a very adequate physical but scribble only a few lines in the chart. The guidelines were published in 1995.

The AMA eliminated the old codes from CPT-4 and replaced them with entirely new codes that described the criteria to be met for that code. Specialists, however, found fault with the 1995 guidelines. For example, an ophthalmologist performs an in-depth exam of the eyes but does not typically perform a complete head-to-toe review of systems. Under the 1995 guidelines, the ophthalmologist would never meet the criteria for higher-level codes. In response, the guidelines were revamped in 1997 and physicians were allowed to use either the 1995 or 1997 guideline, whichever best suited their practice. This chapter uses the 1997 guideline, which is the most recent CMS guideline.

Where the service is rendered is an important consideration as well. There are separate categories of E&M codes for different locations such as office visits, inpatient exams, ER exams, and so on. The guidelines allow for these differences. For example, E&M codes for emergency room services do not have a time component because ER physicians are typically handling multiple patients at once; however, patient acuity and the intensity of service are factors for ER codes. Because the exercises in this book and the Student Edition software are oriented toward EHR in a physician's office, we will use examples of E&M codes for office visits.

Using EHR Software to Calculate the Correct E&M Code

One benefit of EHR systems is that the clinician automatically has a response to the HCFA mandate "if it isn't documented, it wasn't done," because it is always documented. EHR systems that use standardized nomenclatures have a codified record of the encounter, which enables the software to use the records from a patient encounter to calculate the correct E&M code for billing.

In an office using paper records, clinicians often select the E&M code by circling a code on a paper encounter form. These clinicians are at risk. If they select a code that is at a higher level than the paper note justifies, they can be fined. To avoid risk, most practices undercode, taking the attitude "better safe than sorry." This is bad for the practice financially. If the clinicians are choosing a code one level below what they have done, they are losing payment for their work. Mathematically, undercoding by one level is the same as seeing 80 patients and getting paid for seeing 60.

EHR systems can analyze the amount and type of data and accurately determine the correct E&M code at the correct level. Many EHR systems show how the calculation was determined, thus giving the provider confidence that the code is correct and can be substantiated. In addition to E&M codes, cross-reference codes in the Medcin nomenclature can suggest CPT-4 codes for performed procedures as well.

In this chapter, we are going to focus on understanding E&M codes. The Student Edition software contains an E&M code calculator. You are going to use that tool while learning how E&M codes are derived.

Hands-On Exercise 30: Calculating the E&M Code from an Exam

In this exercise, you are going to learn to use two new features of the software: the first is the ability to retrieve patient encounters from a previous visit and the second is to learn how to use the E&M Calculator.

Because your copy of the Student Edition may be shared by students from other classes, your software does not save encounters. However, the real purpose of an EHR is to do exactly that. In an actual office environment, every encounter for every patient seen would be saved and would become part of the patient's electronic medical record. In this exercise, you will learn to retrieve a previously stored encounter that is already in your system. Using a previous encounter will allow you to focus on understanding the E&M codes themselves without worrying about creating the note.

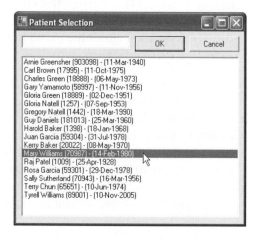

▶ **Figure 5-1 Select Patient Mary Williams.**

Step 1

If you have not already done so, start the Student Edition software.

Click Select on the Menu bar, and then click Patient (as shown in Figure 5-1).

In the Patient Selection window, locate and click on **Mary Williams**.

► Figure 5-2 Select Existing Encounter for May 5, 2006.

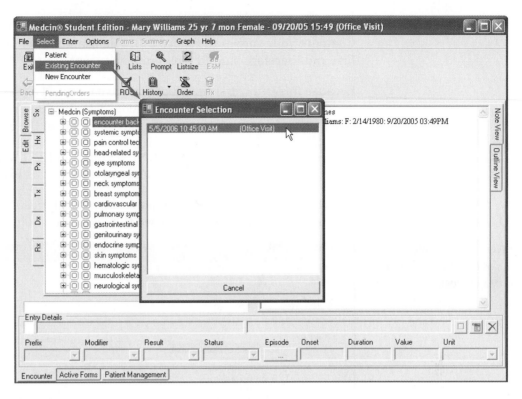

Step 2

Click Select on the Menu bar, and then click **Existing Encounter**.

This is a new feature you haven't used before. A small window of previous encounters will be displayed. Compare your screen to the window showing in the center of Figure 5-2.

Select **5/5/2006 10:45 AM Office Visit.**

The exam note from that date will be displayed.

► Figure 5-3 Patient Exam Note for May 5, 2006 Encounter.

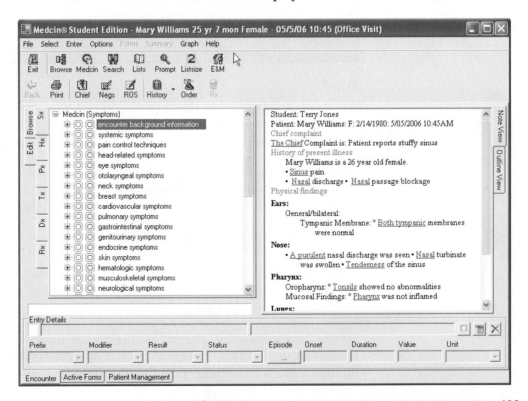

Step 3

Compare your screen to Figure 5-3. The exam was created using the Adult URI List and therefore should look familiar to you.

Because this is the first time that you have retrieved a previous encounter, and as we are going to be using the information from the exam note to calculate the E&M code, take a few minutes to look at the exam note in the right pane of your screen.

Pay attention to the History section. It contains HPI but no Review of Systems nor social history; this will be discussed later in this exercise.

Not all of the note will fit in the pane, so you will need to use the scroll bar on the right to scroll downward to see the rest of the note, as shown in Figure 5-4.

▶ **Figure 5-4 Scrolled Portion of Patient Exam Note for May 5, 2006.**

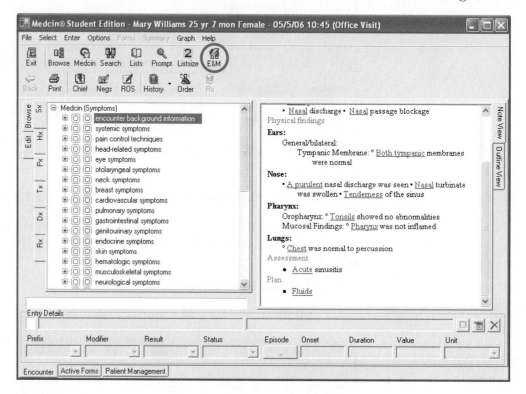

Step 4

When you scroll the note downward, you will be able to compare your screen to Figure 5-4 as well. Note the number of body systems in the Physical Findings section of the note.

When you are sufficiently familiar with the exam note, locate the button labeled "E&M" in the Toolbar at the top of your screen. The icon resembles a horseshoe magnet with a lightning bolt. It is circled in red on Figure 5-4.

Click on the E&M button and the E&M calculator window will be invoked.

Step 5

The fields in this screen will be explained in detail in subsequent steps; for the moment, just calculate the E&M code.

Locate the area labeled "Patient Status" in the upper right corner. If the white circle next to "Existing" is empty, click it once with your mouse. It should then fill with a black center (as shown in Figure 5-5, circled in red).

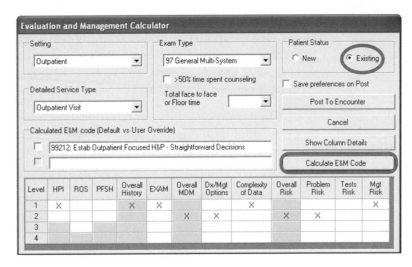

► **Figure 5-5 E&M Calculator for May 5, 2006 Encounter.**

Locate the large button (circled in red) labeled "Calculate E&M Code" and click it.

Compare your screen to the Evaluation and Management Calculator in Figure 5-5. If the field labeled "Calculated E&M code" displays "99212 Estab Outpatient Focused H&P—Straightforward Decisions," you are ready to proceed.

Step 6

You are going to use the E&M calculator window to help you understand the CMS Documentation Guidelines for Evaluation and Management Services.

Look at the bottom of the calculator window where there is a grid. The columns are labeled with terms you may recognize such as HPI and ROS. The rows are numbered 1–4; these are the four levels discussed earlier. Some of the columns have the letter "X" in one of the boxes indicating the level of that type of finding. This will be explained further later in this chapter.

Leave your E&M calculator displayed as you read the following section. Do not click any more buttons until instructed to do so. If you cannot complete the reading in the allotted time, simply repeat steps 1, 2, and 5 to reinvoke the E&M Calculator window when you are ready to resume.

How the Level of an E&M Code Is Determined

Each category of E&M codes (outpatient, inpatient, etc.) has at least four codes representing the four levels of service. Some categories have more than four E&M codes because there are subcategories, for example, new versus established patients; but even in subcategories there are codes for each of the four levels.

There are seven components that are evaluated to determine the level of E&M services. These components include:

◆ History
◆ Examination
◆ Medical Decision Making
◆ Counseling
◆ Coordination of Care
◆ Nature of Presenting Problem
◆ Time

Three components—history, examination, and medical decision making—are the *key* components in determining the level of E&M services. The three key components and their levels are named in the CPT-4 description of an E&M code. For example, code 99212 has the following description: "Established Patient, Focused History and Physical, Straightforward Decision Making."

The key components each have levels numbered 1–4 of their own. However, performing and documenting one key component (e.g., examination) at the highest level does not necessarily mean that the encounter as a whole will qualify for the highest level of E&M service.

The level of E&M code is derived from the highest level of two or three key components. The level of each key component is determined separately. This chapter will explain each of the components, the levels within the key components, and how they are combined to calculate the E&M code.

There is one exception; for services such as psychiatry, which consist predominantly of counseling or coordination of care, time is the key or controlling factor determining the level of E&M service. Time will be covered later in this chapter.

Key Component: History

The History component includes the following elements:

◆ **CC**, which is an acronym for Chief Complaint.

◆ **HPI**, which is an acronym for History of Present Illness.

◆ **ROS**, which is an acronym for Review of Systems.

◆ **PFSH**, which is an acronym for Past History, Family History, and Social History.

The extent of history of present illness, review of systems, and past, family, or social history that is obtained and documented is dependent on clinical judgment and the nature of the presenting problems.

Chief Complaint (CC) Chief Complaint is required for all levels of History. The guidelines state: "The medical record should clearly reflect the chief complaint."[1]

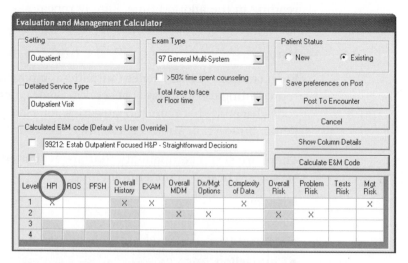

▶ **Figure 5-6 History Section of E&M Calculator with HPI (circled in red).**

---

[1]1997 Documentation Guidelines for Evaluation and Management Services, U.S. Department of Health and Human Services, Health Care Finance Administration, 1997.

Look at the grid section of the E&M Calculator window shown in Figure 5-6. The History section consists of the columns labeled HPI, ROS, PFSH, and Overall History.

Each of the history elements (HPI, ROS, PFSH) has levels that will determine the Overall History level. We will now discuss the history elements and levels.

History of Present Illness (HPI) The HPI is a chronological description of the development of the patient's present illness from the first sign and/or symptom or from the previous encounter to the present. HPI includes the following characteristics:

◆ location

◆ quality

◆ severity

◆ duration

◆ timing

◆ context

◆ modifying factors

◆ associated signs and symptoms

Step 7

The X in a column means there is a sufficient number of findings to meet the guidelines for the level at which it appears. For example, HPI has an X in the row for level 1, meaning HPI has enough findings for level 1 but not enough for level 2. The E&M calculator will allow you to see these findings.

Locate and click on the column label the acronym "HPI" (circled in red in Figure 5-6).

Step 8

A pane has opened in the upper portion of the E&M calculator window to display the findings that were recorded in the exam note for History of Present Illness (HPI) (as shown in Figure 5-7).

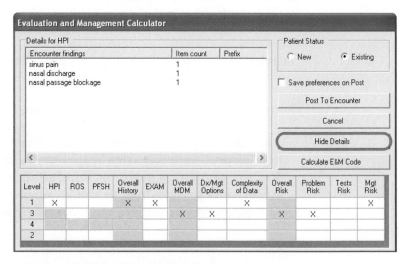

▶ **Figure 5-7 HPI Details in E&M Calculator.**

Each component of HPI, such as history, exam, decision making, and so on, has a numerical level of 1–4. Each level also has a name, such as brief, extended, low, high, simple, or complex.

In this case, HPI has two named levels, brief and extended. However, it also has numbers 1–4, the same as the components do. In this case, levels 1 or 2 both equate to brief. But levels 3 or 4 both equate to extended. The levels are determined by the quantity of findings:

1 or 2. Brief (consists of one to three items in the HPI).

3 or 4. Extended (consists of at least four items in the HPI or the status of at least three chronic or inactive conditions).

There are three findings shown in Figure 5-7; therefore, the HPI level is 1.

Close the Details for HPI pane and return to the previous view, by clicking the button labeled "Hide Details" (circled in red in Figure 5-7). Be careful not to click the Cancel button by mistake, as it will close the E&M calculator instead of hiding the details of HPI.

Step 9

Look at the column under ROS; note that it is empty. In steps 3 and 4, you reviewed the encounter note; you may recall that there was no ROS section in the note.

Review of Systems (ROS) "A ROS is an inventory of body systems obtained through a series of questions seeking to identify signs and/or symptoms which the patient may be experiencing or has experienced." You are familiar with ROS from previous exercises.

The ROS level is determined by the number of systems reviewed. ROS has three levels:

Level 2: Problem Pertinent (ROS inquires about the system directly related to the problems identified in the HPI).

Level 3: Extended (ROS inquires about the system directly related to the problems identified in the HPI and a number of additional systems. Extended level requires two to nine systems be documented).

Level 4: Complete (ROS inquires about the systems directly related to the problems identified in the HPI plus all additional body systems).

For level 4—Complete, the guidelines state:

> **"At least ten organ systems must be reviewed. Those systems with positive or pertinent negative responses must be individually documented. For the remaining systems, a notation indicating all other systems are negative is permissible. In the absence of such a notation, at least ten systems must be individually documented."[2]**

---

[2]Ibid.

Step 10

Look at the column under PFSH, and note that it is empty. In steps 3 and 4, you reviewed the encounter note. You may recall that there was no past medical history, family history, or social history sections in the note.

Past, Family, and/or Social History (PFSH) The PFSH consists of a review of three areas:

◆ Past history (the patient's past experiences with illnesses, operations, injuries, and treatments);

◆ Family history (a review of medical events in the patient's family, including diseases that may be hereditary or place the patient at risk); and

◆ Social history (an age-appropriate review of past and current activities).

PFSH level is determined by the number of findings in these three history types. PFSH has two levels, level 3 and level 4:

Level 3: Pertinent (at least one item in any of PFSH area directly related to the problems identified in the HPI).

Level 4: Complete (a review of two or all three of the PFSH history areas, depending on the category of the E&M service. Complete requires all three history areas for services that include a comprehensive assessment of a new patient or reassessment of an existing patient. A review of two of the three history areas is sufficient for other services).

Table of Elements Required for Each Level of History

	Level of History	CC	History Elements		
			History of Present Illness (HPI)	Review of Systems (ROS)	Past, Family, and/or Social History (PFSH)
1	Problem Focused	*	Brief (1–3 elements)	(No elements required)	(No elements required)
2	Expanded Problem Focused	*	Brief (1–3 elements)	Problem Pertinent (related to HPI)	(No elements required)
3	Detailed	*	Extended (4 or more)	Extended (2–9 body systems)	Pertinent (1 or more)
4	Comprehensive	*	Extended (4 or more)	Complete (10 or more body systems)	Complete (2 areas Past, Family, or Social)

* Chief Complaint is expected for all Types of History.

▶ **Figure 5-8 Elements Required for Each Type of History.**[3]

---

[3]Chart adapted from 1997 Documentation Guidelines for Evaluation and Management Services, U.S. Department of Health and Human Services, Health Care Finance Administration, 1997.

For certain categories of E&M services that include only an interval history, it is not necessary to record information about the PFSH. Those categories are subsequent hospital care, follow-up inpatient consultations, and subsequent nursing facility care.

Step 11

The key component History has four levels:

1. Problem Focused

2. Expanded Problem Focused

3. Detailed

4. Comprehensive

Figure 5-8 shows the elements required for each level of history. The Level of History (shown in the first column) is determined by the levels of the HPI, ROS, and PSFH elements.

Compare Figure 5-8 to the HPI, ROS, and PFSH columns on your screen. The fifth column in the grid, Overall History, is comparable to the first column in Figure 5-8.

Looking at the chart in Figure 5-8, do you see why the overall history is only Level 1? It is because that is the only level at which the ROS and PFSH items are not required.

How History May Be Documented

The guidelines state:

"The CC, ROS and PFSH may be listed as separate elements of history, or they may be included in the description of the history of the present illness.

A ROS and/or a PFSH obtained during an earlier encounter does not need to be re-recorded if there is evidence that the physician reviewed and updated the previous information. This may occur when a physician updates his or her own record or in an institutional setting or group practice where many physicians use a common record. The review and update may be documented by:

♦ describing any new ROS and/or PFSH information or noting there has been no change in the information; and

♦ noting the date and location of the earlier ROS and/or PFSH.

The ROS and/or PFSH may be recorded by ancillary staff or on a form completed by the patient. To document that the physician reviewed the information, there must be a notation supplementing or confirming the information recorded by others.

If the physician is unable to obtain a history from the patient or other source, the record should describe the patient's condition or other circumstance which precludes obtaining a history."[4]

---

[4]1997 Documentation Guidelines for Evaluation and Management Services, U.S. Department of Health and Human Services, Health Care Finance Administration, 1997.

Key Component: Examination

The second key component is the Physical Exam. Examination guidelines have been defined for a general multisystem exam and the following 10 single-organ systems:

◆ Cardiovascular

◆ Ears, Nose, and Throat

◆ Eyes

◆ Genitourinary (Female or Male)

◆ Hematologic/Lymphatic/Immunologic

◆ Musculoskeletal

◆ Neurological

◆ Psychiatric

◆ Respiratory

◆ Skin

A general multisystem examination or a single organ system examination may be performed by any physician, regardless of specialty. The type and content of examination are selected by the examining physician and are based on clinical judgment, the patient's history, and the nature of the presenting problems.

There are four levels of any type of examination:

1. Problem Focused—a limited examination of the affected body area or organ system.

2. Expanded Problem Focused—a limited examination of the affected body area or organ system and any other symptomatic or related body areas or organ systems.

3. Detailed—an extended examination of the affected body areas or organ systems and any other symptomatic or related body areas or organ systems.

4. Comprehensive—a general multisystem examination, or complete examination of a single organ system and other symptomatic or related body areas or organ systems.

The required elements for different levels of single organ system exams and the general multisystem exam vary; therefore, separate tables are published for each type of system. Two of those tables, General Multisystem, and Ears, Nose, and Throat, have been reprinted in Appendix A of this book.

Within the guideline tables, individual elements of the examination pertaining to a body area or organ system are identified by bullets. A bullet is a typographic character that looks like this: • (a solid black circle.)

If you have taken a class in medical coding or read the CPT-4 book you may be familiar with the concept of "the number of bullets required to meet a level of E&M coding." This simply means how many findings in the exam note corresponded to elements in the guideline table with bullet characters printed next to them.

Step 12

Locate and click on the column labeled "Exam" (circled in red in Figure 5-9). The grid has only one column for the Exam component. A pane displaying the exam details will open in the E&M Calculator window.

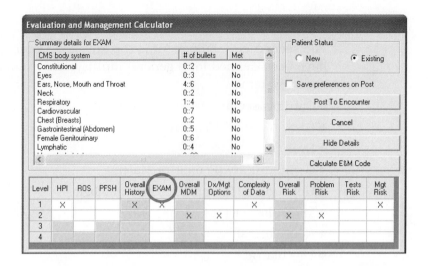

The Summary Details for Exam pane has three columns: CMS body systems, a column labeled "# of bullets," and a column labeled "Met."

Each row under the column labeled # of bullets has a pair of numbers. For example, locate the row for Ears, Nose, Mouth, and Throat; you will see the numbers 4:6. This means the clinician examined four of six elements in that system.

Turn to Appendix A in the back of the book and look at the CMS guideline tables. You can see that the "bullets" referred to in Figures 5-9 and 5-10 are

Table of Elements Required for Each Level of Examination

	Level of Examination	Examination Elements by Type of Exam	
		General Multisystem Examinations	Single Organ System Examinations
1	Problem Focused	1 to 5 elements identified by a bullet (•) in one or more organ systems or body areas.	1 to 5 elements identified by a bullet (•), whether in a box with a shaded or unshaded border.*
2	Expanded Problem Focused	At least 6 elements identified by a bullet (•) in one or more organ systems or body areas.	At least 6 elements identified by a bullet (•), whether in a box with a shaded or unshaded border.*
3	Detailed Examination	At least 6 organ systems or body areas; for each system/area selected at least 2 elements identified by a bullet (•). Alternatively, at least 12 elements identified by a bullet (•) in 2 or more organ systems or body areas.	At least 12 elements identified by a bullet (•), whether in a box with a shaded or unshaded border.* Exception: requirement reduced to 9 elements for Eye and psychiatric examinations.
4	Comprehensive Examination	At least 9 organ systems or body areas; for each system/area selected all elements identified by a bullet (•).	Every element in each box with a shaded border and at least 1 element in each box with an unshaded border; Plus all elements identified by a bullet (•) whether in a box with a shaded or unshaded border.*

* This refers to sections of the printed tables for Single Organ System Exams, which are outlined with a shaded border. See Appendix A for examples.

---

[5]Chart adapted from 1997 Documentation Guidelines for Evaluation and Management Services, U.S. Department of Health and Human Services, Health Care Finance Administration, 1997.

quite literally the typographic characters printed in the tables in Appendix A. Follow the instructions provided in Appendix A for comparing the two tables.

Step 13

Compare your screen with the table in Figure 5-10. You will see from the table that this is Level 1, "Problem Focused Exam," because there are only five elements with bullets documented in the exam (four bullets in Ear, Nose, Mouth, and Throat and 1 bullet in Respiratory). Although the provider can choose General Multisystem or Single organ exam guidelines, in this case you can see from the table that either choice would equate to Level 1 because there are only five bullets.

The Exam level is not determined by the number of findings but by the number of bullets satisfied within a system/body area. However, findings do not have to be abnormal; normal findings count as well.

The guidelines state:

> **"A brief statement or notation indicating "negative" or "normal" is sufficient to document normal findings related to unaffected areas or asymptomatic organ systems.**
>
> **Specific abnormal and relevant negative findings of the examination of the affected or symptomatic body areas or organ systems should be documented. A notation of "abnormal" without elaboration is insufficient."[6]**

Key Component: Medical Decision Making

The third key component is medical decision making. Medical Decision Making (MDM) refers to the complexity of establishing a diagnosis or selecting a management option as measured by these elements:

◆ Number of possible diagnoses or management options that must be considered.

◆ Amount or complexity of medical records, diagnostic tests, or other information that must be obtained, reviewed, and analyzed.

◆ Risk of significant complications, morbidity or mortality, as well as comorbidities, associated with the patient's presenting problems, the diagnostic procedures, or the possible management options.

Each of the elements of medical decision making has four levels, as described in step 14. The overall level of the MDM component is derived from the highest level of two of the three elements.

Step 14

The remaining columns in the E&M Calculator window grid are all concerned with Medical Decision Making.

Locate and click on the column labeled "Dx/Mgt Options" (shown circled in red in Figure 5-11). Dx/Mgt Options stands for Diagnosis and/or Management Options. The pane in the E&M Calculator window will display the Details for Dx/Mgt Options.

---

[6]1997 Documentation Guidelines for Evaluation and Management Services, U.S. Department of Health and Human Services, Health Care Finance Administration, 1997.

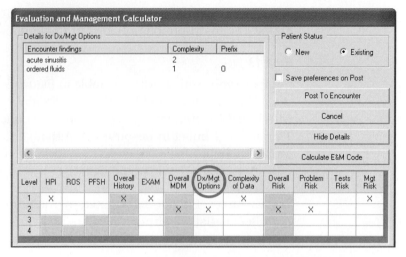

▶ Figure 5-11 Medical Decision Making—Details of Dx/Mgt Options.

The details pane has three columns labeled: Encounter Findings, Complexity, and Prefix. The Complexity column displays a level of complexity associated with the finding. The prefix column contains a code or abbreviation if the finding has a prefix. In this example, the finding "Ordered Fluids" displays the letter "O," which stands for ordered.

Number of Diagnoses or Management Options There are four levels of this element. The level is determined by the number and types of problems addressed during the encounter, the complexity of establishing a diagnosis, and the management decisions that are made by the physician. The levels include:

1. Minimal

2. Limited

3. Multiple

4. Extensive

In addition to the actual number of diagnoses codes selected, the number and type of diagnostic tests employed may be an indicator of the number of possible diagnoses. Problems that were reviewed also are counted. Consulting or seeking advice from others is another indicator of complexity of diagnostic or management problems.

Amount or Complexity of Data to Be Reviewed The amount and complexity of data to be reviewed is based on the types of diagnostic testing ordered or reviewed. A decision to obtain and review old medical records or obtain history from sources other than the patient increases the amount and complexity of data to be reviewed.

Discussion of contradictory or unexpected test results with the physician who performed or interpreted the test is an indication of the complexity of data being reviewed. On occasion, the physician who ordered a test may personally review the image, tracing, or specimen to supplement information from the physician who prepared the test report or interpretation; this is another indication of the complexity of data being reviewed.

There are four levels for this element as well, including:

1. Minimal or None

2. Limited

3. Moderate

4. Extensive

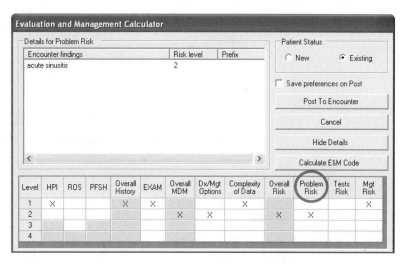

▶ **Figure 5-12 Medical Decision Making—Details of Problem Risk.**

Step 15

The remaining columns in the E&M Calculator window grid are concerned with the medical decision-making element of risk.

Locate and click on the column labeled "Problem Risk" (shown circled in red in Figure 5-12). The pane in the E&M Calculator window will display the Details for Problem Risk.

The details pane has three columns, labeled Encounter Findings, Risk, and Prefix. The Risk column displays a level of risk associated with the finding. The Prefix column was explained in the previous step.

Risk of Significant Complications, Morbidity, or Mortality The final element in Medical Decision Making is the risk of significant complications, morbidity, or mortality, which is based on the risks associated with the presenting problems, the diagnostic procedures, and the possible management options.

Risk also has four levels:

1. Minimal

2. Low

3. Moderate

4. High

Risk has its own table for calculating the level of risk (shown in Figure 5-14). However, risk differs from the other two elements of medical decision making in that risk level is the highest level of any **one** column in the table.

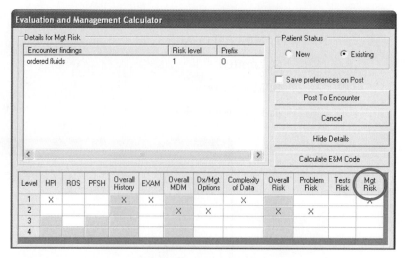

▶ Figure 5-13 Medical Decision Making—Details of Mgt Risk.

Step 16

Locate and click on the column labeled "Mgt Risk" (shown circled in red in Figure 5-13). Mgt is the software abbreviation for Management. The pane in the E&M Calculator window will display the Details for Management Risk.

The details pane has three columns, labeled Encounter Findings, Risk Level, and Prefix. The Risk column displays a level of risk associated with the finding. The Prefix column was explained in the previous step. In this case there is a low risk (Level 1) when ordering fluids.

The E&M calculator also includes a column measuring the risk of tests, but none were ordered during this exam.

Step 17

The table shown in Figure 5-14 may be used to help determine whether the risk of significant complications, morbidity, or mortality is minimal, low, moderate, or high. Because the determination of risk is complex and not readily quantifiable, the table includes common clinical examples rather than absolute measures of risk.

The assessment of risk of the presenting problems is based on the risk related to the disease process anticipated between the present encounter and the next one.

The assessment of risk of selecting diagnostic procedures and management options is based on the risk during and immediately following any procedures or treatment. *The highest level of risk in any one category* (presenting problems, diagnostic procedures, or management options) *determines the overall risk.*

Locate the column in the E&M Calculator window labeled "Overall Risk." Notice that the X is in the row for Level 2. This is because Problem Risk was Level 2, which was the highest risk element. You will see another example of this aspect of Risk in a subsequent exercise.

Table of Risk

Level of Risk	Presenting Problem(s)	Diagnostic Procedure(s) Ordered	Management Options Selected
1 Minimal	• One self-limited or minor problem, e.g., cold, insect bite, tinea corporis	• Laboratory tests requiring venipuncture • Chest x-rays • EKG/EEG • Urinalysis • Ultrasound, e.g., echocardiography • KOH prep	• Rest • Gargles • Elastic bandages • Superficial dressings
2 Low	• Two or more self-limited or minor problems • One stable chronic illness, e.g., well-controlled hypertension, non–insulin dependent diabetes, cataract, BPH • Acute uncomplicated illness or injury, e.g., cystitis, allergic rhinitis, simple sprain	• Physiologic tests not under stress, e.g., pulmonary function tests • Non-cardiovascular imaging studies with contrast, e.g., barium enema • Superficial needle biopsies • Clinical laboratory tests requiring arterial puncture • Skin biopsies	• Over-the-counter drugs • Minor surgery with no identified risk factors • Physical therapy • Occupational therapy • IV fluids without additives
3 Moderate	• One or more chronic illnesses with mild exacerbation, progression, or side effects of treatment • Two or more stable chronic illnesses • Undiagnosed new problem with uncertain prognosis, e.g., lump in breast • Acute illness with systemic symptoms, e.g., pyelonephritis, pneumonitis, colitis • Acute complicated injury, e.g., head injury with brief loss of consciousness	• Physiologic tests under stress, e.g., cardiac stress test, fetal contraction stress test • Diagnostic endoscopies with no identified risk factors • Deep needle or incisional biopsy • Cardiovascular imaging studies with contrast and no identified risk factors, e.g., arteriogram, cardiac catheterization • Obtain fluid from body cavity, e.g., lumbar puncture, thoracentesis, culdocentesis	• Minor surgery with identified risk factors • Elective major surgery (open, percutaneous, or endoscopic) with no identified risk factors • Prescription drug management • Therapeutic nuclear medicine • IV fluids with additives • Closed treatment of fracture or dislocation without manipulation
4 High	• One or more chronic illnesses with severe exacerbation, progression, or side effects of treatment • Acute or chronic illnesses or injuries that pose a threat to life or bodily function, e.g., multiple trauma, acute MI, pulmonary embolus, severe respiratory distress, progressive severe rheumatoid arthritis, psychiatric illness with potential threat to self or others, peritonitis, acute renal failure • An abrupt change in neurologic status, e.g., seizure, TIA, weakness, sensory loss	• Cardiovascular imaging studies with contrast with identified risk factors • Cardiac electrophysiological tests • Diagnostic endoscopies with identified risk factors • Discography	• Elective major surgery (open, percutaneous, or endoscopic) with identified risk factors • Emergency major surgery (open, percutaneous, or endoscopic) • Parenteral controlled substances • Drug therapy requiring intensive monitoring for toxicity • Decision not to resuscitate or to deescalate care because of poor prognosis

▶ **Figure 5-14 Determining Level of Risk.**[7]

---

[7]Chart adapted from 1997 Documentation Guidelines for Evaluation and Management Services, U.S. Department of Health and Human Services, Health Care Finance Administration, 1997.

Determining the Level of Medical Decision Making

There are four levels of Medical Decision Making:

1. StraightForward
2. Low Complexity
3. Moderate Complexity
4. High Complexity

The individual levels from each of the elements we have discussed, number of diagnoses, amount or complexity of data, and the level of risk are used to determine the level for Medical Decision Making.

Step 18

The chart in Figure 5-15 shows for each level of medical decision making, the level of elements required. The level of Medical Decision Making (shown in the first column) is determined by the highest levels of any two of the three elements.

Compare this chart to the E&M Calculator window. Locate the column labeled "Overall MDM", which has an X in the row for Level 2.

Looking at the columns for the individual elements, you see those labeled "Dx/Mgt Options" and "Overall Risk" both have an X in Level 2. Even though "Complexity of Data" is only Level 1, the MDM level is set to the highest of two out of three elements.

Table of Levels of Medical Decision Making				
Level of MDM	Medical Decision Making	Number of diagnoses or management options	Amount and/or complexity of data to be reviewed	Risk of complications and/or morbidity or mortality
1	*Straightforward*	Minimal	Minimal or None	Minimal
2	*Low Complexity*	Limited	Limited	Low
3	*Moderate Complexity*	Multiple	Moderate	Moderate
4	*High Complexity*	Extensive	Extensive	High

▶ **Figure 5-15 Elements Required for Each Level of Medical Decision Making.**[8]

Other Components: Counseling, Coordination of Care, and Time

In the case in which counseling or coordination of care dominates (more than 50%) of the physician/patient or family encounter (face-to-face time in the office or other or outpatient setting, floor/unit time in the hospital or nursing facility), time is considered the key or controlling factor to qualify for a particular level of E&M services.

---

[8]Ibid.

The guideline states:

"If the physician elects to report the level of service based on counseling and/or coordination of care, the total length of time of the encounter (face-to-face or floor time, as appropriate) should be documented and the record should describe the counseling and/or activities to coordinate care."[9]

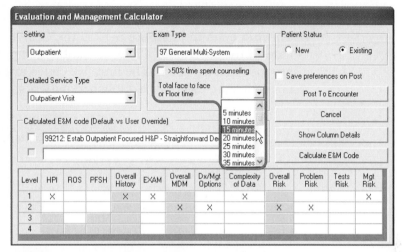

▶ **Figure 5-16 Counseling and Face-to-Face Time.**

Step 19

Click on the button labeled "Hide Details" to return to the E&M calculator screen. (If you have difficulty locating the button, refer to Figure 5-7.)

In the center of the E&M Calculator window are two fields related to time. First is a check box used to indicate that counseling (or coordination of care) exceeded 50% of the face-to-face time for the visit. The second field has a drop-down list used to enter the total face-to-face time.

Face-to-face time incorporates the total time both before and after the visit such as taking patient history, performing the exam, reviewing lab results, planning for follow-up care, and communicating with other providers about the patient's case.

The E&M calculator allows you to record the amount of face-to-face time even when you are not using counseling time as a factor. It is a good practice to record the face-to-face time for each encounter.

Click on the field labeled "Total face-to-face or Floor time" and select **15 min.**

This will not change the E&M code because time does not become a factor until it is more than half of the face-to-face time.

In the next exercise, you will learn to use both of these time-related fields to change the E&M code and to document the results in your exam note.

---

[9]1997 Documentation Guidelines for Evaluation and Management Services, U.S. Department of Health and Human Services, Health Care Finance Administration, 1997.

Putting It All Together

Momentarily leaving the element of time aside, you will see that the levels of each of the three *key components* combine to determine the level of the E&M code.

The chart in Figure 5-17 shows the E&M codes used for the category of outpatient office visits. It will help you to visualize how the relationship of the key components determines the E&M code.

The first column in Figure 5-17 is the CPT-4 code. The second column indicates if the code is for a new or established patient. Note that there are two groups of codes listed. The first five codes are for new patients, then five different codes are listed for established patients.

Relationship of Key Elements to E&M Codes for Outpatient Visits

E&M Code	Type of Patient	# of Key Elements Met	History Level	Exam Level	Medical Decision Making	Face-to-face Time
99201	New	All 3	1	1	1	10 min
99202	New	All 3	2	2	1	20 min
99203	New	All 3	3	3	2	30 min
99204	New	All 3	4	4	3	45 min
99205	New	All 3	4	4	4	60 min
99211	Established	2 of 3	Presentation of Problem Minimal Documentation Req.			5 min
99212	Established	2 of 3	1	1	1	10 min
99213	Established	2 of 3	2	2	2	15 min
99214	Established	2 of 3	3	3	3	25 min
99215	Established	2 of 3	4	4	4	40 min

▶ **Figure 5-17 Relationship of Key Component Levels Determines E&M Code.**

The third column labeled "# of Key Elements Met" indicates how many key components determine the E&M code.

The blue, green, and lavender columns list the levels of the three key components: History, Exam, and Medical Decision Making. The level numbers under each key component are derived from the individual tables in the sections you have just completed. The tables are:

History—Figure 5-8

Exam—Figure 5-10

MDM—Figure 5-15

The final column lists the number of minutes per type of visit used by the E&M calculator. Time will be discussed in a subsequent exercise.

Evaluating Key Components

Once the level of each of the key components is determined, calculating the level of the E&M code is fairly straightforward. The E&M code level is determined by the lowest level of the key components considered. However, there are different requirements for determining the E&M code for New or Established patients.

Scan down the third column of Figure 5-17. Note that the number of key components for New patients is **All 3**. Notice that for Established patients it is **2 of 3**. This doesn't mean that an encounter won't have findings for all three components, but in most cases it will. It means that, for an established patient, the two key components with the highest levels are considered and the lowest level of the two determines the E&M code.

For example, if an encounter has:

History Level 1 (*Problem Focused*)

Exam Level 2 (*Expanded Problem Focused*)

MDM Level 3 (*Moderate Complexity*)

The E&M code for an established patient will be Level 2 because only Exam and MDM are considered and Exam has the lower level.

If the encounter was for a new patient the E&M code would be Level 1 because all three key components are considered and the lowest is History (Level 1).

Look at the section of the table for New Patients. What E&M code would be used when History is Level 1 (*Problem Focused*), Exam is Level 2 (*Expanded Problem Focused*), and MDM is Level 2 (*Low Complexity*)?

If you answered 99201, you are correct. The E&M code for New patients is determined by all three elements. Even though the Exam and MDM components are Level 2, if the History level is not 2, then the lower code must be used.

You can now appreciate the value that an E&M calculator brings to an EHR system. Remember that the level of each of the key components is a combination of elements:

◆ To qualify for a given level of history, the quantity and types of HPI, ROS, and PFSH must be met.

◆ To qualify for a given level of exam, the number of "bulleted" items in the appropriate number of body systems must be met.

◆ To qualify for a given level of medical decision making, two of the three elements (the number of diagnosis, the amount of data, and the Risk Assessment) must be either met or exceeded.

If you can imagine trying to count bullets from your exam notes, calculate the amount of and types of history, and determine the level of decision making in your head, all while you are seeing the patient, you can understand why so many doctors code at the wrong level, just to be safe. You also can appreciate the skill required of medical coders who do this manually.

Step 20

Click the Cancel button to close the E&M calculator window. You may exit the Student Edition software **without printing** an encounter this time because you have not made any changes to the note.

Factors That Affect the E&M Code Set

The beginning of this chapter introduced the idea that there are multiple sets of E&M codes that vary by location and subcategory. Also, Figure 5-17 showed different sets of E&M codes for new and established patients.

The previous exercise demonstrated how the key components determine the level of the E&M code. However, each category of E&M codes has a set of codes representing the four levels. Therefore, once the level has been calculated, it is still necessary to know the location of service, the type of exam, and the type of patient to actually select the right code.

Hands-On Exercise 31: Exploring the E&M Calculator

In this exercise, you are going to learn more about the E&M calculator window. While doing so, you will be able to explore factors that the EHR software uses to select E&M codes from the correct set of CPT-4 codes. The first three steps should be familiar to you, as you performed them in the previous exercise.

Step 1

If you are not already running the Student Edition software, start it at this time.

From the Select Menu, click Patient, and from the Patient Selector window select **Mary Williams**. If you have difficulty, refer to Figure 5-1 at the beginning of this chapter.

Step 2

From the Select Menu, click **Existing Encounter**, and from the Encounter Selector window select **5/5/2006 10:45 AM Office Visit**. If you have difficulty, refer to Figure 5-2 at the beginning of this chapter.

Step 3

Locate and click on the button labeled E&M in the Toolbar at the top of your screen.

The Evaluation and Management Calculator window should be displayed. If you have difficulty, refer to Figure 5-4 at the beginning of this chapter.

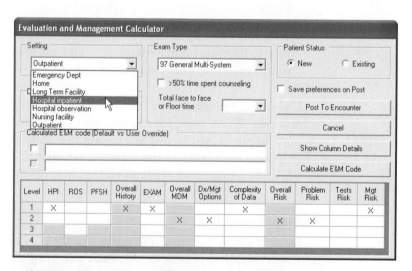

▶ **Figure 5-18 Drop-Down List for the Field Labeled "Setting."**

Step 4

Locate the field labeled "Setting" in the upper left corner of the E&M calculator window. This field allows you to set the location where the service was rendered. The field should already be set to Outpatient.

Click on the button with a down arrow in the field. A drop-down list of Service Locations is displayed. Compare your screen to Figure 5-18.

Locate and click on the location "Hospital Inpatient" in the drop-down list.

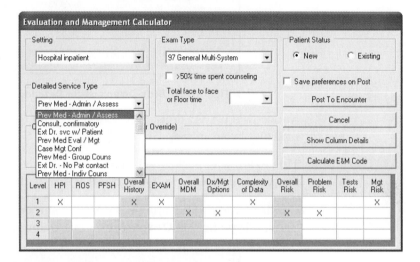

▶ **Figure 5-19 Drop-Down List for Detailed Service Type with Inpatient Setting.**

Step 5

You will recall from earlier in this chapter that within categories of E&M codes for different locations there were also subcategories of the types of services that might be rendered. The Detailed Service Type field is used to indicate the type of service that was performed in a given setting.

Locate the field labeled "Detailed Service Type" on the left of the E&M calculator window. Click on the button with a down arrow in the field. A drop-down list of Service Types is displayed. Compare your screen to Figure 5-19.

Study the Service Types displayed in your drop-down list, but do not make any selection.

Step 6

The "Detailed Service Type" field is related to and dependent on the "Setting" field. To demonstrate that in this step, move your mouse back to the field labeled "Setting" and click on the down arrow button as you did in step 4.

Change the Setting field by locating and selecting "Outpatient" from the drop-down list.

Step 7

Move your mouse back to the field labeled "Detailed Service Type" and click on the down arrow button in the field. Compare your screen to Figure 5-20; a drop-down list of Service Types appropriate to an outpatient setting is displayed.

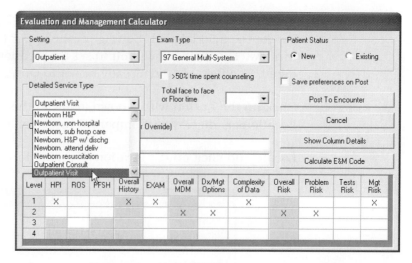

► Figure 5-20 Drop-Down List for Detailed Service Type with Outpatient Setting.

Notice this list is completely different from the drop-down list for inpatient setting displayed in step 5.

This exam was performed in an Outpatient setting. Locate and click on the Detailed Service Type "Outpatient Visit" at the bottom of the list.

Confirm that the Setting field on your screen is **Outpatien**t and the Detailed Service Type field is **Outpatient Visit** before proceeding.

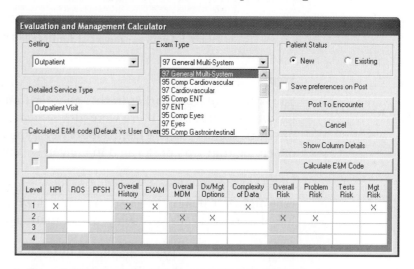

► Figure 5-21 Drop-Down List for Exam Type in E&M Calculator.

Step 8

You will recall that in addition to the General MultiSystem exam, there are guidelines for 10 different specialty exams. Also, clinicians are permitted to use either the 1995 or 1997 guideline, whichever best suits their practice. The field labeled "Exam Type" allows the clinician to select the appropriate guideline for the E&M Calculator to use.

Locate the field labeled "Exam Type" in the upper center of the E&M Calculator window. Click on the down arrow button in the field. The drop-down list not only displays the various exam types, but indicates for each name if it is from the 1995 or 1997 guidelines. Compare your screen to Figure 5-21.

This exercise uses the "97 General Multi-System" exam. Select that exam type.

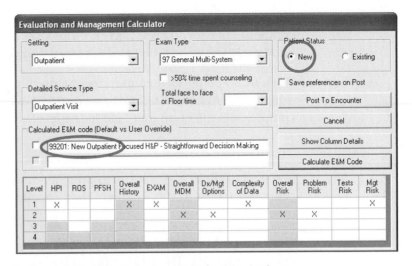

▶ **Figure 5-22 E&M Code Calculated for New Patient.**

Step 9

Some E&M categories, such as outpatient, provide two sets of codes, one for new patients and one for established patients. The Patient Status field allows the E&M calculator to select the appropriate code set for categories that make this distinction. You have used this field in previous exercises and should be familiar with it. In this step, you will see its effect on coding.

Locate the section labeled Patient Status in the upper right corner of the calculator window. Click on the circle next to the label "New" (circled in red.) Then click on the button labeled "Calculate E&M code." Compare your screen to Figure 5-22.

Notice the code and description "99201: New Outpatient Focused H&P—Straightforward Decision Making" (circled in red) are different from the code and description generated in Hands-On Exercise 30. Compare the code currently on your screen with the code shown in Figure 5-16.

Step 10

Click the button labeled "Cancel" to close the E&M Calculator window.

Factors That Increase the Level of Codes

At this point, you should have a good understanding on how an E&M code is determined from the key elements of the encounter. However, what changes the exam to the next level is not always apparent.

The level of E&M code for an established patient is dependent on two of three of the **key components**. Merely adding more findings to any one component may bring that component to a higher-level, but that does not necessarily mean that the visit as a whole will qualify for the higher-level E&M code.

For example, in Hands-On Exercises 30 and 31, an established patient had:

History Level 1 (*Problem Focused*)

Exam Level 1 (*Problem Focused*)

MDM Level 2 (*Low Complexity*)

The E&M code was Level 1 (99212) because the one of the two highest key components was a Level 1. Even if the level of MDM was raised to three, the E&M code would still be Level 1 because the exam component was only Level 1.

Work must be performed and documented in the appropriate areas to result in a higher E&M code. The next exercise will demonstrate how changes to key components affect an increase to the level of an E&M code.

Fraud and Abuse

The goal of these exercises is to provide an experiential understanding of concepts discussed in this chapter. They should not be construed as having any other purpose.

It is unethical and illegal to maximize payment by means that contradict regulatory guidelines. The HHS Office of Inspector General (OIG) investigates allegations of medical billing fraud and abuse. It does not matter if coding errors are made deliberately or inadvertently; OIG still treats it as fraud and abuse.

The student should not get the impression that it is OK to up-code to maximize reimbursement unless legally entitled by documentation and service provided. Similarly, a clinician cannot adjust the time factor unless it is substantiated in the documentation. Diagnoses or procedures should not be inappropriately included or excluded because payment or insurance policy coverage requirement will be affected.

EHR systems support accurate, complete, and consistent coding practices by documenting the encounter with codified nomenclature that can be analyzed and used to determine the levels of billing justified. Medical coders must adhere to the coding conventions, official coding guidelines, and official rules, and assign codes that are clearly and consistently supported by clinical documentation in the health record.

Hands-On Exercise 32: Calculating E&M for a More Complex Visit

In this exercise, you are going to add findings to an existing encounter to study the effects on E&M coding. The goal of this exercise is to provide an experiential understanding of concepts discussed in this chapter. It should not be construed as having any other purpose.

Step 1

If the patient encounter used in the previous exercise is not currently displayed on your screen, start the Student Edition software.

From the Select Menu, click Patient, and from the Patient Selector window select **Mary Williams**. If you have difficulty, refer to Figure 5-1 at the beginning of this chapter.

From the Select Menu, click **Existing Encounter**, and from the Encounter Selector window select **5/5/2006 10:45 AM Office Visit**. If you have difficulty, refer to Figure 5-2 at the beginning of this chapter.

You will recall from Hands-On Exercise 30 that this patient encounter note produces a calculated E&M code of "99212 Established Outpatient Focused H&P—Straightforward Decisions." You do not need to run the E&M calculator yet.

Step 2

The exam note that you have selected was for an Adult URI, and was created using the List feature, which you learned in Chapter 4.

From the Toolbar at the top your screen, click on the button labeled "List." When the Lists Manager window shown in Figure 5-23 is displayed, select **Adult URI** and click the button labeled "Load List."

In the following steps, you are going to use the list to add findings and study their effect on the levels of E&M codes.

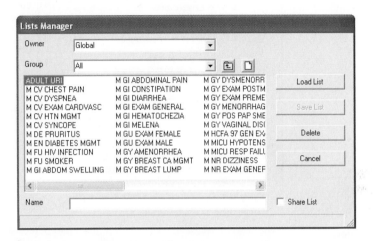

▶ **Figure 5-23 Select the Adult URI List from the Lists Manager.**

History

The History level is determined by the relationship between HPI, ROS, and PFSH. If you refer back to Figure 5-8, you will see the following:

◆ An increase in the number of findings for HPI will only affect the level of history if ROS and PFSH contain data as well.

◆ An increase in the number of body systems in ROS will only affect the level of history if HPI contains at least four findings and PFSH contains at least one.

◆ Adding even one finding for PFSH will only affect the level of history if HPI contains at least four findings and ROS contains at least 2 body systems.

◆ A "Complete" level of PFSH will only affect the overall history level when HPI contains at least four findings and ROS has at least 10 systems.

Step 3

Scroll the exam note, displayed in the pane on the right, upward to view the History section (circled in red in Figure 5-24). Note that there is neither Review of symptoms or PFSH findings in the history section. This means that there is only one of the three History elements in the current calculation.

Locate the button labeled "ROS" (circled in red) on the Toolbar at the top of the screen and click it.

► **Figure 5-24 Upper Portion of Exam Note with ROS Button and History Section (circled in red).**

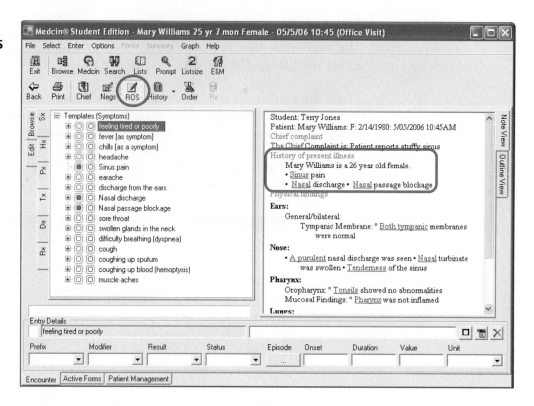

► **Figure 5-25 Review of Systems—No Fever.**

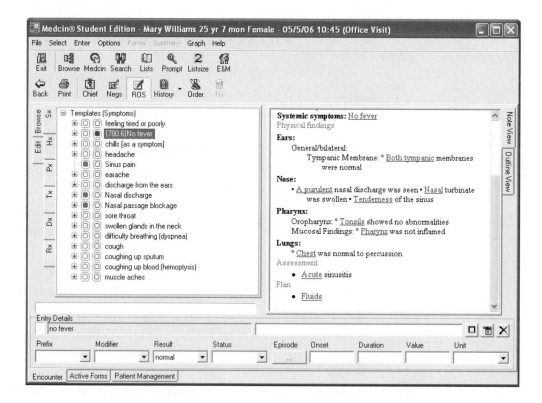

Step 4

Locate and click on the following Symptom finding:

- (blue button) Fever

Compare your screen to Figure 5-25. Note that the HPI findings (with red buttons) were already present.

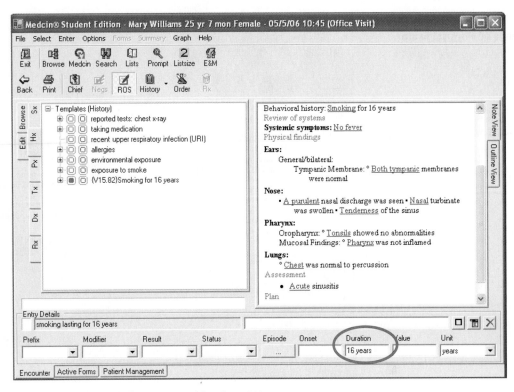

▶ **Figure 5-26 Social History—Smoking for 16 Years.**

Step 5

Click on the Hx tab.

Locate and click on the following History finding:

- (red button) Smoking

In the Entry Details section at the bottom of your screen, type "**16 years**" in the field labeled "Duration."

Compare your screen to Figure 5-26; note that you now have findings in all three History sections: HPI, ROS, and PFSH (behavioral history).

Examination

Exams provide the most direct but not the easiest means to reach a higher-level code. The more systems you examine, or in "single organ" exams the more bullet points you meet in a single area, the more work you are doing and therefore the higher level of code you should be able to bill for.

◆ In a General Multi-System Examination, six or more elements with a bullet are required to reach the second level.

◆ The third level is reached when you have at least two elements in six or more systems/body areas.

◆ The fourth level requires all the bulleted items in at least nine systems/body areas.

Step 6

Click on the Px tab.

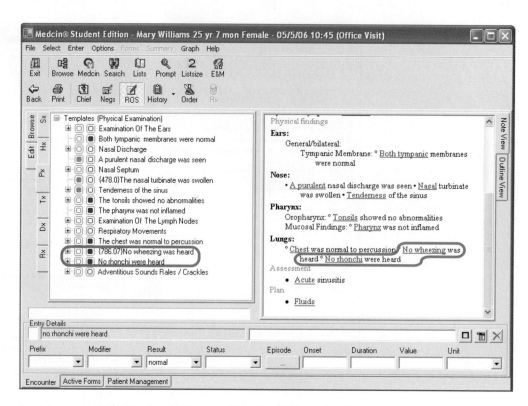

Locate and click on the following Physical Exam findings:

- (blue button) Auscultation Wheezing
- (blue button) Auscultation Rhonchoi

Compare your screen to Figure 5-27.

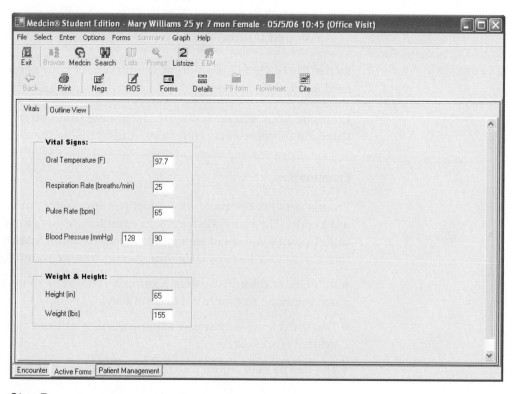

Step 7

Enter the patient's Vital Signs using the Vitals Form located in the Active
Forms tab (as you learned in Chapter 3).

Click on the Active Forms tab at the bottom of your screen. Locate and click on the Forms button on the Toolbar at the top of your screen. A list of Forms will be displayed. Choose the form labeled Vitals.

Enter Ms. Williams's Vital Signs, which are as follows:

Temperature: **97.7**

Respiration: **25**

Pulse: **65**

BP: **128/90**

Height: **65**

Weight: **155**

When you have entered all of the vital signs, compare your screen to Figure 5-28 and then click your mouse on the Encounter tab at the bottom of the screen.

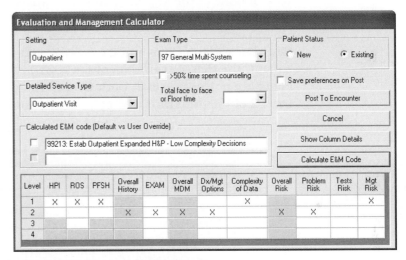

Evaluation and Management Calculator

Level	HPI	ROS	PFSH	Overall History	EXAM	Overall MDM	Dx/Mgt Options	Complexity of Data	Overall Risk	Problem Risk	Tests Risk	Mgt Risk
1	X	X	X					X				X
2					X	X	X		X	X		
3												
4												

▶ **Figure 5-29 Recalculated E&M Code.**

Step 8

Click on the E&M button in the Toolbar at the top of your screen to invoke the Evaluation and Management Calculator window.

Locate the section labeled Patient Status in the upper right corner of the calculator window. Click on the circle next to the label "Existing."

Locate and click on the button labeled "Calculate E&M code."

Medical Decision Making

◆ The level of MDM is determined by two out of three elements in the table shown in Figure 5-15. However, the Risk table in Figure 5-14 indicates that managing prescribed medications raises the Risk to Level 3. Therefore, the MDM level for any patient on medications will usually be determined by the number of diagnosis and the amount or complexity of data reviewed during the visit.

In this exercise, the Medical Decision Making components did not change levels.

Figure 5-29 shows the E&M code generated as a result of the additional findings you have added. The new code is "99213: Estab Outpatient Expanded H&P—Low Complexity Decisions." Figure 5-16 shows the previously calculated E&M code of 99212. Compare the grid at the bottom of your E&M Calculator window to Figure 5-16.

Note that the History sections ROS and PFSH now have an "X" in them. Although none of the history elements moved to Level 2, the Overall History moved to Level 2. This is because of the presence of a "Problem Pertinent" ROS finding, which changed History level from 1–Problem Focused to 2–Expanded Problem Focused. The addition of the PFSH did not, however, affect the Overall History level. Refer to Figure 5-8 Table of History Elements Required for Each Level of History.

Now, notice that the "X" in the grid under the second key component, Exam, has also increased from Level 1 to Level 2. This was a result of the addition of Vital Signs and 2 Physical Exam findings.

Why, if none of the key components changed to Level 3, did the E&M code change from a Level 2 code: 99212 to a Level 3 code: 99213?

Refer back to the Chart in Figure 5-17; you will notice that, for an Established patient, the CPT-4 requirement for 99213 is that two of the three key components are at least Level 2. Both Overall History and Exam now have an "X" in Level 2 of the grid; thus, the encounter justifies a Level 3 E&M code.

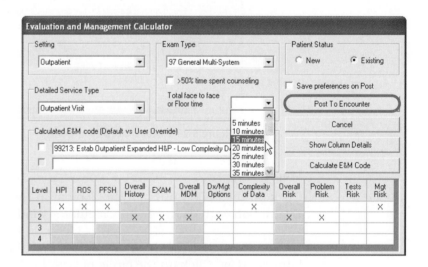

▶ **Figure 5-30 Setting the Face-to-Face Time.**

Time

◆ As you learned earlier, time can be a factor when more than 50% of the face-to-face time is spent counseling the patient. Both the face-to-face time and the counseling time must be documented. This will be covered in Hands-on Exercise 33.

Step 9

It is always a good idea to record the face-to-face time in the exam note. The software allows you to do this when you record the E&M code even if you are not using counseling time as a factor in E&M calculation. Remember face-to-face time is the total time you spent on the visit before, during, and after the patient exam. It is not the time spent counseling the patient.

Click on the button with the down arrow in the field labeled "Face-to-face/Floor time" and select **15 min** (as shown in Figure 5-30).

Recalculate the E&M code by clicking on the button labeled "Calculate E&M Code" again. Note that the time did not change the calculated code, which is still 99213.

Step 10

When a clinician is satisfied with the E&M code that has been calculated, it is posted to the note.

Locate and click on the button labeled "Post To Encounter" (circled in red in Figure 5-30). The E&M Calculator window will close and the E&M code will be added into your note. Compare your screen with Figure 5-31. Notice the procedure and the face-to-face time (circled in red) have been added to the bottom of the exam note.

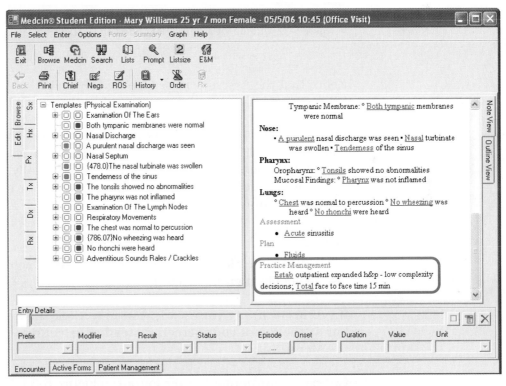

▶ **Figure 5-31 Exam Note with E&M Code and Face-to-Face Time (circled in red).**

Step 11

Locate and click on the tab on the right of the window labeled "Outline View." Compare your screen with Figure 5-32. Locate the Practice Management section near the bottom of the outline view. In outline view, not only is the description information of the calculated E&M code displayed but also the code itself is displayed.

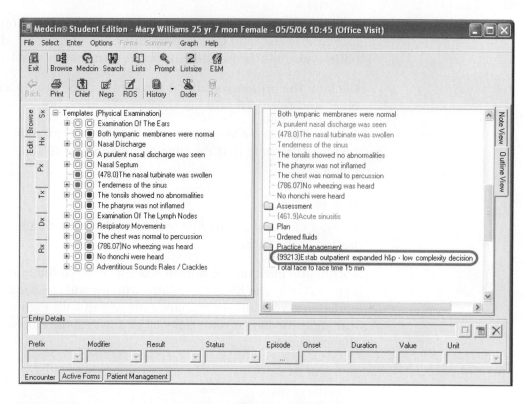

► Figure 5-32 Outline View with E&M Code and Description.

Notice that the Assessment section and several other findings also display ICD9-CM codes in this view. These will be discussed later in this chapter.

In EHR systems that are integrated with Practice Management or billing software, the EHR system transfers the Procedure and Diagnosis (CPT-4 and ICD-9CM) codes to the billing system automatically. The Student Edition does not transfer the codes to a billing system but it does post codes to the patient encounter.

Step 12

Click File on the Menu bar, and then click Print Encounter or Print To HTML (as directed by your instructor).

If you are printing your work, you may click the Print button on the Tool-bar at the top of your screen instead of selecting Print Encounter from the Menu.

Compare your printout or file output to Figure 5-33. If it is correct, hand it in to your instructor. If there are any differences, review the previous steps in the exercise and find your error.

(!) Alert

Do not close or exit the Encounter until you have a printed copy in your hand. You will lose your work if you exit before printing.

Student: Terry Jones
Patient: Mary Williams: F: 2/14/1980: 5/05/2006 10:45AM
Chief complaint
The Chief Complaint is: Patient reports stuffy sinus.
History of present illness
Mary Williams is a 26 year old female.
  • Sinus pain.
  • Nasal discharge o Nasal passage blockage
Personal history
Behavioral history: Smoking for 16 years
Review of systems
Systemic symptoms: No fever
Physical findings
Vital signs:

Vital Signs/Measurements	Value	Normal Range
Oral temperature	97.9 F	97.6 - 99.6
RR	25 breaths/min	18 - 26
PR	65 bpm	50 - 100
Blood pressure	128/90 mmHg	100-120/56-80
Weight	155 lbs	98 - 183
Height	65 in	60.2 - 68.5

Ears:
    General/bilateral:
        Tympanic Membrane: ° Both tympanic membranes were normal
Nose:
  • A purulent nasal discharge was seen • Nasal turbinate was swollen
  • Tenderness of the sinus
Pharynx:
    Oropharynx: ° Tonsils showed no abnormalities
    Mucosal Findings: ° Pharynx was not inflamed
Lungs:
    ° Chest was normal to percussion ° No wheezing was heard ° No rhonchi were heard
Assessment
  • Acute sinusitis
Plan
  • Fluids
Practice Management
    Estab outpatient expanded h&p - low complexity decisions;
    Total face to face time 15 min

▶ Figure 5-33 Printed Exam Note for Mary Williams May 5, 2006 10:45 AM.

Hands-On Exercise 33: Counseling More Than 50% of Face-to-Face Time

When counseling or coordination of care represent more than 50% of the face-to-face time of the visit, time becomes a key or controlling factor to the level of E&M services.

You will recall from the previous exercise that the patient has been smoking since she was a young child. The clinician spent about 10 minutes of time counseling the patient on the need to stop using tobacco and discussing possible strategies she might use to quit. This extra time spent counseling causes the visit take longer. In this exercise you are going to reload the encounter, reenter the history, and recalculate the code using time as a factor.

Step 1

If the Student Edition software is not currently running on your system, start it at this time.

Perform the following tasks *even if* the patient encounter used in the previous exercise is still displayed on your screen. This will refresh the encounter and eliminate the changes you made in the previous exercise.

From the Select Menu, click Patient, and from the Patient Selector window select **Mary Williams**. If you have difficulty, refer to Figure 5-1 at the beginning of this chapter.

From the Select Menu, click **Existing Encounter**, and from the Encounter Selector window select **5/5/2006 10:45 AM Office Visit**. If you have difficulty, refer to Figure 5-2 at the beginning of this chapter.

Do not run the E&M calculator yet.

Step 2

From the Toolbar at the top of your screen, click on the button labeled "List." When the Lists Manager window shown in Figure 5-23 is displayed, select **Adult URI** and click the button labeled "Load List."

Step 3

Click on the Hx tab.

Locate and click on the following History finding:

- (red button) Smoking

In the Entry Details section at the bottom of your screen type "**16 years**" in the field labeled Duration.

If you have difficulty, refer to Figure 5-26 in the previous exercise.

In the next two steps, you are going to experiment with Time, calculating the E&M code 3 times.

Step 4

Locate and click on the E&M button in the Toolbar at the top of your screen to invoke the Evaluation and Management Calculator window.

Locate the Patient Status field and click on the circle labeled "Existing."

Locate and click the button labeled "Calculate E&M Code." Note that the Calculated E&M Code is 99212, the same as it was in the beginning of the previous exercise.

Locate the check box used to indicate that counseling (or coordination of care) exceeded 50% of the face-to-face time for the visit. The box is circled in red in Figure 5-34. Click your mouse on the field and a check mark will appear.

Click your mouse on the down arrow button in the field labeled "Face-to-face/Floor time," and select 10 min from the drop-down list.

Click the button labeled "Calculate E&M Code." The code should still calculate as 99212.

Notice that the code did *not* change, even though the box labeled ">50%" was checked.

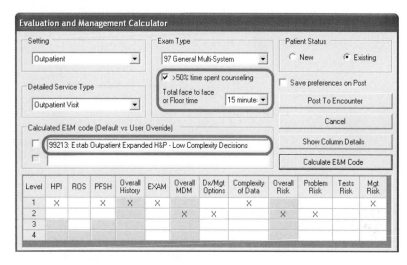

▶ **Figure 5-34 E&M Code Recalculated Using Time as a Factor.**

Step 5

Click your mouse on the down arrow button in the field labeled "Face-to-face/Floor time"; this time select 15 minutes from the drop-down list.

Click the button labeled "Calculate E&M Code." Compare your screen to Figure 5-34. The newly calculated code on your screen should be 99213.

In step 4, the code did not increase to a higher level because the E&M calculator has a minimum amount of time expected to complete each level of exam. Refer back to the table in Figure 5-17. In the right column, the standard amount of time is shown for each code. The E&M code 99212 has a minimum face-to-face time of 10 minutes, whereas the next higher-level E&M code 99213 has a minimum face-to-face time of 15 minutes.

When the face-to-face time for this exam was set at less than 15 minutes, the E&M calculator did not increase the code to the next level. Once you increased the amount of time, and checked the box labeled ">50% time spent counseling," time became the controlling or key component.

Locate and click on the button labeled "Post To Encounter."

Step 6

Remember you can only use time to increase the level of E&M code when the clinician has spent more that 50% of the face-to-face time in counseling or co-ordination of care. In Mary's case, the clinician spent 10 minutes of the total 15 minutes in counseling.

Remember that the guideline also states:" . . . the record should describe the counseling and/or activities to coordinate care."[10]

This means that whenever you use this feature in a medical office, you must add free-text to describe the counseling.

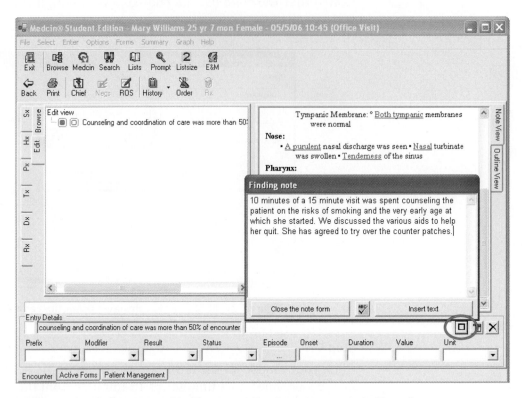

▶ **Figure 5-35 Finding Note Added for Counseling (note button circled in red).**

Locate the finding labeled "Counseling" in the Practice Management section of the right pane.

Click on the word "Counseling" to enter Edit mode.

Add free-text to adequately describe the counseling. Because you need to provide a fairly detailed description it is better to use the Finding Note window (which you previously learned in Chapter 3).

Click on the Note button (circled in red in Figure 5-35) to open the Finding Note window. Type the following text:

> **"10 minutes of a 15 minute visit was spent counseling the patient on the risks of smoking and the very early age at which she started. We discussed the various aids to help her quit. She has agreed to try over the counter patches."**

When you finish typing, click on the button labeled "Close the Note Form."

---

[10]Ibid.

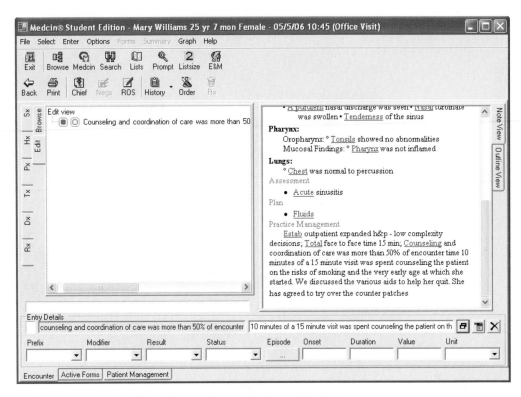

▶ **Figure 5-36 Mary Williams's Exam Note with Counseling Note.**

Step 7

Compare your screen to the right pane in Figure 5-36. If there are any differences, review the previous steps in the exercise and find your error. If it is correct, follow the directions below to print your work.

Click File on the Menu bar, and then click Print Encounter or Print To HTML (as directed by your instructor).

If you are printing your work, you may click the Print button on the Toolbar at the top of your screen.

Compare your printout to Figure 5-37. Hand your printout or HTML file in to your instructor.

> **(!) Alert**
>
> ***Do not close or exit the Encounter until you have a printed copy in your hand.* You will lose your work if you exit before printing.**

ICD-9CM Codes Justify Billing

In addition to CPT-4 codes for procedures, health care claims require diagnosis codes as well. Currently, ICD-9CM is the required code set for reporting diagnoses on insurance claims. CMS has published guidelines for using ICD-9CM codes on claim forms. Chapter 2 discusses the history and structure of ICD-9CM codes, which you can review if necessary.

Although ICD-9CM is a classification system for mortality and morbidity studies, it is used daily by clinicians and billing staff for insurance claims. The use

```
Mary Williams                                                    Page 1 of 1

Student: Terry Jones
Patient: Mary Williams: F: 2/14/1980: 5/05/2006 10:45AM
Chief complaint
The Chief Complaint is: Patient Reports stuffy sinus.
History of present illness
     Mary Williams is a 26 year old female.
     • Sinus pain.
     • Nasal discharge o  Nasal passage blockage
Personal history
Behavioral history:  Smoking for 16 years
Physical findings
Ears:
General/bilateral:
     Tympanic Membrane: ° Both tympanic membranes were normal
Nose:
     • A purulent nasal discharge was seen o Nasal turbinate was swollen o Tenderness of
the sinus
Pharynx:
     Oropharynx: ° Tonsils showed no abnormalities
     Mucosal Findings: ° Pharynx was not inflamed
Lungs:
     ° Chest was normal to percussion
Assessment
     The doctor made the following assessments
     • Acute sinusitis
Plan
     The doctor ordered the following therapy
     • Fluids
Practice Management
     Estab outpatient expanded h&p - low complexity decisions;  Total face to face time
15 min;  Counseling and coordination of care was more than 50% of encounter time 10
minutes of a 15 minute visit was spent counseling the patient on the risks of smoking
and the very early age at which she started. We discussed the various aids to help
her quit. She has agreed to try over the counter patches
```

▶ **Figure 5-37 Printed Exam with Counseling Note for Mary Williams.**

of the correct ICD-9CM code on a claim serves to explain or justify the medical reason for the procedure being billed.

However, many of the patients seen in an outpatient setting come for reasons other than a specific illness. To submit claims for these encounters, diagnosis codes that do not involve disease or death are necessary.

A supplemental section of the ICD-9CM titled "Factors Influencing Health Status and Contact with Health Services" provides codes for many reasons that patients come to the doctor other than illness or injury. These include "Wellness" visits (used for checkups and physicals), as well as vaccinations, maternity care, screening for diabetes, and so on. The codes are called "V Codes" as they begin with the letter "V" and are followed by two numbers, a decimal point, and a fourth or fifth digit to distinguish specificity (discussed below). Some examples of "V codes" include:

V20.2 Well Visit—Child

V22.1 Pregnancy—First Normal

V22.2 Pregnancy—Normal

V70.2 Well Visit—Adult

Another supplemental section of ICD-9CM is used for "External Causes of Injury and Poisoning." These are called "E Codes," as they begin with the letter "E" followed by three numbers, a decimal point, and a single digit to distinguish specificity. E Codes cover injuries ranging from beestings to war. E Codes serve to codify the *cause* of an injury or adverse effect. They are used in conjunction with the main ICD-9CM codes, never alone. Some examples of "E Codes" include:

E812.0   Motor vehicle accident—injury to driver

E812.1   Motor vehicle accident—injury to passenger

E881.0   Fall from a ladder

E905.3   Beestings

Determine the Level of Specificity

ICD-9CM codes are from three to five digits long. The codes for illness and disease begin with three digits called the "rubric," followed by a decimal point and up to two numerals, which serve to further specify or refine the description of the condition. The fourth and fifth digits add specificity as you can see in the example of asthma in Figure 2-9.

Insurance billing rules require clinicians to code to the most specific level. Three-digit (rubric) codes are no longer accepted on claims and if used as the primary diagnosis the claim may get rejected. Most EHR systems contain a "cross-walk" or internal reference table that can produce ICD-9CM codes at the fourth- or fifth-digit specificity automatically.

Offices without an EHR often print a list of diagnosis codes on the paper encounter form. The clinician indicates the diagnosis by checking or circling a code on the form. However, the preprinted codes on the form may not be as specific as the clinician's assessment. The clinician must then be careful to use the same terminology in the dictation as the ICD-9CM description, or the billing for the visit may not match the transcribed exam note.

The advantage of using an EHR with a codified nomenclature is that the codes billed will always be in sync with the note that is produced. Another advantage is that the EHR allows the clinician to record nuances that are beyond the scope of ICD-9CM such as "mild" or "improving." The EHR software will automatically translate the assessment to the correct diagnosis code, which then may be used for billing.

Multiple Diagnosis Codes Per Visit

Multiple diagnoses codes can be assigned to a single encounter. A paper claim form is limited to four diagnosis codes per procedure code, but electronic claims allow seven or more.

Multiple diagnoses occur mainly in patients with ongoing or chronic conditions requiring regular visits. It is correct and appropriate to continue to use diagnosis codes from past visits for as long as the patient continues to have the illness or condition and that condition is clearly documented in the record. For example, a patient with *diabetes mellitus—poorly controlled* might be seen regularly. With

A Real-Life Story

A New Level of Efficiency in Addition to Improved E&M Coding

Philip C. Yount, M.D.

Ashe Medical Associates

Every medical doctor in America reviews the patient's past medical problems, medication list, social history, and so on, but do they always document that? I think it is safe to say that doctors, who dictate after the visit, actually get more information, examine more of the patient, and say things to the patient that they do not recall when they dictate later. Certainly when I was dictating or writing notes I didn't always remember to document all that I did. To be safe I tended to undercode; I am sure most everybody else does, too.

Our practice has been using an electronic medical record for almost 3 years. I would never go back to a paper-based system again. But back when I was dictating, the workflow with the paper system was to finish the visit, mark the charge and the E&M code on a paper encounter form, and then dictate it later. This was really hard because during dictation I was trying both to remember the visit accurately and to make sure I dictated enough to support the level of the E&M code already selected. Now that we use an EMR both things are done simultaneously.

These days I finish the documentation before the patient leaves. I review it, verify my documentation, and then I E&M code it. I am much more accurate and I think I code higher. I think the tendency on a paper system is to always downcode rather than risk getting yourself in trouble.

I practice Family Medicine with two other physicians and a PA. One thing we do in our quarterly meetings is to review each other's charts to see if we agree with the level of E&M coding that the other provider has charged. Our office manager randomly selects three patients' charges for each of us and prints out the exam notes for peer review. Since we have been on the electronic system we have had very few discrepancies. Not only is the coding very accurate with the EMR, but the quarterly review itself is facilitated by the electronic records. If you had to dig up charges and pull records from a paper file system . . . well, with electronic medical records it's a lot simpler.

Did switching to electronic records increase our level of coding? I think we are all doing a much better job of coding than we were in the past and we have definitely stopped downcoding but it is difficult to compare the coding of visits prior to the EMR because you would have to analyze all those old charts. I have a sense that our documentation went up 15%–20% in terms of levels, but we actually chose to measure something else. We wanted something easy to track so we tracked the number of patient encounters instead of the coding levels.

In the first year of using the EMR as compared to the previous year we went up 15% in number of visits so it really improved our efficiency to that extent. The second year we were up 17% and this year we are up 5% above that; and that's with no additional providers, no longer hours open or anything else. In addition, we get done on time. I am rarely at the office after 5:00 P.M. anymore. I finish the patient's chart while the patient is still there. So there is a lot of efficiency in addition to the improved E&M coding.

The system we use does have an E&M coder that will count the points of history, review of systems, exam, and so on, and then suggest a code. Like most other EMR systems, it calculates and suggests the E&M code but the software developer doesn't want the responsibility for actually posting it. It is up to the doctor to actually decide to use the code.

Most EMR systems have templates, but there are two types. One type uses checklists of problems: "You're here for a cold; you have an earache, a cough, and a sore throat." The other type of template fills blanks in a narrative: "30-year-old male presents to the office with a history of cough, cold, fever." The ability of the system to calculate the E&M code depends on whether the template uses discrete items or sentences, because it can't count the status in those narrative sentences. However, even without using the E&M coder, the coding becomes more accurate because the electronic record is capturing the exam more accurately. A doctor can look at a finished EMR note and see the data points.

Our software uses templates and I designed the history items right into them. We don't miss documenting them now and that lends significant points to the E&M coding. But there is something else our templates do that is perhaps more toward the issue of quality of care than just coding, and that is in the plan. By building templates for certain diagnoses we include all the things we might choose in the plan. This not only helps document simple things that might have been overlooked in the old dictation method, like telling the patient to take Tylenol, but it also gives us a complete checklist of things to consider when concluding the visit.

During the first year, we built templates and customized the software to suit our practice's needs. We worked evenings at the office to overcome a steep learning curve and technological obstacles. With the system finally in place and reaching comfortable levels of proficiency, we have now come to realize a new level of efficiency in our practice.

Our workflow has improved markedly since the implementation of an electronic medical record system, allowing us to do more work in less time with the same sized staff. We are now able to accommodate more patients in a day; able to access our system from home; fax prescriptions to pharmacies from our computers; scan and add outside reports to our records; and we have reduced paperwork and increased staff efficiency. Our medical recordkeeping has improved exponentially and we have added at least 20 percent to our bottom line.

---

this disease, on some visits the patient will likely have other problems as well. Therefore, the diagnosis 250.2 Diabetes Mellitus should be included in every visit note and on insurance claims for those visits.

Multiple diagnoses per visit do not necessarily increase the clinician's payment, but the number of diagnoses is one of the factors in calculating the level of the key component: Medical Decision Making. Multiple diagnoses also usually involve an examination of more body systems. This, too, will affect the level of the Exam element.

Primary and Secondary Diagnoses

The concept of the Primary Diagnosis is also important. The primary diagnosis is the reason why the patient came to the office. Other conditions that are addressed during the visit are listed as secondary diagnoses. Any conditions that exist concurrently with the primary diagnosis should be reviewed, examined, or treated and documented in the exam note. Often this is facilitated by a "Problem List," which is a summary of ongoing or previous conditions. The problem list helps the clinician keep track of the patient's needs beyond the scope of the Chief Complaint for today's visit. You will see an example of a problem list in Chapter 6.

Medical Necessity

When a medical office produces an insurance claim, the claim form indicates for each procedure the ICD-9CM codes associated with the procedure. Claim processors use sophisticated computer systems to validate the codes on submitted claims. The computer determines the Medical Necessity of each procedure in part by comparing the CPT-4 code with the associated ICD-9CM codes. Only certain diagnosis codes are allowed by the computer as justification for the necessity of that procedure. The Student Edition software does not automatically create this association or validate that the codes are allowed, but most commercial EHR and practice management systems do.

Ordering Tests to Confirm or Rule Out Diagnosis

One idiosyncrasy in the ICD-9CM guidelines concerns "probable" or "possible" diagnosis codes. The guidelines differ in this respect between Inpatient and Outpatient services. The ICD-9CM code set has neither specific codes nor modifiers to use with diagnosis codes to communicate the concept of "ruling out" a disease or condition. Inconsistently, services performed in Inpatient settings do support the concept of "Rule-out," but the Outpatient setting does not.

The diagnosis for a patient may take more than one visit to be determined or confirmed but the outpatient visit guidelines do not allow for "possible," "probable," "suspected," "rule-out," or similar diagnoses. Although the prefix "possible" may be appropriate and necessary in the exam note, the insurance claim for an outpatient visit should not be coded with a diagnosis for the suspected disease.

This creates a dilemma when ordering diagnostic tests from outside facilities. Reference laboratories cannot bill for the test unless it has a diagnosis. Only the clinician ordering the test is allowed to assign the diagnosis; the reference lab cannot. Therefore, the labs require an order for a test to include a diagnosis code, even though the purpose of the test is only to determine if the patient in fact has the disease. An example of this occurred in Hands-On Exercise 25 (Chapter 4), in which you practiced ordering tests for Gary Yamamoto, a patient with the diagnosis **possible angina pectoris**.

Although the use of a diagnosis code for the condition or disease is currently unavoidable on physician orders, patients object to it on their insurance claims because claim systems often keep the code as part of the patient's history. The patient's concern is the risk of being assigned to a higher risk-pool, because the insurance computer is assuming the patient has a disease, when in fact he may not.

When the medical office bills for an office visit with a "possible" or "probable" diagnosis, the diagnosis code from the assessment should *not* be used. Instead the claim should use diagnoses codes from one or more of the symptom or exam findings.

EHR systems often have cross-reference codes for all findings that have a corresponding ICD-9CM code, not just the assessment findings. Some EHR systems allow the provider to choose from all diagnosis codes associated with the exam note; other systems may allow a person, such as a billing code specialist, to change the diagnosis code before sending the claim.

Clinicians should be aware of this idiosyncrasy in the coding rules. If presented with a choice of ICD-9CM codes when posting the E&M and other procedure codes for an outpatient visit to "rule-out" possible diseases, the clinician should choose the diagnosis codes related to the symptom or exam findings rather than an assessment with the prefix such as "possible."

How the ICD-9 Code Influences Orders and Treatment

Beyond their billing and statistical analysis functions, ICD-9CM codes can be used as a key to problems, protocols, and treatment plans. Many professional journals, associations, and practices create protocols for treating certain diseases. These may consist of specific regimens such as an oncologist might use to treat a particular form of cancer, or they might consist of a list of all possible antibiotics known to be effective for a certain type of infection. In either case, the protocol or plan of treatment can be easily communicated to other clinicians by linking it to the diagnoses for which it is effective.

Disease-based protocols can help the clinician write the orders and document the exam more quickly. Instead of searching through a list of a thousand prescription drugs, the clinician can access a short list of drugs that are regularly prescribed for a particular type of infection. These lists can be created for individual prescribing clinicians, for the practice as a whole, or by some recognized authority such as a medical association.

Similarly, the clinician can create a specific group of orders used to test for certain conditions. When a diagnosis is suspected, the list can be quickly located and the clinician can order tests, consults, or radiological studies all at once.

Even without creating specific protocols, the diagnosis can be used to help locate orders and treatment plans. Hands-On Exercise 25 in Chapter 4 demonstrated this with Gary Yamamoto's encounter. Once you found the diagnosis 413.9 Angina Pectoris, the Prompt feature was able to find a list of appropriate test orders related to the condition.

Hands-On Exercise 34: Orders Based on Diagnosis

In the next two exercises, you will learn to use multiple diagnoses and to create different sets of orders based on established plans associated with each diagnosis. You must complete *both* Exercise 34 and Exercise 35 *in one session*. Do not begin this exercise unless there is enough class time remaining to complete both.

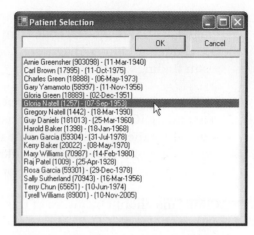

▶ Figure 5-38 Select Patient Gloria Natell.

Step 1

If you have not already done so, start the Student Edition software.

Click Select on the Menu bar, and then click Patient.

In the Patient Selection window, locate and click on **Gloria Natell.**

Step 2

Click Select on the Menu bar, and then click New Encounter.

Select the date **May 8, 2006**, the time **1:30 PM**, and the reason **Office Visit**.

Make certain you set the date and reason correctly. Compare your screen to Figure 5-39 before clicking on the OK button.

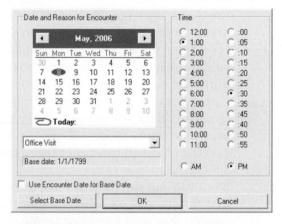

▶ Figure 5-39 Select New Encounter for May 8, 2006 1:30 PM Office Visit.

Step 3

Enter the Chief complaint by locating the button in the toolbar labeled "Chief" and clicking on it.

In the dialog window which will open, type: "Patient reports jaw pain."

Compare your screen to Figure 5-40 before clicking on the button labeled "Close the Note form."

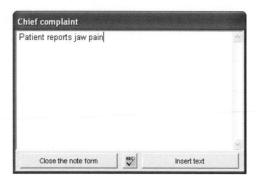

Chief complaint

Patient reports jaw pain

| Close the note form | | Insert text |

▶ **Figure 5-40 Chief Complaint Dialog for Patient Reports Jaw Pain.**

Step 4

In this exercise, the nurse will begin the visit by taking Gloria's Vital Signs.

Use the form labeled "Vitals," which you will select from the Forms Manager, invoked on the Active Forms tab (as you have done in previous exercises).

Enter Gloria's Vital Signs in the corresponding fields on the Form as follows:

Temperature:	**99**
Respiration:	**27**
Pulse:	**70**
BP:	**115/70**
Height:	**70**
Weight:	**150**

When you have finished, compare your screen to Figure 5-41 and, when it is correct, click on the Encounter tab at the bottom of the screen.

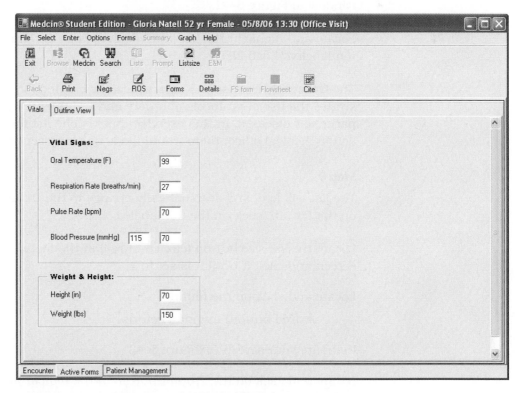

▶ **Figure 5-41 Vital Signs Form for Gloria Natell.**

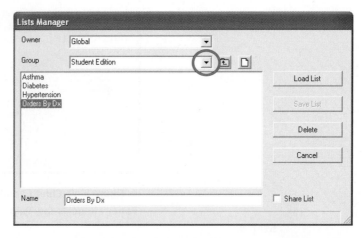

▶ **Figure 5-42 Load Orders by Dx List (down arrow for group circled in red).**

Step 5

Locate and click on the Lists button in the toolbar at the top of your screen. The List Manager window will be invoked.

As you learned in the previous chapter, the List Manager displays the various Lists available to providers in the practice. Two fields at the top of the screen organize the display of List names, filtering them by Owner and Group.

The Group field allows a user to quickly find a list by limiting the display to a desired group. The Student Edition has two groups: "All" and "Student Edition." In this step, you are going to change the lists displayed from All to Student Edition.

Locate and click on the button with a down arrow in the Group field; a dropdown list will be displayed. Select Student Edition. Compare your List Manager window to Figure 5-42.

Locate and highlight the list labeled "Orders By Dx" and then click on the button labeled "Load List."

The Orders By Dx List has been especially created for this exercise. It demonstrates the use of protocols of orders and treatments by associating them with particular diseases. In this exercise there is one list for several diseases. In an actual medical office, there would likely be many separate lists.

Step 6

The list will load and automatically change to the Dx tab. If the left pane is not on the Dx tab, click on the tab labeled "Dx."

Locate the list size button (circled in red) in the toolbar at the top of your screen and click it until it is set to 2.

Locate and click on the finding:

- (red button) Angina Pectoris

Compare your screen to Figure 5-43.

Locate and click on the Prompt button in the toolbar at the top of your screen (circled in red in Figure 5-43).

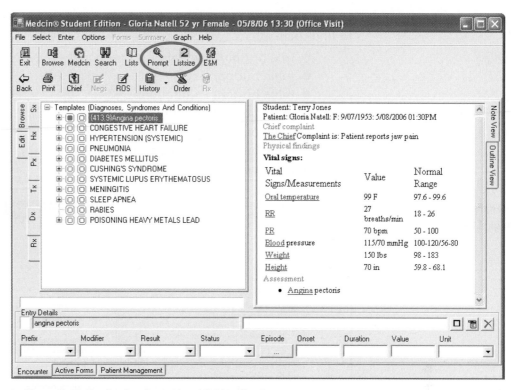

▶ **Figure 5-43 Dx Angina Pectoris with List Size 2.**

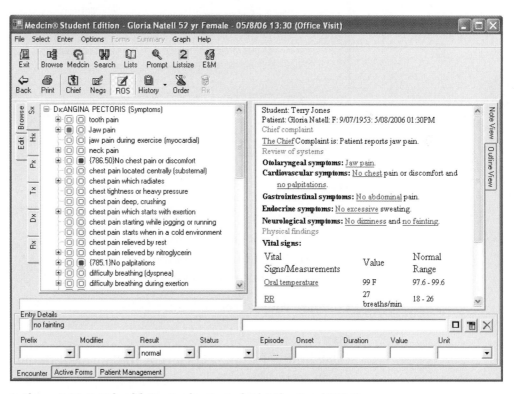

▶ **Figure 5-44 Sx Tab with Dx: Angina Pectoris List Size 2 and ROS On.**

Step 7

Click on the Sx tab.

Locate the ROS button in the toolbar at the top of your screen and click it. It should appear depressed (as shown in Figure 5-44).

Locate and click on the following findings (you will need to scroll the left pane to find them all):

- (red button) Jaw pain (in Jaw bone)
- (blue button) Chest Pain
- (blue button) Palpitations
- (blue button) Abdominal Pain
- (blue button) Excessive Sweating
- (blue button) Dizziness
- (blue button) Fainting

▶ **Figure 5-45 Hx Tab with Dx: Angina Pectoris List Size 2.**

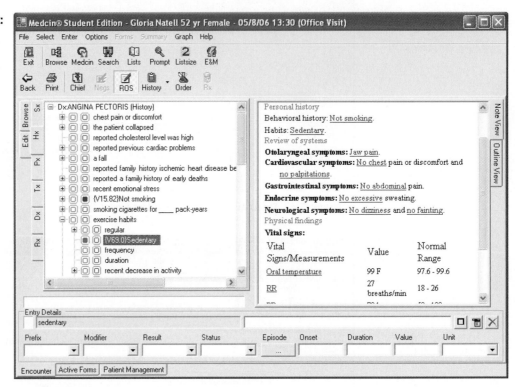

Step 8

Click on the Hx tab. Locate and expand the tree for Exercise Habits.

Locate and click on the following findings:

- (blue button) Smoking
- (red button) Sedentary

Compare your screen to Figure 5-45.

Step 9

Click on the Px tab. Notice that the physical findings from Vitals are already recorded.

Locate and click on the following findings:

- (blue button) Heart Sounds S3
- (blue button) Heart Sounds S4
- (blue button) Heart Sounds Gallop
- (blue button) Pallor, Generalized

Compare your screen to Figure 5-46.

▶ Figure 5-46 Px Tab with Dx: Angina Pectoris List Size 2.

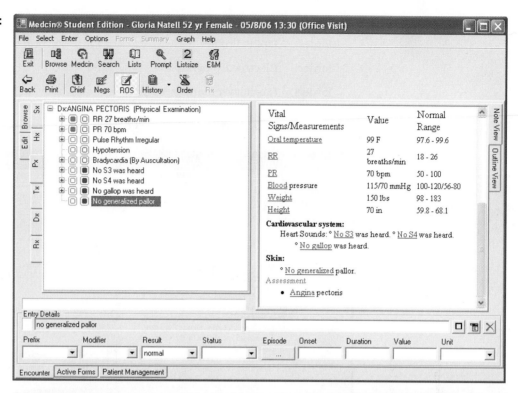

▶ Figure 5-47 Tx Tab with Dx: Angina Pectoris List Size 1.

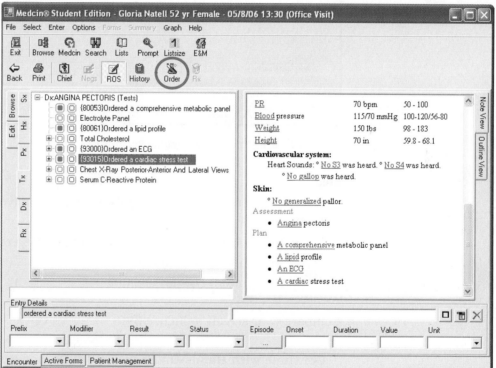

Step 10

Locate the list size button in the toolbar and click it until it is set to 1.

Click on the Tx tab.

Locate the Order button in the toolbar at the top of your screen (circled in red).

Highlight each of the following findings and then click on the order button. Do not click on the red or blue buttons beside these findings. The order button will set them once they are ordered.

(order)	Comprehensive Metabolic Chem Panel
(order)	Lipids Profile
(order)	Electrocardiogram
(order)	Cardiovascular Stress Test

Compare your screen to Figure 5-47.

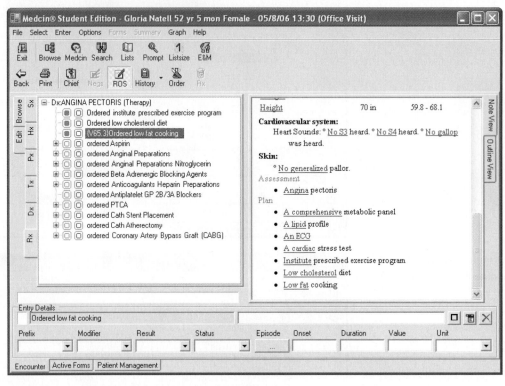

▶ **Figure 5-48 Rx Tab with Dx: Angina Pectoris List Size 1.**

Step 11

Click on the Rx tab. Click on the following findings (you do not need to use the order button):

● (red button) Institute Prescribed Exercise Program
● (red button) Low cholesterol diet
● (red button) Low fat cooking

Compare your screen to Figure 5-48.

> **Continue with Hands-On Exercise 35. Do not exit the Student Edition software or you will lose your work.**

Hands-On Exercise 35: Multiple Diagnoses

It is not unusual during the course of an office visit for a patient to bring up additional problems or provide a piece of information to the clinician that suddenly brings focus on another area of the patient's health.

In this example, Gloria Natell mentions that she has been scraping a lot of old layers of paint off the walls of her childhood home. The clinician realizes that the patient was born in 1953 and there is a possibility that she is being exposed to lead-based paints. This fact alters the direction of inquiry and of the exam.

Step 12

Locate the List button in the toolbar at the top of your screen and click it to invoke the List Manager window.

Reload the List "Orders By Dx" by selecting it and clicking the button labeled "Load List." If you have difficulty, see Figure 5-42 and review step 5 above.

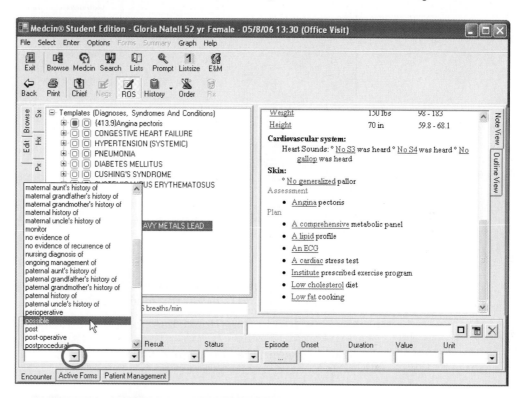

▶ **Figure 5-49 Dx Tab with Heavy Metals Highlighted—Select "Possible" from List.**

Step 13

The list will be reloaded and the Dx tab will be displayed.

Verify the List Size is 1. If it not, then locate and click on the button labeled "List Size" in the Toolbar until it is set to 1.

Locate and highlight the finding "Poisoning Heavy Metals Lead."

Locate the field labeled "Prefix" in the Entry Details section of your screen. Click the button with the down arrow in the Prefix field (circled in red). A drop-down list of Prefix terms will be displayed.

Scroll the list of prefixes. Locate and click on the term "Possible."

The finding will automatically be recorded and the text of the finding will change to "Possible poisoning by lead."

Locate the list size button in the toolbar at the top of your screen; if it is not currently set to 1, click it until it is set to 1.

With the finding "Possible Poisoning by Lead" still highlighted, locate and click on the Prompt button in the toolbar at the top of your screen.

► **Figure 5-50 Hx Tab with List from Dx: Poisoning Heavy Metals Lead.**

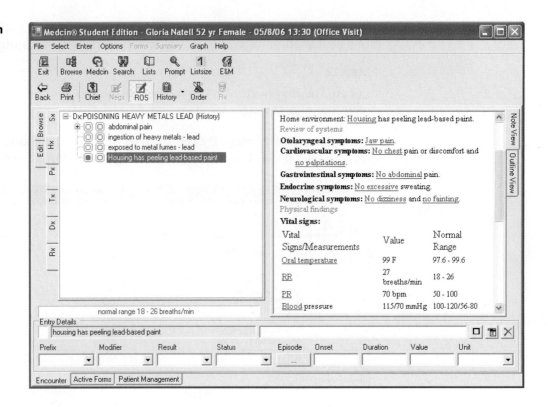

Step 14

The clinician is going to first record this new piece of information. Click on the Hx tab. Locate and click on the following finding:

● (red button) House has peeling paint which is lead based

Compare your screen to Figure 5-50.

► **Figure 5-51 Sx Tab with List from Dx: Poisoning Heavy Metals Lead.**

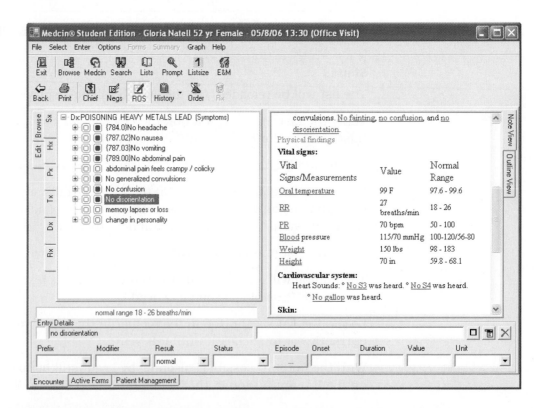

Step 15

Click on the Sx tab. Verify the ROS button in the toolbar at the top of your screen is still depressed. If it is not, then click it.

Locate and click on the following findings:

- (blue button) Headache
- (blue button) Nausea
- (blue button) Vomiting
- (blue button) Convulsions, generalized
- (blue button) Confusion
- (blue button) Disorientation

Compare your screen to Figure 5-51.

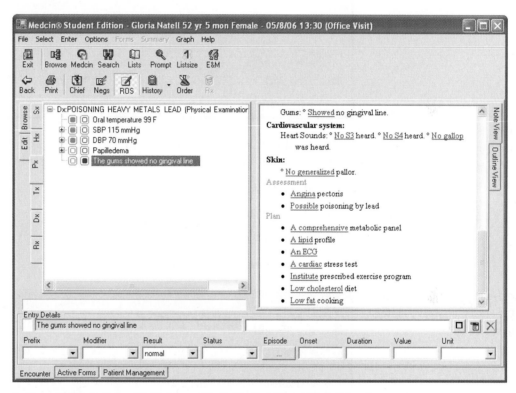

▶ **Figure 5-52 Px Tab with List from Dx: Poisoning Heavy Metals Lead.**

Step 16

Click on the Px tab. Note some findings are already selected (from the previous exercise).

Locate and click on the following finding:

- (blue button) Gums gingival line

Compare your screen to Figure 5-52.

Step 17

Click on the Tx tab.

Locate the Order button in the toolbar at the top of your screen.

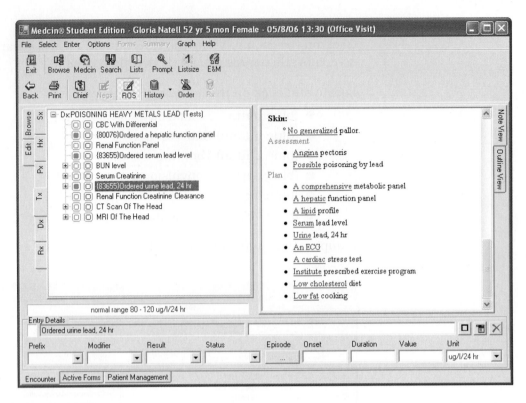

Locate and highlight each of the following findings and then click on the order button. Do not click on the red or blue buttons next to these findings.

(order)   Hepatic Function Panel

(order)   Serum Lead Level

(order)   Urine Lead 24 hour

Compare your screen to Figure 5-53.

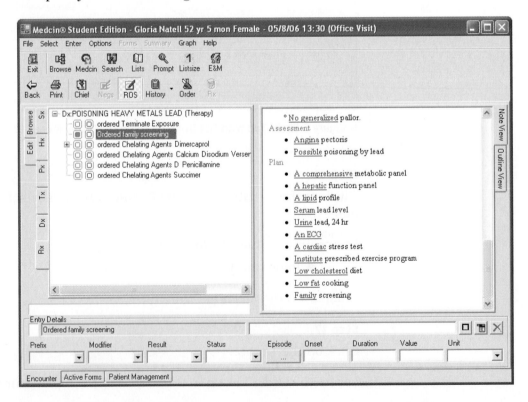

Step 18

The clinician is also concerned about others who might be in the home and will need to be screened for lead poisoning as well.

Click on the Rx tab.

Locate and click on the following findings (you do not need to use the order button):

- (red button) Screen Family

Compare your screen to Figure 5-54.

```
Gloria Natell                                          Page 1 of 1

Student: Terry Jones
Patient: Gloria Natell: F: 9/07/1953: 5/08/2006 01:30PM
Chief complaint
The Chief Complaint is: Patient reports jaw pain
Personal history
Behavioral history:  Not smoking
Habits:  Sedentary
Home environment:  Housing has peeling lead-based paint
Review of systems
Head symptoms: No headache.
Otolaryngeal symptoms: Jaw pain.
Cardiovascular symptoms: No chest pain or discomfort and no palpitations.
Gastrointestinal symptoms: No nausea, no vomiting, and no abdominal pain.
Endocrine symptoms: No excessive sweating.
Neurological symptoms: No dizziness and no generalized convulsions. No fainting,
no confusion, and no disorientation.
Physical findings
Vital signs:
Vital Signs/Measurements               Value             Normal Range
Oral temperature                       99 F              97.6 - 99.6
RR                                     27 breaths/min    18 - 26
PR                                     70 bpm            50 - 100
Blood pressure                         115/70 mmHg       100-120/56-80
Weight                                 150 lbs           98 - 183
Height                                 70 in             59.8 - 68.1
Oral cavity:
    Gums: ° Showed no gingival line
Cardiovascular system:
    Heart Sounds: ° No S3 was heard ° No S4 was heard ° No gallop was heard
Skin:
    ° No generalized pallor
Assessment
    • Angina pectoris
    • Possible poisoning by lead
Plan
    • A comprehensive metabolic panel
    • A hepatic function panel
    • A lipid profile
    • Serum lead level
    • Urine lead, 24 hr
    • An ECG
    • A cardiac stress test
    • Institute prescribed exercise program
    • Low cholesterol diet
    • Low fat cooking
    • Family screening
```

▶ **Figure 5-55 Printed Exam Note—Gloria Natell 05/08/2006 1:30 PM Office Visit.**

Step 19

This exercise has shown how a diagnosis can be used to find and display lists of orders and treatments for particular conditions.

Click File on the Menu bar, and then click Print Encounter or Print To HTML (as directed by your instructor).

If you are printing your work, you may click the Print button on the toolbar at the top of your screen instead of selecting Print Encounter from the Menu.

Compare your printout or file output to Figure 5-55. If it is correct, hand it in to your instructor. If there are any differences, review the previous steps in the exercise and find your error.

> **! Alert**
>
> ***Do not close or exit the Encounter until you have a printed copy in your hand.* You will lose your work if you exit before printing.**

Chapter Five Summary

CPT-4 and ICD-9CM codes are national standards that are required on insurance claims for outpatient and other services.

A group of the CPT-4 codes called Evaluation and Management (E&M) codes is used to bill for nearly every kind of patient encounter. There are separate categories of E&M codes for different locations such as outpatient, inpatient hospital exams, nursing home visits, consults, emergency room doctors, and so on. There are also four levels of E&M codes within each category. The levels represent the least complicated exam (Level 1) to the most complex exam (Level 4), with higher levels paying the provider more.

HCFA (now CMS) developed guidelines for determining what level of service justified what level of E&M code. The guidelines were published in 1995 and revised in 1997. Providers are permitted to use either version, but the medical record for the encounter must support the level of E&M code billed with documented findings. Using an EHR makes it possible for software to calculate the correct level of E&M code from the findings that are documented.

There are seven components that are used in defining the level of E&M services. These components are:

- History
- Examination
- Medical Decision Making
- Counseling
- Coordination of Care
- Nature of Presenting Problem
- Time

The first three of these components, History, Examination, and Medical Decision Making, are called *key* components. Each of the key components has subcomponents called elements that determine the level of the component. Once the level of each of the key components is determined, the results are evaluated to calculate the correct level of E&M code. The additional factor of Time can be used to adjust the level of the E&M code only when counseling/coordination of care exceeds 50% of the face-to-face time.

The key component History encompasses History of Present Illness, Review of Systems, and Past, Family, and Social History. The extent to which these are documented in the exam note determines the level of History. There are four possible levels of History:

1. Problem Focused
2. Expanded Problem Focused
3. Detailed
4. Comprehensive

The key component Examination is based on the number of systems examined or the depth of examination in single-organ systems. The guidelines provide tables for a General Multi-System Examination and 10 Single Organ System Exams. The tables list elements of the examination for each body system with a typographic character called a bullet (•) beside them. The number of items with a bullet (•) that have been examined and are documented in the exam note determines the level of Examination. There are four possible levels of Examination:

1. Problem Focused
2. Expanded Problem Focused
3. Detailed
4. Comprehensive

The key component Medical Decision Making refers to the number of diagnoses, the complexity of establishing a diagnosis or selecting a management option, and risk of significant complications, morbidity, or mortality.

The level of Medical Decision Making is measured by two out of three of the following: the number of diagnoses or management options, the amount or complexity of data, and the level of risk. There are four possible levels of Medical Decision Making:

1. Straightforward
2. Low Complexity
3. Moderate Complexity
4. High Complexity

Within MDM, the subcomponent Risk has its own levels, 1–4, which are determined by the presenting problem, diagnostic procedures ordered, and management options selected. Risk is assessed at the highest level of any one of these.

Once the level of each of the key components is determined, calculating the level of the E&M code is fairly straightforward. The E&M code level is determined by the lowest level of the key components considered. However, there are different requirements for determining the E&M code for New or Established patients.

Review the chart in Figure 5-17, which illustrates how the levels of the key components determine the E&M code.

For an established patient, the two key components with the highest level are considered and the lowest level of the two determines the E&M code. For a New patient, all three key components are considered. Therefore, the E&M code level is the lowest level of any of the three key components.

Because the level of E&M code is dependent on the levels of multiple *key components*, merely adding more findings to only one key component may bring that component to a higher level, but that does not necessarily mean that the visit as a whole will qualify for the higher-level E&M code.

The factor of Time can change the level of the E&M code but only when time spent on counseling or coordination of care is greater than 50% of the total face-to-face time; in such cases, the counseling time, face-to-face time, and an explanation of the counseling activities must be documented in the chart. Face-to-face time incorporates the total time both before and after the visit such as taking patient history, performing the exam, reviewing lab results, planning for follow-up care, and communicating with other providers about the patient's case.

Health care claims not only require CPT-4 or HCPCS procedure codes but also diagnosis codes. Currently, ICD-9CM is the required code set for reporting diagnoses on insurance claims.

ICD-9CM codes are from three to five digits long. The fourth and fifth digits add specificity. Insurance billing rules require that clinicians code to the most specific level. Three-digit codes are no longer accepted on claims and, if used as the primary diagnosis, may get the claim rejected. EHR systems automatically reference ICD-9CM codes at the fourth- or fifth-digit specificity.

A supplemental section of ICD-9CM titled "Factors Influencing Health Status and Contact with Health Services" provides codes for many reasons that patients come to the doctor other than illness or injury. These codes are called "V Codes" and start with the letter "V." They are used for checkups, physicals, vaccinations, maternity care, screening is for diabetes, and so on.

Another supplemental section of codes is titled "External Causes of Injury and Poisoning." These codes begin with the letter "E." E Codes cover injuries ranging from beestings to war; other examples include falling and vehicle accident injuries. E Codes are use in addition to the numeric ICD-9CM codes, never alone. E Codes are used to codify the *cause* of an injury or adverse event.

Multiple diagnoses codes can be assigned to a single encounter. This occurs mainly because patients with ongoing or chronic conditions require regular visits. It is correct and appropriate to continue to use diagnosis codes from past visits for as long as the patient continues to have that illness or condition. Multiple diagnoses per visit do not necessarily increase the clinician's payment. However, the number of diagnoses is one of the factors in calculating the level of Medical Decision Making; thus, multiple diagnoses may increase the level of MDM.

Diagnosis codes also are used in billing to justify the medical necessity of a test or procedure. The association of the correct ICD-9CM code with the test justifies the need for the test to the insurance carrier. Unfortunately, when a test is ordered from an outside laboratory, a diagnosis must be included because the reference lab is required to have it for insurance billing even though the clinician may be ordering the test only to rule out the condition. When billing for an office visit which the assessment diagnosis has a prefix such as "possible" or "suspected," the ICD-9CM codes for the symptoms or exam findings should be used for billing instead of the assessment code.

ICD-9CM codes also are used as a key to problems and protocols in health care. Examples of protocols might be a specific set of tests used to monitor a particular disease or a list of antibiotics known to be effective for a certain type of infection. Creating protocols and finding them based on the assessment can help the clinician write orders and document the exam quickly.

The codified nomenclature of an EHR system records findings with medical terms the clinician uses allowing the addition of nuances that are beyond the scope of ICD-9CM or CPT-4. However, to get paid, these two important billing code sets must be used. EHR systems based on Medcin can automatically resolve the assessment to the most specific level of diagnosis code and automatically calculate the correct E&M code from the bullets performed in the exam.

Testing Your Knowledge of Chapter 5

1. What does the acronym E&M stand for?
2. How many levels are there for a category of E&M code?
3. Name the three key components of an E&M code.
4. How many levels are there for each key component?
5. How many key components determine the level of E&M code for an established patient?
   Write the definitions for the following History acronyms:
6. HPI   _____
7. ROS   _____
8. PFSH   _____
9. Explain how the level of a General Multisystem Exam is determined.
10. What determines the level of Risk?
11. How many subcomponents (elements) of Medical Decision Making determine its level?
12. What makes up face-to-face time?
13. When does time become a factor in determining the level of E&M code?
14. What does the E&M button on the toolbar do?
15. How do you record an E&M code in the Patient Exam Note?

Comprehensive Evaluation of Chapters 1–5

This comprehensive evaluation will enable you and your instructor to determine your understanding of the material covered so far. Complete both the written test and the hands-on exercise provided below. Depending on the time provided, it may be necessary to do this in two separate sessions. Your instructor will advise you. Do not begin the hands-on exercise if there will not be enough class time to complete it.

Part I–Written Exam

You may run the Student Edition software and use your mouse on the screen to answer the following questions:

Give a brief description of the purpose of each of the following coding systems:

1. Medcin

2. CPT-4

3. ICD-9CM

4. Explain the difference between an EHR nomenclature and a Billing code set.

5. Describe how to retrieve a previous patient encounter.

6. Which screen do you use to set the reason for the visit?

7. How do you load a list?

8. How do you enter Vital Signs?

Write the meaning of each of the following medical abbreviations:

9. ROS _____

10. Hx _____

11. HEENT _____

12. Dx _____

13. PFSH _____

14. URI _____

15. E&M _____

16. Describe how to record a test that was performed.

17. How many levels are there for a category of E&M codes?

18. Name the key components of an E&M code.

19. What Entry Details field is used with a finding to indicate a "possible" diagnosis?

20. What determines the E&M level of risk?

21. Where are "bullets," used in E&M calculation?

Describe the purpose of the following buttons on the Medcin Toolbar:

22. Prompt   _____

23. Order   _____

24. ListSize   _____

25. Rx   _____

26. Search   _____

27. Negs   _____

28. ROS   _____

29. E&M   _____

30. Explain the difference in calculating the E&M level of a General Multisystem exam and a single organ exam.

Part II–Hands-On Exercise

The following exercise will use features of the software with which you have become familiar. Complete each step in sequential order using the instructions and other information provided.

When you have finished the complete exercise, print out the exam note and hand it to your instructor. Do not begin the hands-on exercise if there will not be enough class time to complete it.

Hands-On Exercise 36: Examination of a Patient with Asthma

Carl Brown is a 30-year-old established patient with possible mild asthma who comes to the office complaining of awakening in the night short of breath. Carl does not smoke, but he is exposed to second-hand smoke and has pets in the house.

In this exercise, you use the skills you have acquired to document this exam.

Step 1

If you have not already done so, start the Student Edition software.

Click Select on the Menu bar, and then click Patient.

In the Patient Selection window, locate and click on **Carl Brown**.

Step 2

Click Select on the Menu bar, and then click New Encounter.

Select the date **May 9, 2006**, the time **9:15 AM**, and the reason **10 Minute Visit**.

Make certain that you set the date and reason correctly. Compare your screen to the date, time, and reason printed in bold type before clicking on the OK button.

Step 3

Enter the Chief Complaint by locating the button in the toolbar labeled "Chief" and clicking on it.

In the dialog window that will open, type "**Patient reports waking at night short of breath**."

When you have finished typing, click on the button labeled "Close the note form."

Step 4

Begin the visit by taking Carl's Vital Signs and Medical History.

Use the form labeled "Vitals," which you will select from the Forms Manager, invoked on the Active Forms tab (as you have done in previous exercises).

Enter Carl's Vital Signs in the corresponding fields on the Form as follows:

Temperature: **98.6**

Respiration: **28**

Pulse: **78**

BP: **120/80**

Height: **71**

Weight: **175**

When you have finished, check your work. If it is correct, proceed to step 5.

Step 5

Remain on the Active Forms tab. Take the patient's medical history by using the Short Intake form.

Locate and click on the button labeled "Forms" in the toolbar at the top of your screen to invoke the Forms Manager window again.

Locate and click on the Form labeled "Short Intake" as you have done in previous exercises.

Step 6

When the Short Intake form is displayed, locate and click on the tab labeled "Medical History."

Enter the Dx History and Family History by clicking on the Y (yes) check box or the N (no) check box for the following items:

Diagnosis	Dx Hist	Family Hist
Angina	✓ N	✓ N
Asthma	✓ Y	✓ N
Bronchitis	✓ Y	✓ N
Cancer	✓ N	✓ N
Congestive Heart Failure	✓ N	✓ N
Coronary Artery Disease	✓ N	✓ N
Diabetes	✓ N	✓ N
Heart Attack	✓ N	✓ N
Hypertension	✓ N	✓ N
Migraine Headache	✓ N	✓ N
Peptic Ulcer	✓ N	✓ N
Reflux	✓ N	✓ N
Stroke	✓ N	✓ N

Complete the rest of his Medical History on the right side of the form by locating and clicking on the check boxes as follows:

Currently Taking Medication	✓ N
Recent Exposure (Contagious Disease)	✓ N
Recent History of Travel	✓ N
Recent Medical Examination	✓ Y
Recent X-Ray	✓ N
Recent ECG	✓ N
Allergies	✓ Y
Allergy to Drugs	✓ N
Tobacco	✓ N
Alcohol	✓ Y

When you have finished, check your work. If it is correct, click on the Encounter tab at the bottom of the screen.

Step 7

Locate and click on the Lists button in the toolbar at the top of your screen. The List Manager window will be invoked.

Two fields at the top of the List Manager window organize the display of List names, filtering them by Owner and Group. The Student Edition has two groups, "All" and "Student Edition."

Click on the down arrow in the Group field and select the Group "Student Edition," as you have done in Chapter 5.

Locate and highlight the list named Asthma. Click your mouse on the button labeled "Load List."

Step 8

The left pane should be on the Sx tab and the title of first line should be "Templates (Symptoms)." If it is not, click on the tab labeled "Sx."

Locate and click on the following symptom findings:

- ● (red button) awaking in night short of breath

The text will change to Paroxysmal Nocturnal Dyspnea.

Step 9

Locate and click on the ROS button in the toolbar at the top of your screen.

Verify that the ROS button is depressed.

Locate and click on the button labeled "Negs" in the toolbar at the top of your screen.

All unselected symptoms findings will be set by Auto Negative.

Step 10

Next, click on the Hx tab to enter the patient's history. Note that "No family history of Asthma" was already set via the Short Intake form.

Locate and click on the following findings:

- (blue button) Previous Hospitalization for pulmonary problem
- (red button) Exposure to Secondhand Cigarette Smoke
- (red button) Exposure to Dust Mites
- (red button) Exposure to Animal Dander

Step 11

Click on the Px tab to document the physical exam. Notice that the findings from the vitals form are already displayed.

Locate and highlight the finding: **Intranasal polyp _____ cm**

In the Entry Details section of your screen, locate the field labeled "Value," and enter the numeric value **0.2** (two tenths). Then press the enter key.

The finding text should change to read "An .2 cm intranasal polyp was found."

Step 12

Locate the button labeled "Negs" in the toolbar and click it once.

Px findings not previously set will be set by Auto Negative.

Step 13

Click on Tx tab.

Locate and highlight **CBC with Differential**, and click on the order button.

Expand the tree of findings for Pulmonary Function Tests.

Locate and highlight **Spirometry** and click on the order button.

Verify that both tests appear in the plan before proceeding.

Step 14

Click on the Dx tab.

Locate and click on the following finding:

- (red button) Asthma mild intermittent

Click the down arrow button in the prefix field. Select the prefix "**possible**" from the drop-down list displayed.

Step 15

Click on the Rx tab.

Expand the tree for Environmental Control Measures.

Locate and click on the following finding:

- (red button) Frequent vacuuming
- (red button) Avoid Allergens
- (red button) Patient Education—Asthma
- (red button) Follow-up visit

Step 16

Enter a prescription.

Expand the tree for Bronchodilators.

Locate and highlight **Albuterol**.

Click on the Rx button in the toolbar. The prescription writer window will be invoked.

Step 17

In the Rx Dosage Inquiry window, locate and click on the following Sig:

90 microgram puffs 1 inh prn DSP1

When the Rx Brand Inquiry window is displayed, position your mouse over the brand **Proventil** and click your mouse button.

Locate the field labeled "Generic Allowed."

Click your mouse in the white circle next to **Yes**. It should then be filled in.

Review the completed prescription. If anything is incorrect, click on the button labeled "Rx Inquiry" to correct it.

Locate and click on the button labeled "Save Rx."

Step 18

Locate and click on the button labeled "E&M" in the toolbar at the top of your screen.

The E&M Calculator window should be invoked.

Step 19

Locate the Patient Status section in the upper right corner of the E&M Calculator window. Click your mouse in the white circle next to **Existing**. It should then be filled in.

Locate and click your mouse on the down arrow button in the field labeled "Face to Face or Floor time." Select **10 minutes** from the drop-down list.

Locate and click on the button labeled "Calculate E&M Code." The Calculated E&M Code field should display "99213: Estab Outpatient Expanded H&P—Low Complexity Decisions."

If this is the code displayed in your window, locate and click on the button labeled "Post To Encounter." If this is not the code calculated, click on the Cancel button, and review the previous steps to find your error.

Step 20

Click File on the Menu bar, and then click Print Encounter or Print To HTML (as directed by your instructor).

If you are printing your work, you may alternatively click the Print button on the toolbar at the top of your screen.

Hand the completed printout or HTML file to your instructor.

! **Alert**

Do not close or exit the Encounter until you have a printed copy in your hand. **You will lose your work if you exit before printing.**

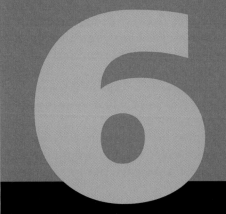

Chapter Six

Advanced Techniques Speed Data Entry

Learning Outcomes

After completing this chapter, you should be able to:

- ◆ Understand and use Patient Management
- ◆ Understand and use problem lists
- ◆ Cite information from previous visits in a new encounter
- ◆ Explain how vital signs and diagnostic tests can be recorded in the EHR
- ◆ Describe the workflow of electronic lab orders and results
- ◆ View pending orders and lab results
- ◆ Create a graph of lab results
- ◆ Describe triage by a nurse
- ◆ Discuss patient entry of symptoms and previous history

ACRONYMS USED IN CHAPTER 6	
Acronyms are used extensively in both medicine and computers. Following are acronyms that are used in this chapter.	
ECG	Electrocardiogram
FVC	Forced Vital Capacity
H&P	History and Physical
HDL	High Density Lipoprotein
JCAHO	Joint Commission on Accreditation of Healthcare Organizations
LDL	Low Density Lipoprotein
LIS	Laboratory Information System
MVV	Maximal Voluntary Ventilation
VC	Vital Capacity
Wi-Fi	Wireless Fidelity (wireless computer networking)

Important Information about the Student Edition Patient History Program

The classroom environment provides a challenge for computer programs because the exercises require multiple students to simultaneously retrieve patient charts and enter findings for the same patient, without disturbing the sample data for the next class.

Thus far, you have worked with only one encounter at a time. In the next two chapters, you will work with patients' complete medical history using information from years of previous encounters for some patients.

To accommodate this, a special software program loads previous patient history into the computer's memory just for these exercises. The program must be running during the time you are performing the exercises in Chapter 6 and Chapter 7.

Warnings at key steps in the exercises will explain how to detect if the History Program needs to be restarted before you can continue. Instructions for starting this special software are provided in Appendix B.

If your classroom is part of a school network, the program is probably already running. If you reach a point in an exercise when you believe the History Program is not running, alert your instructor and refer to Appendix B in the back of this book.

Improved Data Entry

In Chapter 4, you learned to speed up data entry at the point of care using Lists, Prompts, and Forms as shortcuts. While doing so, a medical practice automatically builds codified medical data about each patient.

In Chapter 5, you learned to use existing encounters, when you selected a single previous encounter. However, EHR software can use data from all previous encounters for research, analysis, graphing, or to follow up on previous conditions.

In this chapter, you will learn how to use the information from multiple past encounters to both manage the patient's health and speed up documenting the current visit. This chapter also will explore different ways to populate key portions of the patient chart without repetitious rekeying of data that is available elsewhere.

Management of Patients' Health

Primary care practices (and some specialty practices) see a patient regularly over an extended period of time. In this way, the provider comes to know the patient and helps to monitor and hopefully improve the patient's health. To do so, the clinician must review the records from the patient's past visits and recheck problems noted on previous encounters.

Providers also must keep track of what medications the patient is currently taking, which tests have results, and any other orders that have been issued. A clinician would always check the medications list before writing a new prescription, as well as to renew any that were about to expire.

In a world of paper charts, this is done by flipping through the papers in the chart and skimming the previous notes. In some offices, current medications and current problems are copied by hand to a list in the front of the paper chart. In other cases, the clinician simply makes a mental note of them while skimming the chart, keeping a mental list as he or she reads the chart.

In a codified electronic chart, the software itself can dynamically locate the necessary information and organize it for quick review. Additionally, the clinician can note the items reviewed, make updates to the problems, and then record them in the current encounter. The clinician does not have to search for findings in the system because the findings are already identified in the previous exam notes.

The Student Edition software includes a Patient Management feature that will allow you to explore some of these concepts. Although commercial EHR vendors use national standard nomenclatures such as Medcin, they differentiate their software with unique visual styles to present patients' charts. Software you will use in a medical office will have concepts and features for Patient Management similar to the Student Edition, but the presentation of the information is likely to have a different appearance.

Understanding Problem Lists

Clinicians of all levels are trained to work with problem lists and depend on the information contained in the problem lists when providing care. Furthermore, maintaining a problem list is a requirement for accreditation by organizations such as the Joint Commission on Accreditation of Healthcare Organizations (JCAHO).

Problem lists are used to track both acute and chronic conditions related to the care of the patient. Clinical staff should be able to easily see the active problems for a patient and also view the history of problems. Most clinical information recorded in the chart will be related to one or more problems.

The relationship between diagnoses and problems is very close. In most EHR software, they are synonymous. However, the concept of a primary diagnosis used for billing does not apply to a problem list. Although chronic diseases that are poorly controlled or malignancies take precedence in clinical decision making over mild conditions that are not life-threatening, the idea of a problem list is to make sure everyone who touches the patient knows what conditions are present.

The concept of a "problem-oriented" view is to organize entries in a patient record by problem. The problem list provides an up-to-date list of the diagnoses and conditions that affect that particular patient's care. Typically, it links the data from all encounters, orders, and prescriptions to the respective problem. This problem-oriented view allows the clinician to quickly see the patient's problems and what has been done thus far.

Problem lists usually have an onset date, indicate Chronic or Acute, and show whether or not the problem is active. Problems are removed from the list or set inactive once the patient is "cured" or the problem is "resolved." Some problems have a natural period of time in which they normally resolve themselves. These problems are called Acute Self-Limiting.

In some systems, problem lists can include findings that are not disease related but, rather, are *wellness conditions*. Wellness conditions are based on the age and sex of the patient and used in health maintenance and preventative screening programs to keep healthy patients healthy. Both disease conditions and wellness conditions have activities that are typically performed for patients with that condition, including:

◆ an annual EKG for a person with congestive heart failure;

◆ a quarterly blood sugar test for a patient with diabetes;

◆ a mammogram for a healthy woman over 35; and

◆ immunizations for a healthy infant.

These recommendations can be driven by the data in the problem list. Health Maintenance will be discussed more fully in Chapter 7.

In many EHR systems, a problem is added to the problem list either manually or automatically from the Assessment in the exam note. Some clinicians prefer to add the problems manually so that diagnoses for "possible" and "rule-out" conditions do not appear on the problem list until the diagnosis is confirmed. Manually adding a problem to the problem list is especially useful when the problem is being treated by a specialist at another office, but the clinician wants to remain aware of the condition. It is also possible to manually add findings to the problem list that would normally be in other sections of the narrative, such as Past Medical History or Symptoms.

Hands-On Exercise 37: Exploring Patient Management

The Patient Management tab is used to manage a patient's problems over time. It presents a Clinical Summary View of the patient's previous visits. The view presents historical data that is obtained from findings recorded in past encounters. The view can be updated from the current encounter or, conversely, the exam note for the current visit can be created using data from Patient Management.

In the next two exercises, a patient who has been treated previously is returning for a follow-up visit. Instead of retrieving any previous encounters, you are going to start a new encounter. You will subsequently learn to *cite* information from previous encounters into the current exam note. For the first exercise, you are just going to become familiar with this aspect of the software, Patient Management.

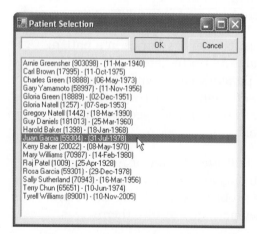

▶ **Figure 6-1 Selecting Juan Garcia from the Patient Selection Window.**

Step 1

If you have not already done so, start the Student Edition software.

Click Select on the Menu bar, and then click Patient.

In the Patient Selection window, locate and click on **Juan Garcia**.

Step 2

Click Select on the Menu bar, and then click New Encounter.

Select the date **May 10, 2006**, the time **3:00 PM**, and the reason **Office Visit**.

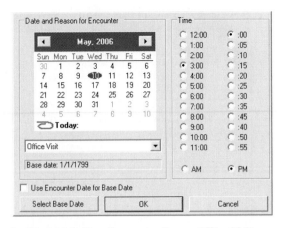

▶ **Figure 6-2 New Encounter for an Office Visit, May 10, 2006 3:00 PM.**

Make certain you set the date, time, and reason correctly. Compare your screen to Figure 6-2 before clicking on the OK button.

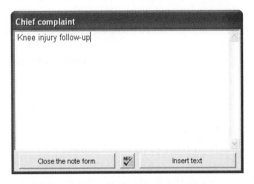

▶ **Figure 6-3 Chief Complaint Dialog for Knee Injury Follow-Up.**

Step 3

Enter the Chief complaint by locating the button in the toolbar labeled "Chief" and clicking on it.

In the dialog window, type "Knee injury follow-up."

Compare your screen to Figure 6-3 before clicking on the button labeled "Close the note form."

Step 4

Locate and click on the tab labeled "Patient Management" at the bottom of your screen. It is circled in red in Figure 6-4.

Compare your screen to Figure 6-4. The Medcin nomenclature normally displayed in the left pane of your screen has been replaced by an information window displaying information from previous encounters.

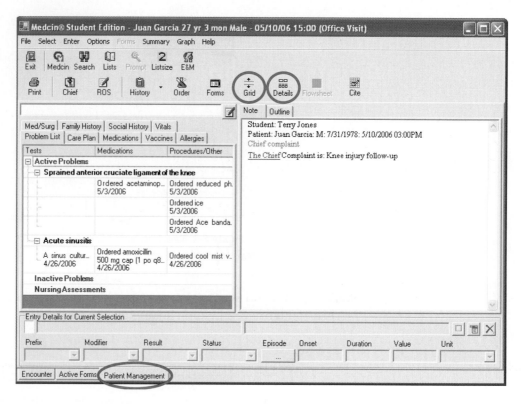

▶ Figure 6-4 Patient Management Tab (circled in red).

When you are on the Patient Management tab, the toolbar (at the top of the screen) has some additional buttons. Two of these are "Grid" and "Details" (circled in red).

Locate the button in the toolbar labeled "Details." This button allows you to see more of patient management by hiding the Entry Details section at the bottom of the screen. Click on the button until the Entry Details section is hidden. The Entry Details section can be restored if it is hidden by clicking the Details button again.

Look at the left pane of your screen. Note that the pane contains nine tabs:

◆ Problems (The patient management feature opens on the Problem List tab.)

◆ Care Plan

◆ Medications

◆ Vaccines

◆ Allergies

◆ Past Medical/Surgical History (Med/Surg)

◆ Family History

◆ Social History

◆ Vitals

In the following steps, you will examine each tab.

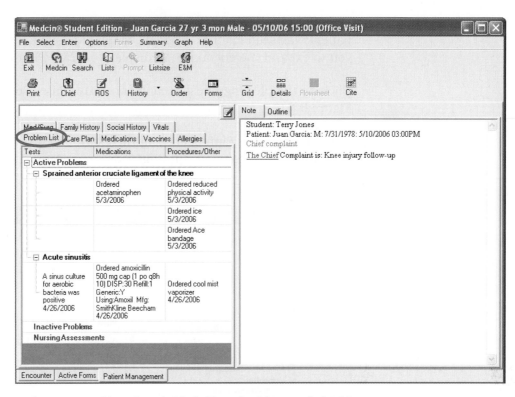

▶ **Figure 6-5 Problem List Tab (circled in red) with Expanded Grid.**

Step 5

The patient management feature opens on the Problem List tab (circled in red). The problem list includes a view of both active and inactive problems, as well as nursing assessments. This example has two active problems.

Locate and click on the button labeled "Grid" in the toolbar at the top of your screen. (It is circled in red in Figure 6-4). The Grid button expands the rows of information displayed in the problem list, allowing you to see more about each item ordered for each problem. Clicking on the Grid button again will compress the rows.

Compare your screen to Figure 6-5. Within the problem list, there are three columns: Tests, Medications, and Procedures/Other. The most recent active findings (from the Tx and Rx sections of previous encounters) are listed in these columns for each problem.

If tests have been ordered, they appear in the first column. If the test has results, the name of the test is displayed in **bold**. Any medications prescribed for the problem appear in the second column. The last column lists any other orders or procedures from past encounters related to this problem.

The clinician also can focus on a particular problem by closing the others. A small plus or small minus sign next to a problem description allows you to open and close the details of the problem in the same way you expand or contract the tree structure when browsing the Nomenclature list. You will work more with the Problem List in the next exercise.

Step 6

Locate and click on the tab labeled "Care Plan" in the information pane on the left of your screen.

The Care Plan tab displays each problem, followed by each encounter date the patient was seen for that problem. Small plus signs next to the encounter allow you to expand the encounter to display the Care Plan for that date.

Click on the plus sign beside each encounter date. Compare your screen with Figure 6-6.

Findings from the Plan section of the exam note are displayed beneath the encounter date; however, findings from any group can be manually added to the care plan.

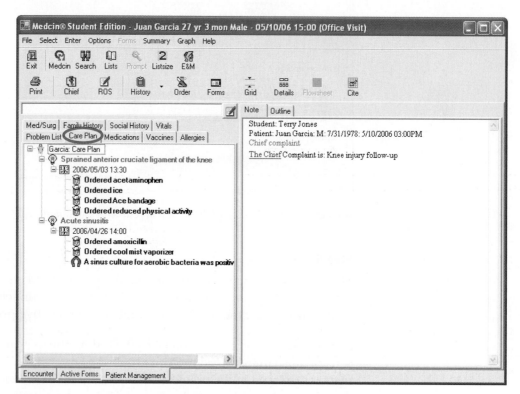

▶ **Figure 6-6 Care Plan Tab (circled in red)**

Step 7

Locate and click on the tab labeled "Medications" in the information pane on the left of your screen. Compare your screen to Figure 6-7.

The Medications tab provides a traditional medications list. Although the two previous tabs (problems and care plan) listed the medications ordered for each problem, the Medications tab displays all medications ordered by any clinician in the practice and those reported by the patient.

Step 8

Locate and click on the tab labeled "Vaccines" in the information pane on the left of your screen. Compare your screen to Figure 6-8.

The tab displays the patient's history of vaccines. Note that vaccines also appear in the medications list; these are not duplicate findings. The software deliberately shows vaccines in both lists.

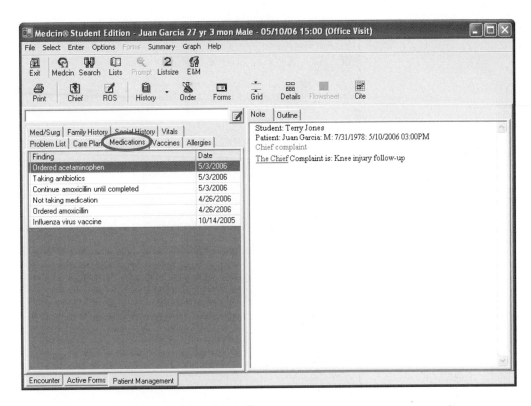

▶ **Figure 6-7 Medications Tab (circled in red).**

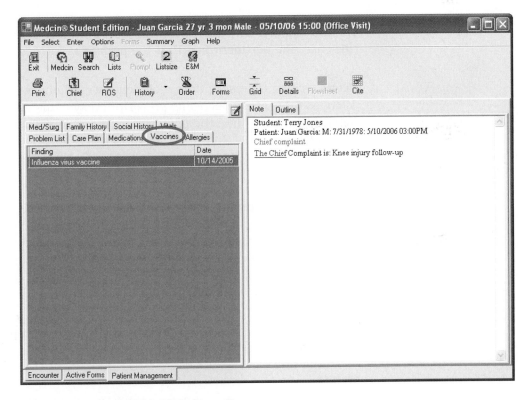

▶ **Figure 6-8 Vaccines Tab (circled in red).**

Step 9

Locate and click on the tab labeled "Allergies" in the information pane on the left of your screen. Compare your screen to Figure 6-9.

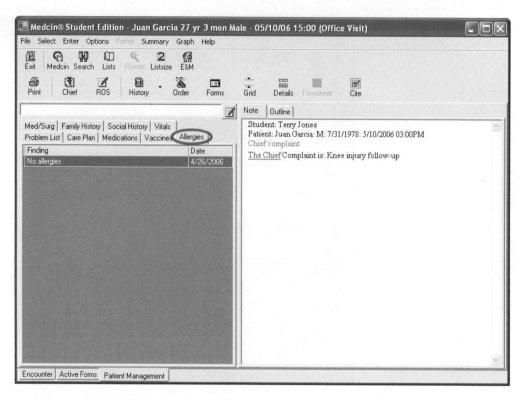

► Figure 6-9 Allergies Tab (circled in red).

The tab displays any allergy information from any of the patient encounters. In this case, the pertinent fact that the patient reports is "No Allergies."

Before writing a prescription, a clinician would check both the Medications and Allergies tabs. Most electronic prescription systems also check allergy data automatically at the time the prescription is written. This will be discussed further in Chapter 7.

Step 10

Locate and click on the tab labeled "Med/Surg" in the information pane on the left of your screen. Compare your screen to Figure 6-10. Note that the tabs in the left pane are arranged in two rows; when you click any tab in the upper row, the entire row moves down. The tab for the data currently displayed in the left pane is always in the (bottom) row of tabs closest to the grid.

"Med/Surg" stands for Medical and Surgical History and displays all findings that have been recorded in the Past History section of previous encounters. The date column displays the date the finding was recorded.

Step 11

Locate and click on the tab labeled "Family History" in the information pane on the left of your screen. Compare your screen to Figure 6-11.

The tab displays all findings that have been recorded in the Family History section of previous encounters. The date column displays the date that the finding was recorded.

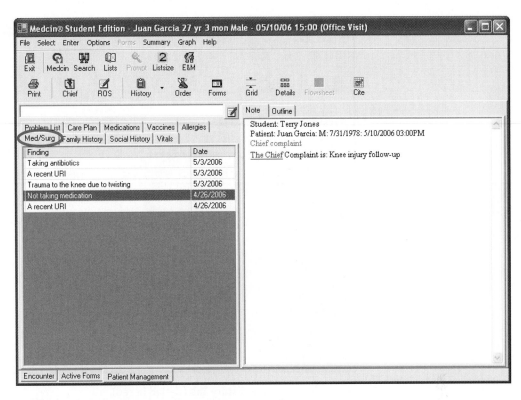

▶ **Figure 6-10 Past Medical and Surgical History Tab.**

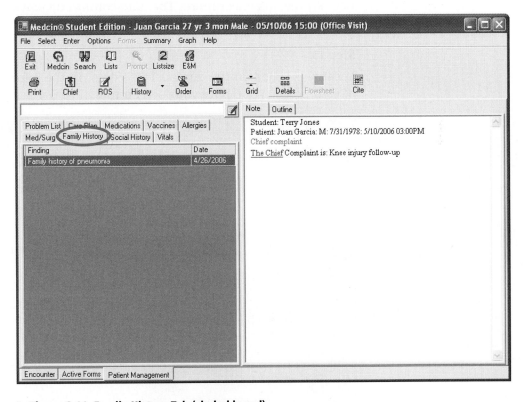

▶ **Figure 6-11 Family History Tab (circled in red).**

Step 12

Locate and click on the tab labeled "Social History" in the information pane on the left of your screen. Compare your screen to Figure 6-12.

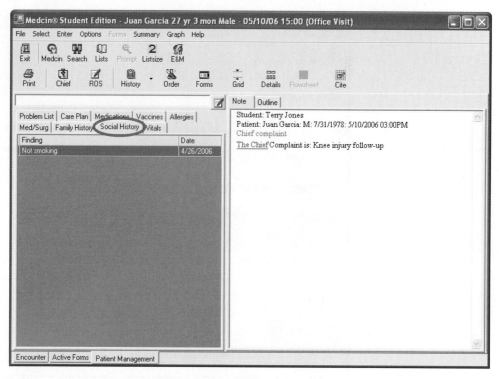

▶ **Figure 6-12 Social History Tab (circled in red).**

The tab displays all findings that have been recorded in the Social History section of previous encounters. The date column displays the date that the finding was recorded.

Step 13

Locate and click on the tab labeled "Vitals" in the information pane on the left of your screen. Compare your screen to Figure 6-13.

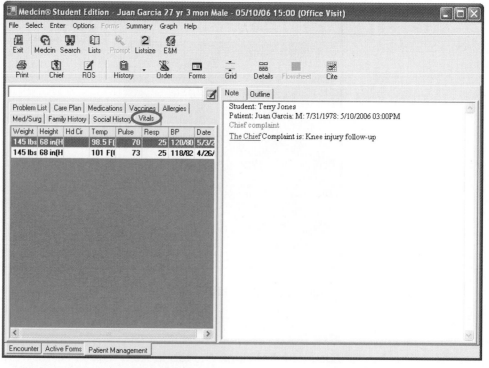

▶ **Figure 6-13 Vitals Signs Tab (circled in red).**

The tab displays the Vital Signs findings that have been recorded in multiple encounters.

▶ **Figure 6-14 Vital Signs Sorted by Patient Temperature.**

Problem List	Care Plan	Medications	Vaccines	Allergies			
Med/Surg	Family History	Social History	Vitals				
Weight	Height	Hd Cir	Temp	Pulse	Resp	BP	Date
145 lbs	68 in(H		101 F((	73	25	118/82	4/26/
145 lbs	68 in(H		98.5 F(	70	25	120/80	5/3/2

Step 14

In each of the tabs the data can be sorted. This is done by clicking on the labels over the columns of data. For example:

Locate and click on the column labeled "Temp" within the Vitals tab. Compare the Vitals tab on your screen with Figure 6-14. You will notice that the rows of vital signs data changed places and the date that Juan had a temperature of 101° is now the top row. When sorting, the entire row stays together. To restore the Vitals tab to its original order, click on the column labeled "Date."

This example used the Vitals tab, but the data in any tab of Patient Management can be sorted by clicking on the column labels.

If there is not enough class time remaining to complete the next exercise, you may stop at this point. You do not need to print the encounter.

Citing Previous Visits from Problem Lists

Patient Management is an excellent tool for reviewing information from the patient's previous encounters without having to open and read each one individually. Presenting the information in a "problem-oriented" view and having the previous findings at hand enable the clinician to record the reexamination of each area examined during the previous visits quickly. However, it is much more than just a review tool; it also is a very efficient method of documenting a follow-up exam.

In an EHR, citing from a previous exam note means to bring a finding into the current encounter, usually as a follow-up to a previous visit.

Hands-On Exercise 38: Following Up on a Problem

Juan Garcia has returned for a follow-up on his previous knee injury. Using Patient Management, you will see how easy it is to document this type of visit.

You will recall from a previous chapter that the mouse typically has at least two buttons, a Left button and a Right button. In this exercise, when instructed, you are going to be using the Right button on the mouse as well as the Left button.

Step 1

If you are continuing from the previous exercise, proceed to step 4.

Otherwise, start the Student Edition software.

From the Select Menu, click Patient, and from the Patient Selector window select **Juan Garcia** (see Figure 6-1).

Step 2

From the Select Menu, click New Encounter. Use the date **May 10, 2006**, the time **3:00 PM**, and the reason **Office Visit**.

Make certain you set the date, time, and reason correctly before clicking on the OK button (see Figure 6-2).

Step 3

Enter the Chief complaint by locating the button in the Toolbar labeled "Chief" and clicking on it.

In the dialog window, type "**Knee injury follow-up**."

When it is correct, click on the button labeled "Close the note form" (see Figure 6-3).

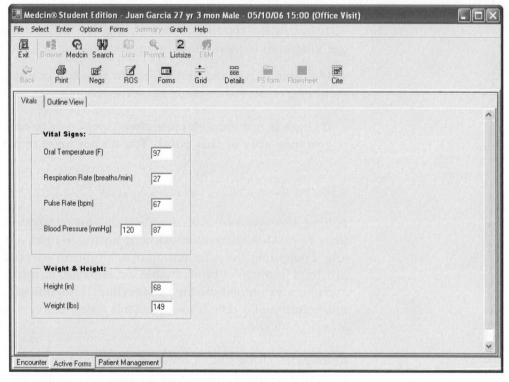

▶ **Figure 6-15 Vital Signs Form for Juan Garcia.**

Step 4

Enter Juan Garcia's Vital Signs using the Vitals Form located in the Active Forms tab (as you have done in the previous exercises).

Enter Mr. Garcia's Vital Signs in the corresponding fields as follows:

Temperature: **97**

Respiration: **27**

Pulse: **67**

BP: **120/87**

Height: **68**

Weight: **149**

When you have finished, compare your screen to Figure 6-15. If it is correct, click on the tab labeled Patient Management at the bottom of the window. (If you have difficulty locating Patient Management, refer to Figure 6-4.)

Step 5

Verify that you are on the Patient Management tab.

If the information pane on the left of your screen is not already displaying the Problem List, click on the tab labeled "Problem List" (circled in red in Figure 6-5).

If the Entry Details section is currently covering the bottom of your screen, locate the button labeled "Details" in the toolbar at the top of your screen and click it until the Entry Details section is hidden.

If the full Order information under each problem is not fully displayed, locate the button labeled "Grid" in the toolbar at the top of your screen and click it to expand the Grid.

Position the mouse pointer over the first problem, "Sprained anterior cruciate ligament of the knee," and click the **Right** button on your mouse. A drop-down list will be displayed, as shown in Figure 6-16.

If the drop-down list does not match the list shown in Figure 6-16, your mouse was not positioned correctly on the problem description. Reposition your mouse and click the **Right** mouse button again.

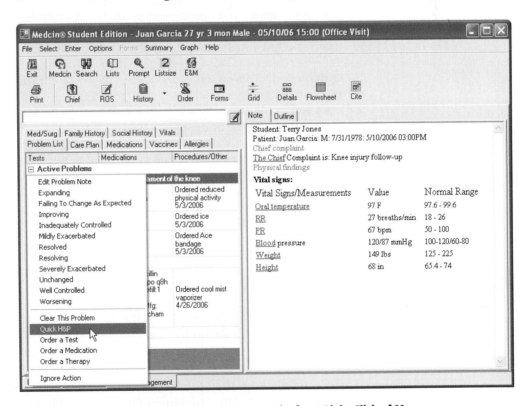

▶ **Figure 6-16 Problem List Tab with Drop-Down List from Right Click of Mouse.**

Without clicking on any of the options, study the options on the drop-down list. Most of these options are used to cite updated findings into the new encounter. Do not select any option until directed to do so. The following is a brief explanation of each option in the drop-down list:

> **Edit problem note:** Allows you to edit a free text note that is attached to the problem.

The next 11 options are used to record the status of the problem. Selecting any of the following items from the drop-down list will add a new finding to today's encounter. The finding will have a status set with one of the following:

Expanding

Failing to change as expected

Improving

Inadequately controlled

Mildly exacerbated

Resolved

Resolving

Severely exacerbated

Unchanged

Well controlled

Worsening

The remaining options allow the clinician to take multiple actions quickly. They are as follows:

Clear this problem: Clears all test orders, discontinues medications related to the problem, clears therapy orders, and sets the problem as Inactive.

Quick H&P: This option invokes a data entry window that lists symptoms, history, and physical findings as they appeared in the most recent encounter for this problem. The clinician can quickly review the last History and Physical (H&P) taken for this problem and update the new encounter with any findings in the Quick H&P window. The Quick H&P window will be shown in the next step.

Order a test: This option is provided to allow the clinician to order a new test for this problem. When the option is selected, the right pane will temporarily display a list of tests you would normally see in Tx tab. When the Tx list is displayed, you can order directly from the list in the right pane.

Order a medication: This option is provided to allow the clinician to order a new Medication for this problem. When the option is selected, the right pane will temporarily display the Rx list of Medications. When the Rx list is displayed, you can order directly from the list in the right pane. If the drug selected requires a prescription, the prescription writer will be invoked automatically.

Order a therapy: This option is provided to allow the clinician to quickly order any type of therapy other than medications. As with the previous two options, a list of therapies will temporarily display in the right pane. You can order directly from the displayed list.

Ignore action: This option cancels the drop-down list without recording anything. You also can cancel the drop-down list by clicking anywhere else on the screen.

Step 6

Locate and click on the Quick H&P option in the drop-down list (shown highlighted in Figure 6-16). The Quick History and Physical window will be invoked.

Compare your screen to Figure 6-17. The window displays findings from the previous exam for this condition.

Using the findings in the list, the clinician can be certain to update anything that was observed in the previous visit. Items that have already been entered in today's encounter appear on the Quick H&P list in gray. Examples in this exercise include Chief complaint and Vital Signs.

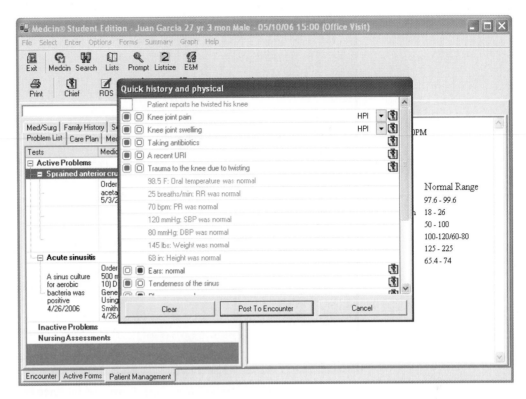

▶ **Figure 6-17 Quick History and Physical for Knee Injury.**

The patient reports that his knee is better. Locate and click on the following findings (you will need to scroll the window to get them all):

- (blue button) Knee joint pain
- (blue button) Knee joint swelling
- (blue button) Taking antibiotics
- (blue button) Localized swelling of the right knee
- (blue button) Warmth of the right knee
- (blue button) Pain was elicited by motion of the right knee

Important—do not click every finding that is listed. Click only those indicated above.

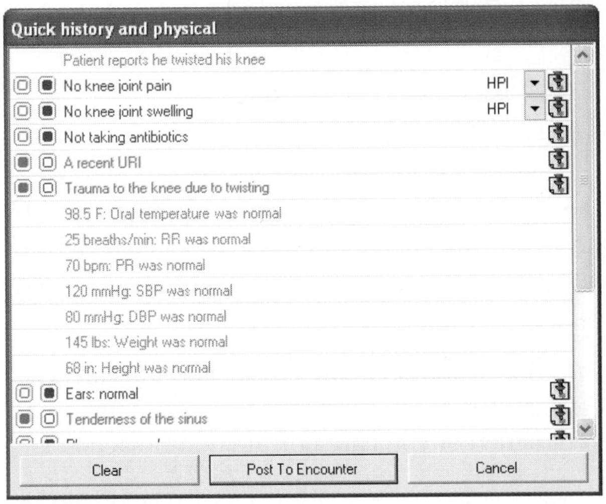

Step 7

Compare your screen to Figure 6-18. Scroll the window and verify that you have selected only the items listed in step 6. If you find an error, click on the button labeled "Cancel," and repeat steps 5 and 6.

When all the findings have been selected correctly, click on the button labeled "Post To Encounter."

Step 8

The findings you selected in the Quick H&P window should now be displayed in the patient exam note (as shown in the right pane of Figure 6-19).

The problem is resolved. To indicate this in today's exam note, position the mouse over the first problem, "Sprained

▶ **Figure 6-18 Knee Injury Findings Set to Normal—Post To Encounter.**

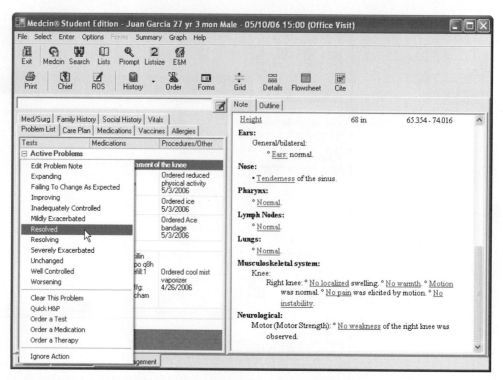

▶ **Figure 6-19 Select "Resolve" from Drop-Down List for Knee Problem.**

anterior cruciate ligament of the knee," and click the **Right** button on your mouse. Again the drop-down list will be displayed, as shown in Figure 6-19.

Locate and click on the option labeled "Resolved." The window shown in Figure 6-20 will be invoked.

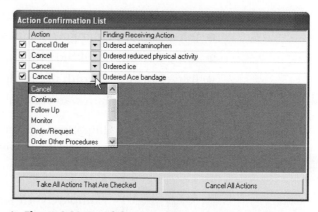

▶ **Figure 6-20 Resolving a Problem—Action Confirmation List.**

Step 9

When a problem is resolved, there are certain actions you may want to take: canceling previous orders, discontinuing any medications, or setting the problem as inactive. The Resolved option invokes a window of all active orders related to the problem and sets appropriate default actions.

A check box next to each item indicates that you wish to take the action indicated. A drop-down list of possible actions is available for each order, as shown in Figure 6-20. You can use the list to select a different action or you can indicate that no action is to be taken by unchecking the box.

Do not make any changes to the default list. When you have reviewed the list, locate and click the button labeled "Take All Actions That Are Checked."

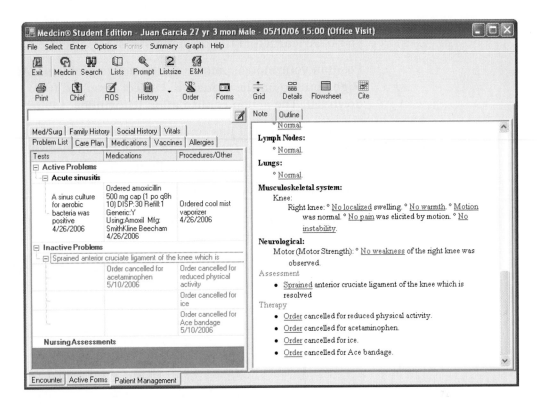

▶ **Figure 6-21 Inactive Problem on Problem List.**

Step 10

Compare your screen with Figure 6-21. Note in the left pane that the knee problem has moved to the section labeled "Inactive Problems." Note in the right pane that the previous therapy orders have been canceled.

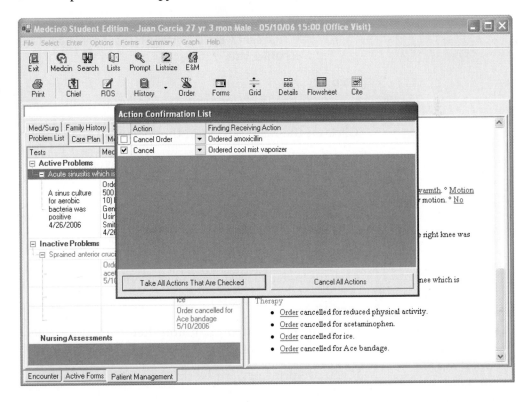

▶ **Figure 6-22 Resolve Acute Sinusitis Action Confirmation List.**

Step 11

The problem list also listed a second problem, Acute Sinusitis, for which the patient was recently treated. The patient reports that his Sinusitis has cleared up and that he has finished the prescribed course of antibiotics. Using what you have learned in the previous steps, Resolve the Acute Sinusitis problem.

Position your mouse pointer on the active problem, "Acute Sinusitis." Click the **Right** button on the mouse and select Resolved from the options on the drop-down list. The action confirmation list window will be invoked.

Because the patient has reported taking all the amoxicillin, there is no reason to cancel the order. Click on the check box to clear it. Compare your screen to the Action Confirmation List in Figure 6-22.

Click on the button labeled "Take All Actions That Are Checked."

When you have completed this step, you will notice that both problems are now in the inactive problem list.

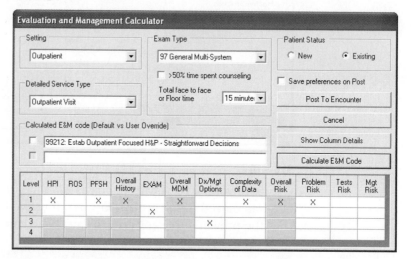

▶ **Figure 6-23 Evaluation and Management Code Calculator for Juan Garcia Office Visit.**

Step 12

Locate and click on the Encounter tab at the bottom of your screen.

Click on the E&M button in the toolbar at the top of your screen.

When the E&M Calculator window is invoked:

Set Face-to-face time at 15 Minutes.

Locate Patient Status and click on the circle next to Existing.

Click the button labeled "Calculate E&M Code."

Compare your screen to Figure 6-23.

Click the button labeled "Post To Encounter."

Step 13

Click File on the Menu bar, and then click Print Encounter or Print To HTML (as directed by your instructor.)

If you are printing your work, you may click the Print button on the Toolbar at the top of your screen.

Compare your printout or file output to Figure 6-24. If it is correct, hand it in to your instructor. If there are any differences, review the previous steps in the exercise and find your error.

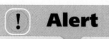

! Alert

Do not close or exit the Encounter until you have a printed copy in your hand. You will lose your work if you exit before printing.

Student: Terry Jones
Patient: Juan Garcia: M: 7/31/1978: 5/10/2006 03:00PM
Chief complaint
The Chief Complaint is: Knee injury follow-up.
History of present illness
    Juan Garcia is a 27 year old male.
    ° No knee joint pain ° No knee joint swelling
Past medical/surgical history
Reported History:
    Reported medications: Not taking antibiotics.
    Medical: A recent URI.
    Physical trauma: Trauma to the knee due to twisting.
Physical findings
Vital signs:

Vital Signs/Measurements	Value	Normal Range
Oral temperature	97 F	97.6 - 99.6
RR	27 breaths/min	18 - 26
PR	67 bpm	50 - 100
Blood pressure	120/87 mmHg	100-120/60-80
DBP	80 mmHg	60 - 80
Weight	149 lbs	125 - 225
Height	68 in	65.4 - 74

Ears:
    General/bilateral:
       ° Ears: normal.
Nose:
    • Tenderness of the sinus.
Pharynx:
    ° Normal.
Lymph Nodes:
    ° Normal.
Lungs:
    ° Normal.
Musculoskeletal system:
    Knee:
    Right knee: ° No localized swelling. ° No warmth. ° Motion was normal. ° No pain
      was elicited by motion. ° No instability.
Neurological:
    Motor (Motor Strength): ° No weakness of the right knee was observed.
Assessment
    • Acute sinusitis which is resolved
    • Sprained anterior cruciate ligament of the knee which is resolved
Therapy
    • Order canceled for cool mist vaporizer.
    • Order canceled for reduced physical activity.
    • Order canceled for acetaminophen.
    • Order canceled for ice.
    • Order canceled for Ace bandage.
Practice Management
    Estab outpatient focused h&p - straightforward decisions; Total face to face
      time 15 min

► **Figure 6-24 Printed Exam Note for Juan Garcia.**

EHR Data from External Sources

Data in the patient chart can often be captured directly from modern medical instruments. This saves the time of rekeying readings from the equipment being used and improves accuracy by reducing the risk of transcription errors. Many of the devices being used in your office may already have a capability to transfer readings into the EHR. Many of the newer devices also have Wi-Fi

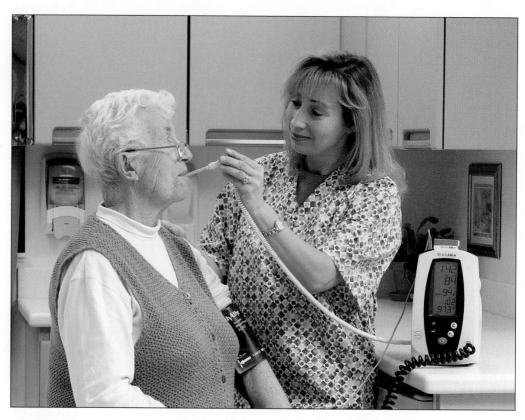

Photo Courtesy of Welch Allyn.

▶ **Figure 6-25 Nurse Taking Vital Signs Using Welch Allyn® Spot Vitals Signs®.**

capability, which enables the data transfer to the EHR without wires. (See Chapter 9 for a further discussion of Wi-Fi.)

Even though the transfer capability may be present in these devices, it may require interface software or mapping tables on the part of the EHR vendor. These will likely cost more. The medical practice must weigh the extra cost of the interface with the improved accuracy and time savings for nurses and other providers, as well as the value of the additional data in the EHR.

Three examples of instruments that can send data to the EHR are shown here.

Vital Signs

Most offices today use an electronic thermometer to take the patient's temperature, but the newest instruments from manufacturers such as GE, Welch Allyn, and others can do much more. Figure 6-25 shows a nurse taking the patient's vital signs using an instrument from Welch Allyn that takes the temperature, blood pressure, pulse rate, and mean arterial pressure, and then transfers the data wirelessly to the EHR. The unit is lightweight, operates on a rechargeable battery, and can be carried from room to room.

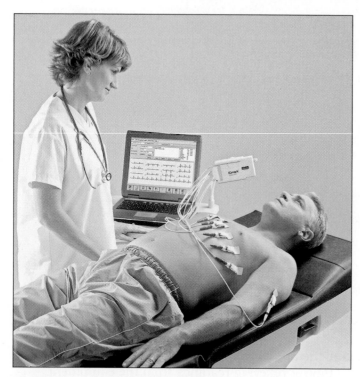

Photo Courtesy of Midmark Diagnostics Group.

▶ **Figure 6-26 Technician Using IQmark™ Digital ECG Saves Results into EHR.**

Diagnostic Tests

Computerized equipment now makes it possible to perform diagnostic tests in the medical office and capture the results into the EHR. These include ultrasound equipment, ECG, Holter monitors, spirometers, as well as lab equipment used for blood and urine analysis.

Figure 6-26 shows a computer-based ECG device that captures 10-second strips of a patient's ECG data, which can then be transferred into the patient's EHR.

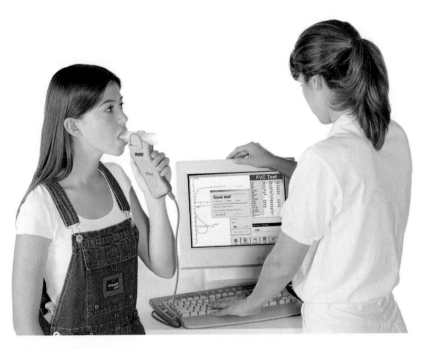

Photo Courtesy of Midmark Diagnostics Group.

▶ **Figure 6-27 Nurse Performing Spirometry Using IQmark™ Digital Spirometer.**

Figure 6-27 shows a patient using a digital spirometer. Spirometers perform FVC (forced vital capacity), VC (vital capacity), and MVV (maximal voluntary ventilation) tests. This instrument is used for pre- and postbronchodilator tests. The data is helpful for pulmonary conditions and asthma patients. Digital spirometry has been used in smoking cessation programs as well.

Electronic Lab Orders and Results

Digital laboratory test instruments also can communicate with the EHR. Primary care clinics and medical specialists frequently have one or more instruments to perform in-office a few key lab tests rather than send the patient to a reference lab. Nearly all lab instruments link to a computer called a Laboratory Information System (LIS), which can be interfaced to the EHR. The results from the LIS are merged into the EHR when the test is complete; the clinician is then automatically alerted that results are ready to review.

Virtually all national and regional reference laboratories offer medical practices the ability to receive lab results electronically. Most also offer the practice the ability to submit the orders electronically.

The main advantage of an electronic laboratory system interface is that it speeds the arrival of results and transmits them in a format that allows them to be merged as data into the EHR. The ability to electronically order also adds several improvements to the process. When orders are written electronically, they are immediately part of the patient's chart and the exam note. This means that other providers in the clinic who may see the patient are aware of what has already been ordered, saving unnecessary duplication of tests.

Electronic orders also prevent potential transcription errors that could be caused when a lab technician must rekey a paper requisition into the lab system. The electronic order has a unique requisition number that serves as a placeholder in the EHR for tracking tests that are pending results. When lab data is received by the EHR system, this number helps to automatically match the results to the original order.

Chapter 2 discussed the advantages of having electronic records with codified results as opposed to electronic records that are scanned images of printed reports. Nowhere is that more evident than with lab result reports. One important thing clinicians want to do for their patients is "trending," which is comparing the change of certain test components over a period of time.

In a paper chart, the trend is observed by paging through past tests, locating the desired component on each report, and making a mental comparison. However, when the lab results are stored as data in the EHR, the computer can instantly find all instances of any component the clinician wishes to consider. Additionally, with computerized data, graphs and charts can be easily created for any finding that has numerical results.

Workflow of Electronic Lab Orders and Results

For some types of visits, medical offices order tests ahead so the results can be ready before the clinician sees the patient. This is especially true of tests that can be performed at the medical office. Other tests, which require more time to result or which require the capabilities of an outside lab, also may be scheduled before the visit.

Having the results ready when the clinician sees the patient allows the results to be considered during the exam, used in the current assessment, and used to educate and counsel the patient. However, many tests are ordered when examining the patient. If a test is ordered when the clinician is creating the encounter note, the order is automatically documented as part of the plan.

Figure 6-28 illustrates the workflow of electronic lab orders.

1. The workflow begins when the clinician decides a lab test will be useful and writes an order. Whether this occurs before or during the exam, the starting point of the workflow is the doctor's order.

2. In most medical offices the clinician does not complete the actual requisition form. The lab order initiates a "task" for someone in the office to act on. The task involves at least two actions: completing the requisition and obtaining a specimen.

   A nurse, phlebotomist, or other staff person will complete the electronic requisition to be transmitted to the laboratory. Electronic orders are trans-

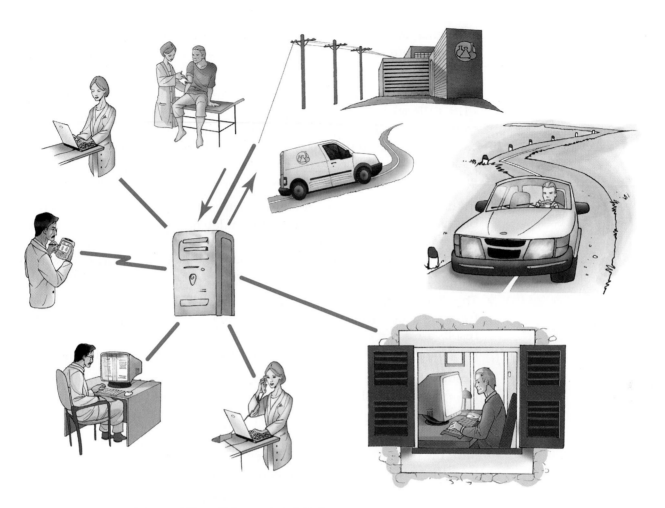

▶ **Figure 6-28 Diagram of the Workflow of Electronic Lab Orders.**

mitted to the lab either in real time as each order is written or in batches throughout the day.

The specimen to be tested is taken either at the practice or at an outside lab.

3. If the specimen is taken at the practice, for example, for a blood test, a phlebotomist or nurse will take a specified amount of blood from the patient. If a test requires a urine sample or other specimen, this is almost always taken at the medical office.

A clinician usually only takes the specimen when it is part of the exam or procedure; for example, taking a swab for a throat culture, or removing a mole that is to be sent to pathology.

4. Specimens taken at the medical office for tests performed at an outside lab are picked up by a courier and transported to the lab one or more times a day.

5. If the patient is sent to an outside lab for a blood test, a phlebotomist or lab technician will draw the blood. Because the order has been sent electronically, the requisition is already waiting in the lab system when the patient arrives.

6. The lab performs the requested tests. Labs may sometimes send "preliminary" results to give the clinician an early indication of the test and then send "final" results once the test has been repeated for verification.

For example, a bacterial culture's preliminary results may appear after 24 hours, but the culture may be monitored for 72 hours before the final results.

As soon as any results are ready, they are made available to the medical office EHR. EHR systems may connect to the lab system frequently as new orders are written or at predefined intervals throughout the day. Whenever a connection is established between the two systems, all available results for all of the clinic's patients are downloaded to the EHR. Software then matches each result to the original order and notifies the clinician that the results are ready.

In the EHR system, all orders have a status. Lab orders that have been sent but have no results are "pending." When lab data is received, most systems merge the data instantly into the patient's chart. The status will then be preliminary, final, or corrected, as designated by the lab. The EHR system also keeps track of which results have not yet been reviewed by the clinician.

7. The clinician reviews the lab results and "signs" them. Clinicians typically have two ways of managing the results. If they are looking at the patient chart, lab results are a part of the chart and therefore are easily seen and reviewed. For example, results available before the exam are reviewed during the exam.

   Results that arrive at other times are presented to the clinician in a "task" list. A task list facilitates reviewing the results for multiple patients quickly by eliminating the need to retrieve and open each patient chart individually.

   The clinician may order follow-up tests, a follow-up visit, send a "task" to have the patient called, add comments or annotations to the test, and compare the results to previous similar tests' results.

8. A nurse or other staff member calls the patient with the results.

9. Alternatively, some practices allow the patient to view the test results online via a medical office Web site.

Electronic lab orders and results benefit both the patient and the practice. Waiting for the results of an important test is stressful to patients. Electronic laboratory interfaces help expedite the process ensuring the provider knows about the results as soon as they are ready at the lab. Whether the patient is subsequently contacted by the phone or has access to lab results via the Web, the waiting time (and accompanying anxiety) is reduced.

The other benefit of electronic lab results is the codified data. Most practices cannot afford the personnel to have lab data keyed into the computer. Thus, without an electronic laboratory interface, the practice and the patient both miss the advantages that codified lab data provides.

Hands-On Exercise 39: Viewing Pending Orders and Lab Results

The Student Edition software does not contain an electronic laboratory order and result system. It would be inappropriate to order tests from a classroom. Because the Student Edition does not contain the electronic lab interface, the following two exercises have been created solely to demonstrate how useful it is to have lab data at hand while seeing the patient. The features you will find in commercial EHR software automate the lab order/result workflow differently and more elegantly than this simple exercise.

In Exercise 35 in Chapter 5, this patient's mother reported the possible exposure to lead-based paints while remodeling their older home. You will recall the plan recommended screening other family members. The clinician ordered tests for her son Gregory and he has already visited the lab before his appointment. Today is his office visit for examination and to review the test results.

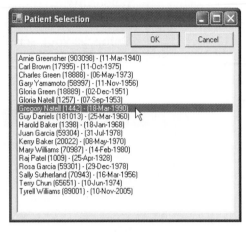

▶ Figure 6-29 Selecting Gregory Natell from the Patient Selection Window.

Step 1

If you have not already done so, start the Student Edition software.

Click Select on the Menu bar, and then click Patient.

In the Patient Selection window, locate and click on **Gregory Natell** as shown in Figure 6-29.

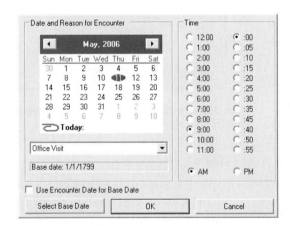

▶ Figure 6-30 New Encounter for an Office Visit, May 11, 2006 9:00 AM.

Step 2

Click Select on the Menu bar, and then click New Encounter.

Select the date **May 11, 2006**, the time **9:00 AM**, and the reason **Office Visit**.

Make certain you set the date, time, and reason correctly. Compare your screen to Figure 6-30 before clicking on the OK button.

In the next two steps, the nurse enters the Chief complaint and Vital Signs.

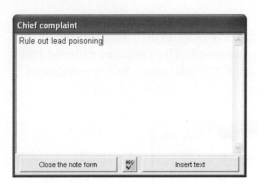

Chief complaint

Rule out lead poisoning

| Close the note form | | Insert text |

► **Figure 6-31 Chief Complaint Dialog for "Rule Out Lead Poisoning."**

Step 3

Enter the Chief complaint by locating the button in the toolbar labeled "Chief" and clicking on it.

In the dialog window that will open, type "Rule out lead poisoning."

Compare your screen to Figure 6-31 before clicking on the button labeled "Close the note form."

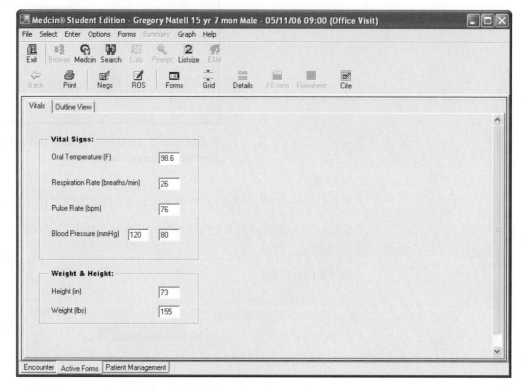

► **Figure 6-32 Vital Signs Form for Gregory Natell.**

Step 4

Enter the patient's Vital Signs using the Vitals Form located in the Active Forms tab (as you have done in previous exercises). Vital Signs for Gregory Natell are as follows:

Temperature: **98.6**

Respiration: **26**

Pulse: **76**

BP: **120/80**

Height: **73**

Weight: **155**

When you have finished, compare your screen to Figure 6-32. If it is correct, click on the tab labeled Encounter at the bottom of the window.

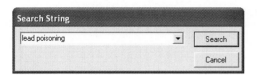

▶ **Figure 6-33 Search for Lead Poisoning.**

Step 5

Click on the Dx Tab.

Click on the button labeled "Search" on the toolbar near the top of the screen. (The Search button icon resembles a small pair of binoculars.) The Search String window will be invoked.

Enter the search string "Lead poisoning" and click on the button labeled "Search" in the window, as shown in Figure 6-33.

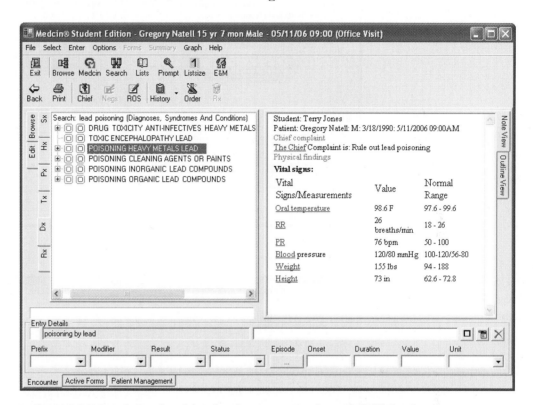

▶ **Figure 6-34 Search Results with Poisoning Heavy Metals Lead Highlighted.**

Step 6

Locate and highlight the finding "Poisoning Heavy Metals Lead."

Click on the List Size button until the list size is **1**.

Compare your screen to Figure 6-34, and then click on the button labeled "Prompt" on the toolbar near the top of the screen.

Step 7

Click on the Sx tab.

Verify that List Size is set to 1.

Click on the button labeled "ROS" on the toolbar near the top of the screen.

Click on the button labeled "Negs" (auto negative) on the toolbar near the top of the screen.

Compare your screen to Figure 6-35.

► **Figure 6-35 Symptoms for Heavy Metal Poisoning Lead.**

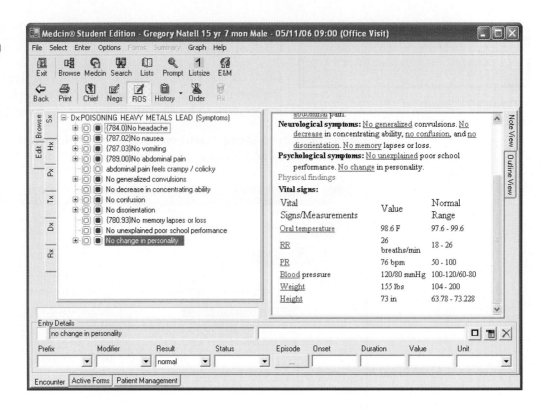

► **Figure 6-36 History for Heavy Metal Poisoning Lead.**

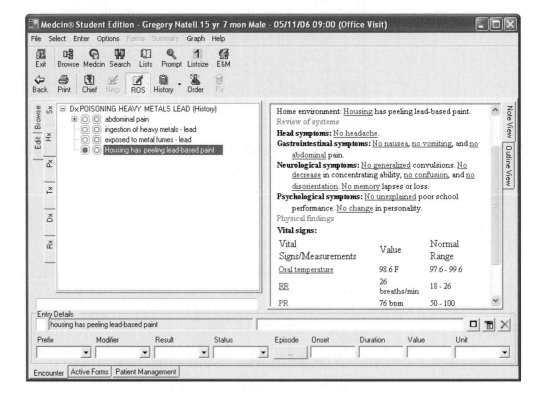

Step 8

Click on the Hx tab. Locate and click on the following finding:

● (red button) House has peeling paint which is lead based

Compare your screen to Figure 6-36.

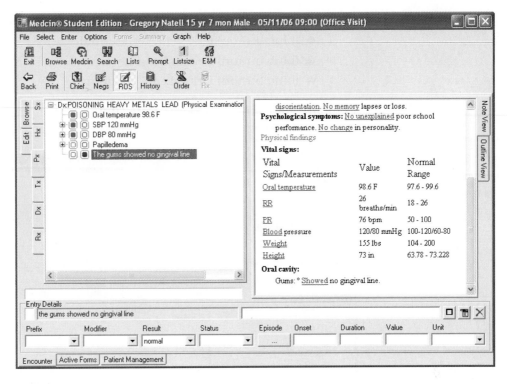

Step 9

Click on the Px tab. Locate and click on the following finding:

● (blue button) Gums gingival line

Compare your screen to Figure 6-37.

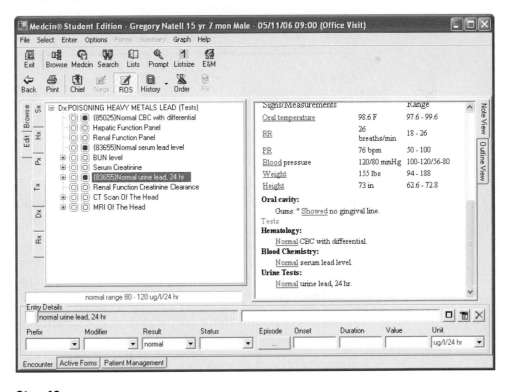

Step 10

As discussed at the beginning of the exercise, the patient has had several lab tests performed before the office visit. The results were within normal limits. The clinician will review results of the tests and document them in the exam note.

Click on the Tx tab. Locate and click on the following finding:

- (blue button) CBC with differential
- (blue button) Serum Lead Level
- (blue button) Urine Lead, 24 hour

Compare your screen to Figure 6-38. If it is correct click on the tab labeled **Patient Management** at the bottom of the window.

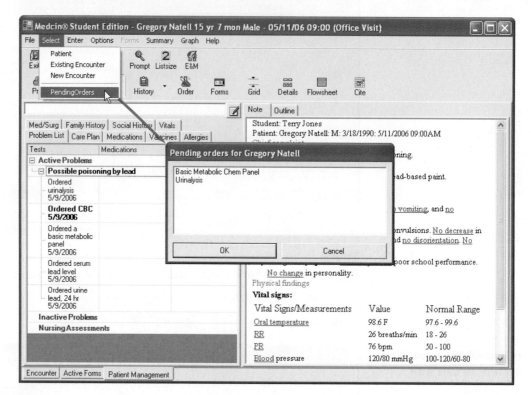

▶ **Figure 6-39 Patient Management—Pending Orders Window.**

Step 11

Your screen should display the problem list. If the information pane on the left of your screen is not already displaying the Problem List, click on the tab labeled "Problem List."

If the Entry Details pane is covering part of your list, locate and click on the button labeled "Details" in the toolbar at the top of your screen.

If the full order information under each problem is not fully displayed, locate the button labeled "Grid" in the toolbar at the top of your screen and click it.

Knowing which orders are still pending results is especially useful in offices in which multiple clinicians share patients because it prevents duplicate orders. A clinician can see what orders are outstanding on a patient, including those ordered by another provider.

Click Select on the Menu bar, and then click **Pending Orders**. A window of pending orders will be displayed.

Compare the window in your screen labeled "Pending Orders for Gregory Natell" to Figure 6-39. This window contains a list of tests that have been ordered but for which results have not yet been entered.

Close the window by clicking on the Cancel button. Note: If you click OK by mistake, you will invoke a results entry window. Simply click the Cancel button in that window, and proceed to the next step.

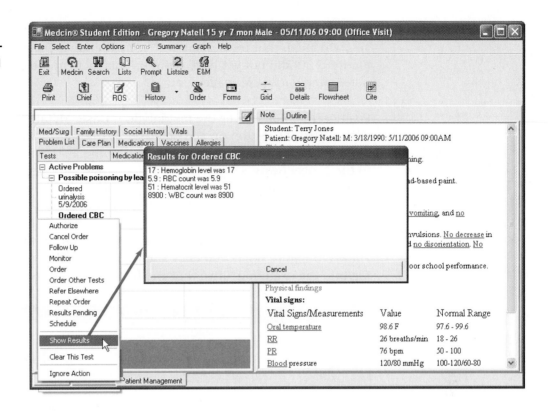

Step 12

From the Patient Management tab, you also can see the results of any tests that have been entered. As we discussed earlier, EHR systems can receive results from the lab electronically and merge them directly into the patient's chart. Typically, the ordering clinician is notified that results are ready for review.

Look at the Problem list in the left pane of your screen, under the test column.

Test names that are in bold type in the list indicate those that have results in the system.

Position the mouse over the test labeled "CBC Ordered" and click the **Right** button on your mouse. A drop-down list will be displayed.

If the drop-down list does not match the list shown in Figure 6-40, your mouse was not positioned correctly on the test. Reposition your mouse and click the right mouse button again.

Locate the option to Show Results and click the left mouse button. A window displaying the "Results for Ordered CBC" will be displayed, as shown in Figure 6-40.

The clinician can review the actual test results. Click the Cancel button to close the results window.

> **!** **Alert**

Important!

If the option "Show Results" in the drop-down list is displayed in gray text, the Student Edition Patient History program is not running. *Stop the exercise and notify your instructor.* Refer to Appendix B, Information about the Student Edition History Program, at the end of this book.

Step 13

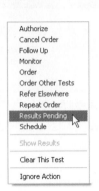

You will recall that tests displayed in the Pending Orders window (shown in Figure 6-39) did not yet have results. This fact can be easily noted in the exam note using Patient Management.

Position the mouse over the test labeled "Basic Metabolic Panel Ordered" and click the **Right** button on your mouse. A drop-down list will be displayed. Without clicking on any of the options, look at the list that is displayed. In addition to the "Show Results" option, used in the previous step, the drop-down list options include the ability to reorder a test, order additional follow-up tests, or to enter the status of a test into the current encounter.

▶ Figure 6-41 Select Option Pending Results for Basic Metabolic Panel.

Locate and highlight the option "Pending Results" in the drop-down list (as shown in Figure 6-41) and click the left mouse button. This will record a finding into the exam narrative that the test results are pending.

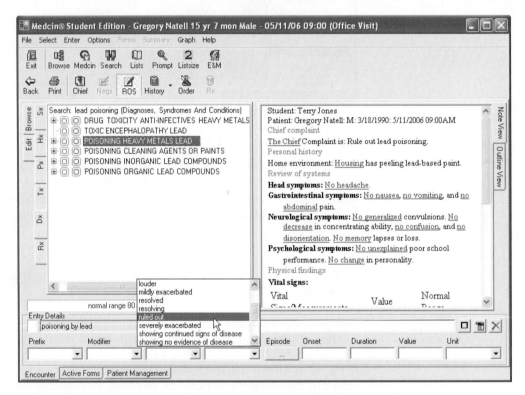

▶ Figure 6-42 Dx Tab—Select the Status Ruled Out for Poisoning Heavy Metals Lead.

Step 14

Locate and click on the **Encounter** tab at the bottom of your screen.

Click on the Dx tab (which has now returned to the full list of findings).

Again, click on the Search button in the toolbar at the top of your screen.

The Search String window will be invoked and should still contain the words "lead poisoning." If it does not, type them again.

Click on the button in the window labeled Search. (If you need help, refer to Figure 6-33.)

When the list of diagnoses is displayed, locate and highlight the finding "Poisoning Heavy Metals Lead." (If you need help, refer to Figure 6-34.)

In the Entry Details section at the bottom of your screen, locate the Status Field and click on the down arrow button in it.

Scroll the drop-down list that is displayed to locate and click on "ruled out" as shown in Figure 6-42.

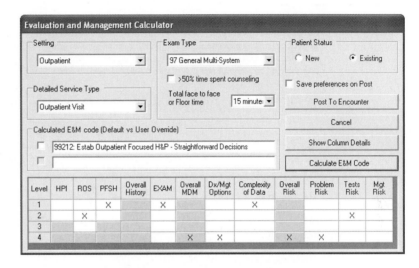

▶ **Figure 6-43 Evaluation and Management Calculator.**

Step 15

Click on the E&M button in the toolbar at the top of your screen. When the E&M Calculator window is invoked:

Set face-to-face time at 15 Minutes.

Locate Patient Status and click on the circle next to Existing.

Click the button labeled "Calculate E&M Code."

Compare your screen to Figure 6-43.

Click the button labeled "Post To Encounter."

Step 16

Click File on the Menu bar, and then click Print Encounter or Print To HTML (as directed by your instructor).

If you are printing your work, you may click the Print button on the toolbar at the top of your screen instead of selecting Print Encounter from the Menu.

Compare your printout or file output to Figure 6-44. If it is correct, hand it in to your instructor. If there are any differences, review the previous steps in the exercise and find your error.

> **! Alert**
>
> **Do not close or exit the Encounter until you have a printed copy in your hand. You will lose your work if you exit before printing.**

```
Student: Terry Jones
Patient: Gregory Natell: M: 3/18/1990: 5/11/2006 09:00AM
Chief complaint
The Chief Complaint is: Rule out lead poisoning.
Personal history
Home environment: Housing has peeling lead-based paint.
Review of systems
Head symptoms: No headache.
Gastrointestinal symptoms: No nausea, no vomiting, and no abdominal pain.
Neurological symptoms: No generalized convulsions.  No decrease in concentrating ability,
    no confusion, and no disorientation.  No memory lapses or loss.
Psychological symptoms: No unexplained poor school performance.  No change in personality.
Physical findings
Vital signs:
```

Vital Signs/Measurements	Value	Normal Range
Oral temperature	98.6 F	97.6 - 99.6
RR	26 breaths/min	18 - 26
PR	76 bpm	50 - 100
Blood pressure	120/80 mmHg	100-120/56-80
Weight	155 lbs	94 - 188
Height	73 in	62.6 - 72.8

```
Oral cavity:
    Gums: ° Showed no gingival line.
Tests
Hematology:
    Normal CBC with differential.
Blood Chemistry:
    Pending results for a basic metabolic panel.
    Normal serum lead level.
Urine Tests:
    Normal urine lead, 24 hr.
Assessment
    • Poisoning by lead which is ruled out
Practice Management
    Estab outpatient focused h&p - straightforward decisions; Total face to face time
    15 min
```

▶ **Figure 6-44 Printed Exam Note for Gregory Natell.**

Graphing Lab Results from the Chart

As we have discussed earlier in this section, one of the advantages of having lab results in the EHR as codified data instead of as scanned or text reports is the ability to graph a trend of lab values. This provides the clinician with a quick picture of the changes over time. It is sometimes used for patient education and counseling.

Hands-On Exercise 40: Graphing Lab Results

An EHR system can graph any component of a lab test that has numerical values. To create a meaningful graph, the test must have been performed multiple times. In this exercise, the clinic has been helping Sally Sutherland monitor her cholesterol by testing her at each annual exam. You are going to create a graph of Sally's total cholesterol.

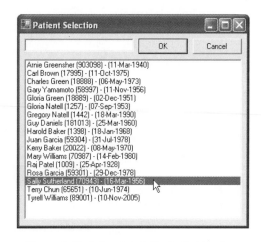

▶ **Figure 6-45 Selecting Sally Sutherland from the Patient Selection Window.**

Step 1

If you have not already done so, start the Student Edition software.

Click Select on the Menu bar, and then click Patient.

In the Patient Selection window, locate and click on **Sally Sutherland**.

▶ **Figure 6-46 Select Existing Encounter for May 11, 2006 10:00 AM.**

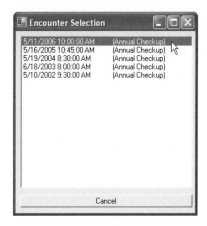

Step 2

A nurse has already started the encounter; the Chief complaint and the Vital Signs have already been entered, and you are going to retrieve and work with an encounter already in progress.

Click Select on the Menu bar, and then click Existing Encounter.

Position your mouse pointer on the first encounter in the list, dated **May 11, 2006 10:00 AM** and click on it (as shown in Figure 6-46).

Step 3

Click on the Tx Tab.

Click on the button labeled Search on the toolbar near the top of the screen. The Search String window will be invoked.

Type the search string "Total cholesterol" and click on the button in the window labeled Search as shown in Figure 6-47.

▶ **Figure 6-47 Search for Total Cholesterol.**

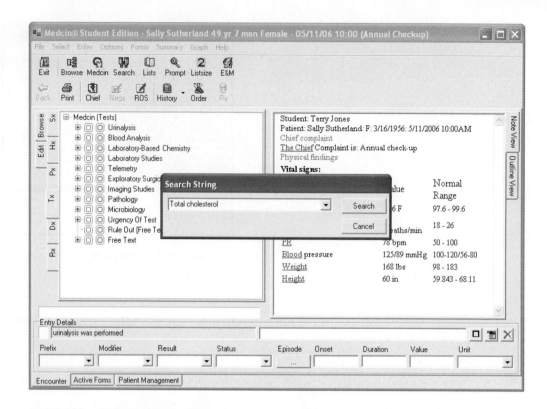

▶ **Figure 6-48 Select Graph Current Finding from the Menu.**

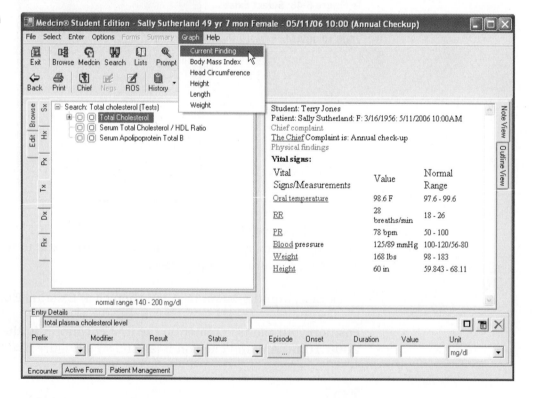

Step 4

Your should be in the Tx tab with the finding Total Cholesterol highlighted.

Click Graph on the Menu bar, and then click "Current Finding" from the drop-down list (as shown in Figure 6-48.)

The Medcin Graph window will be invoked.

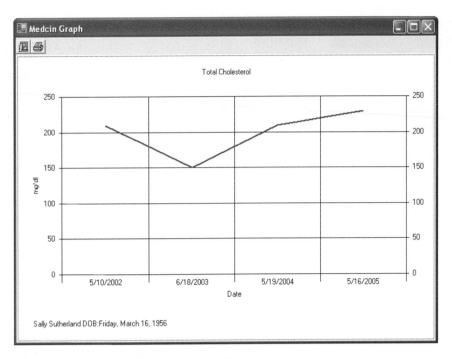

► Figure 6-49 **Graph of Sally Sutherland's Total Cholesterol.**

Step 5

The software will find and graph Sally's cholesterol over the last 4 years. Compare your screen to Figure 6-49.

This example shows the changes in Total Cholesterol. Similar graphs could have been created for any component of the cholesterol lab results, such as HDL or LDL.

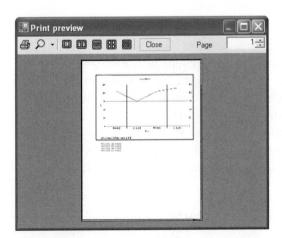

The Graph window has two buttons in the upper left corner that are identical in appearance and purpose to the corresponding buttons in the toolbar. The first button is Exit, which closes the graph window. The second button is the Print button, which prints your graph.

Locate the Print button in the upper left corner of the Graph window and click on it.

Step 6

A Print Preview window for graphs will be invoked. This window allows users to see what the printout will look like before it is printed.

► Figure 6-50 **Print Preview Window for Graphs.**

Locate the Print button in the upper left corner of the Preview window and click on it.

When your graph has printed successfully, click on the button labeled "Close" to close the Print Preview window.

Write your name on your printout and hand it into your instructor.

Quick Access to Frequent Orders

One time-saving feature that is typical in all commercial EHR systems is the concept of keeping a quick pick-list of a clinician's frequently used orders. The student edition emulates this by displaying a list of Rx Sig information for each medication you have ordered thus far. However, commercial EHR systems provide a much more robust application of the concept, in many cases allowing the clinician to write the entire prescription or lab order with a single click of the mouse.

With thousands of tests that could be ordered and thousands of drugs to choose from, a clinician doesn't have the time to go through a search of medications or tests to write an Rx or order a lab. Many clinicians find that they order a fairly narrow range of tests (appropriate to their specialty and patient population) and write prescriptions for only a small group of medications.

It makes sense for clinicians to keep a list of the items they most frequently use from which they can select when writing the order. Commercial EHR systems handle this in different ways; some automatically create the list by memorizing what the clinician has been ordering, whereas others allow the clinicians to build their own lists. Most EHR systems offer a combination of both.

The EHR system you will use in a medical office will most certainly have this type of feature. Making use of the feature is definitely a good way to speed up data entry at the point of care. Creating or customizing your Rx and orders lists will certainly save time when you are with the patient.

Patient Entry of Symptoms and Previous History

Contributed by Allen R. Wenner, M.D.[1]

EHR systems facilitate documentation at the point of care, but only the patient has the information about what symptoms were present at the outset of the illness and what the outcome of medical treatment of those symptoms was. The patient is also typically the source of past medical, family, and social history. Up to 67% of the nurse or clinician's time with the patient is spent entering the patient's symptom into the visit documentation. Because in this chapter we are exploring methods to speed up data entry at the point of care, let us consider a technique that frees up the clinicians' time while improving the depth and quality of the information gathered.

---

[1]Courtesy of Primetime Medical Software and Instant Medical History, used by permission.

Triage

Patient screening occurs in all health care settings to determine the level of care needed so that each patient is given the highest quality of care in the most efficient fashion. In different settings, the screening is managed differently, but careful attention to the patient's chief complaint and reason for visit is common to all health care facilities.

In emergency rooms, specially trained "triage nurses" are the first responders to patients. Their job is to quickly decide which patients need priority. The review is often a simplified, organ-specific review of systems determined by the presenting complaint. The emergency room triage nurse helps to decide how long treatment can be delayed without deterioration of the condition. The Emergency Department physician uses this screening to begin determining the diagnosis. Although the nurse never tells a doctor the diagnosis, he or she has pregathered information that helps the physician decide what is wrong more quickly.

Similarly, both receptionists and nurses in primary care offices function as physician extenders. When the patient calls on the telephone, the receptionist determines when the patient's appointment is made. The determination, based on rules such as the duration of the illness, is proportional to the urgency of the appointment. When patients arrive at the medical office, nurses sometimes use their considerable clinical experience and personal knowledge of the patients to elicit a history of the present illness often while they record the vital signs. Before the encounter with the clinician, the nurse reviews the pertinent organ system, follows up each positive with additional questions, checks the pertinent negatives, and inquires about other issues such as stress, diet, and so on. If time permits and staffing is adequate, the nurse performs a repetitive, yet necessary, labor-intensive task for the physician and documents this as quickly as she can. In doing so, the nurse aids the physician assessment by presenting critical information to the physician for review.

The Clinicians' Dilemma

A day in a medical clinic is a busy stream of patients ranging in age from newborn to geriatric. Their presenting complaints are as varied as their age range. Because patients may have a minor illness or a life-threatening condition, it is very hard to predict exactly how long each patient will take. Doctors run behind as a result. Patients from the morning often spill over into lunch, which often becomes abbreviated.

In contrast, to the hectic pace of the clinicians, time seems to drag for the patients who are waiting. A major challenge for the staff is keeping the patients from waiting too long in the waiting room or exam rooms.

In a traditional paper-based office, by the time the physician enters the examination room and greets the patient, there is still little or no information about the patient except for a few notes from the nurse. The physician has to begin asking why the patient has sought care. After briefly listening to the patient describe a complaint, the typical clinician interrupts the patient after 18 seconds to clarify the story, often cutting off the patient's natural flow of narration.

Physicians are pressed for time and need to get to the point quickly. Then there are the CMS requirements to document the encounter (discussed in Chapter 5), which sap time away from patient care.

An experienced physician can make a preliminary assessment after a few minutes of the interview. The physician uses the bulk of the visit confirming this hypothesis by querying the patient about symptoms, history of present illness, review of systems, and then performing the physical exam. Because of time pressures or fatigue as the day wears on, the physician may forget to ask about vital pieces of data including essential symptoms, family or social history, or habits such as alcohol or drug use.

With the pressures of patients waiting, after completing the physical exam, assessment, and writing a prescription, the clinician may not have enough time to provide patient education. Instead of answering questions about the treatment and care plan, the clinician relies on a nurse or receptionist to educate the patient. In the traditional paper office, the clinician leaves the exam room, and goes to a private area to complete the patient's chart by dictating or handwriting his or her recollection of the history as told by the patient, any other relevant data remembered from the encounter and the physical exam, as well as the diagnosis, prescription, and treatment plan.

Triage by Computer

In the late 1980s, Allen Wenner, M.D., a physician in Columbia, South Carolina, wondered if history couldn't be taken by a computer. The medical literature was replete with academic efforts at patient computer dialog beginning with Warner Slack at Harvard[2] and John Meyne at Mayo Clinic.[3] If the patients entered their own data, it would free up clinical staff and allow more of the physician's time to be focused directly on the important issues identified by patient. Dr. Wenner confirmed the theories of the academics that given the opportunity to add information to their medical chart, while waiting was readily accepted by most patients. Working with his colleagues at Primetime Medical Software, he developed Instant Medical History™, an automated patient data-entry component for the EHR. It is available in many commercial EHR systems today.

Dr. Wenner decided that the computer could ask all the necessary questions intelligently if it was given a limited set of initial information. A nurse would start the interview by entering the patient's age, sex, and selecting the symptoms and organ systems for review. At that point, the computer could pose questions that simulated a live patient interview. The knowledge-based approach of the computer's artificial intelligence changed the questions based on the patient's answers, simulating a live clinical interview. The software sought to collect the necessary prerequisite data for the clinical interview.

Another important element of history taking is the depth to which a patient is asked questions. Dr. Wenner found the use of computer interviews improves the quality of the information presented by the patient because it is more complete since the computer never forgets details. It allows a physician to converse

---

[2]Slack, WV, Hicks GP, Reed CE, et al. A computer-based medical-history system. *N Engl J Med.* 1966;274;194–198.

[3]Mayne, JG, Weksel W, Sholtz PN. Toward automating the medical history. *Mayo Clin Proc.* 1968;43;1–25.

casually with a patient while clarifying the objective information needed to make a confident diagnosis. For example, an ideal interview about the upper respiratory tract and sinuses should include questions about unusual causes such as *psittacosis*, an infection acquired from raising birds, query about prevention such as use of tobacco, and consideration of the risk for pregnancy in determining treatment options. The clinician may forget or just not have enough time to ask these questions; the computer will not forget.

Because patients want their physicians to arrive at the best diagnosis, Dr. Wenner found they are willing to answer questions. Also, because the physician can review the information entered by the patient, more time is available for explaining the diagnosis and educating the patient; the patient's time and effort to enter the data are rewarded.

In the earliest days of computers, a study at Cornell University had patients answer questions on a punch card that was processed by a computer. The study found that "... it collects for appraisal a large and comprehensive body of information about the patient's medical history at no expenditure of the physician's time; it facilitates interview by making available to the physician a preliminary survey of the patient's total medical problems; its data, being systematically arranged, are easier to review than those on conventional medical histories, and, by calling attention to the patient's symptoms and significant items of past history, it assures that their investigation will not be overlooked because the physician lacked time to elicit them."[4]

Workflow Using Patient-Entered Data

There are several workflows that illustrate Instant Medical History in use. Depending on the workflow of the office, Instant Medical History can be administered on a kiosk or pen-tablet device in the waiting room, in a subwaiting area, in the exam room, or at home via the Web.

Figure 6-51 shows an interview screen of Instant Medical History. To the patients, it represents a replacement of the clipboard with questions that the receptionist handed to patients on arrival at medical offices. The difference is that the questions are asked one at a time and can dynamically branch to other question sets based on the answers provided by the patient.

Patients complete the computer program at their own pace. The computer calculates well and can use the answers to several questions to branch to standardized screening instruments published in the medical literature. Patients have an opportunity to change their answers.

Patients can review their histories (as shown in Figure 6-52) and are better prepared to interact with the physician.

The computer produces legible output. Once the patient has answered the questions, the information is organized for the provider in a succinct and easy-to-read format that becomes the starting point for the encounter. The clinician can review this output either on a computer screen or as a printout (shown in Figure 6-53).

---

[4]Brodman K, Erdmann AJ Jr, Lorge I, et al. The Cornell Medical Index: An adjunct to medical interview. *JAMA* 1949;140:530–534.

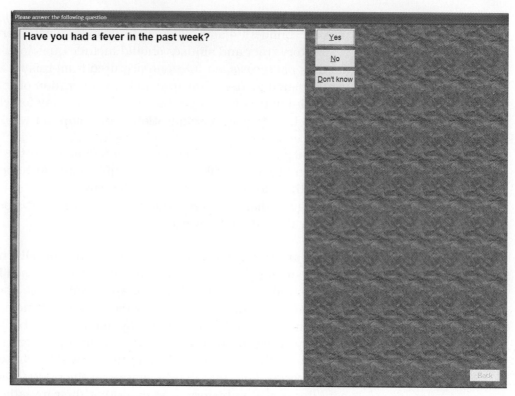

Courtesy of Primetime Medical Software & Instant Medical History.

▶ Figure 6-51 Instant Medical History™ on a Kiosk in the Waiting Room.

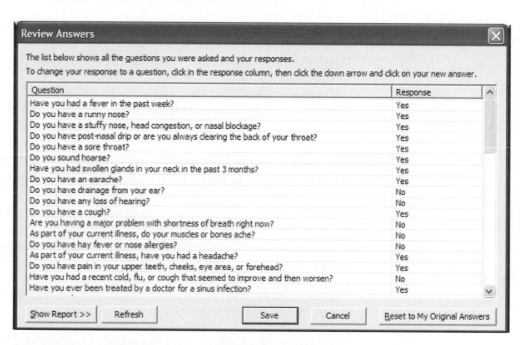

Courtesy of Primetime Medical Software & Instant Medical History.

▶ Figure 6-52 Summary Screen Allows Patient to Review Answers.

This output can be reviewed before going into the exam, so that the clinician is armed with a great deal of useful information to begin making the proper diagnosis and considering appropriate treatment. For example, from the output shown in Figure 6-53, the clinician knows that the patient has a sinus infec-

CHIEF COMPLAINT
Mary Williams is a 25 year old female. Her reason for visit is "upper respiratory infection".
HISTORY OF PRESENT ILLNESS
#1. "URI"
　　She reported: Sore throat. Rhinorrhea 1-2 days. Nasal congestion 5-6 days. Bilateral nasal congestion.
　　Post nasal drip. Facial pain worsened by bending over. Yellow and thick nasal drainage.
　　She denied: Dyspnea.
　　DURATION
　　　　She reported: Cough 4-6 da.
　　TIMING
　　　　She denied: Nocturnal cough.
　　CONTEXT
　　　　She reported: Non-productive cough.
　　ASSOCIATED SIGNS AND SYMPTOMS
　　　　She denied: Recent coryza improved then worsened.
PAST, FAMILY, AND SOCIAL HISTORY
　PAST MEDICAL HISTORY
　　History of: Sinusitis.
　SOCIAL HISTORY
　　PREGNANCY HISTORY
　　Menses within last week.
　　TOBACCO USE
　　　　History of: Smoking cigarettes. Smoked 6-8 yrs. 21-30 cigarettes (1 and a half packs) smoked per day.
　　　　Plans to quit smoking within month. Advised to quit smoking within 12 mos.
REVIEW OF SYSTEMS
CONSTITUTIONAL
　　She reported: Fever associated with cough. Did not measure temperature. Fever 1-2 days. Fever w/rigor.
EAR, NOSE, AND THROAT
　　She denied: Hoarseness. Cervical adenopathy. Otalgia. Otorrhea. Auditory loss. Seasonal allergies.
　　Chronic nasal congestion. Seasonal rhinorrhea.
　　DENTAL HEALTH
　　　　She denied: Recent dental therapy.
MUSCULOSKELETAL
　　She denied: Myalgias.
NEUROLOGICAL
　　She reported: Headache assoc w/illness.
　　She denied: HAs assoc/w vomiting. Severe HA. Neck stiff w/HA. Severe pain bending chin to chest.
SELF-ASSESSMENT SCALES
　　Title: **Fagerstrom Tolerance Test - Addiction**
　　Description: 8 questions determining nicotine dependence with higher scores indicating more addiction.
　　Patient Score: **8 - Highly dependent on nicotine**
　　Scoring Key and Interpretation:
```
     0 - 6 : Low to moderate nicotine dependence
     7 - 9 : Highly dependent on nicotine
```
　　Title: **Fagerstrom Tolerance Test - Motivation**
　　Description: 2 questions indicating motivation and determination to successfully quit smoking.
　　Patient Score: **6 - Good motivation to quit smoking**
　　Scoring Key and Interpretation:
```
     0 - 2 : No motivation to quit smoking
     3 - 4 : Some motivation to quit smoking
     5 - 6 : Good motivation to quit smoking
```
　　Reference: *Glynn T.J., Manley M.W., How to Help Your Patients Stop Smoking, American Cancer*
　　Society/National Cancer Institute; April 1990 NIH Publication 90-3064

Courtesy of Primetime Medical Software & Instant Medical History.

▶ **Figure 6-53 Output from Patient Entered Data for an Upper Respiratory Infection.**

tion that is likely to have been caused by tobacco abuse. Having a complete history in advance of the visit allows the physician to ask fewer questions about the diagnosis and more about the effects of the illness on the patient. It also allows the clinician to discuss the treatment plan with the patient. In this example, the clinician can spend time at this visit discussing smoking cessation because the patient has indicated a desire to quit smoking soon.

Jack Gould of Columbia, South Carolina, became the first person in medical history to save his own life with software he operated himself.

One day, Mr. Gould came to his physician's office to pick up a prescription renewal for his wife who also was a patient there. In the waiting room was a computer kiosk running Instant Medical History, a patient-operated medical expert system. A sign posted near the system read "Stay Healthy: Take Our Prevention Questionnaire." While waiting for the prescription refill to be authorized, he decided to try it out.

In addition to eating and exercise recommendations, the software suggested that he needed the standard procedure to check for colon cancer because he could not recall having been checked within the time frame suggested by standard guidelines. Normally, after the patient completes the questionnaire, the physician reviews the information with the patient. Because in this case he was not there to see the physician, he spoke with the triage nurse, who confirmed it was a wise preventive action to take and scheduled an appointment.

A few weeks later, the patient returned for his appointment. The doctor was surprised that the patient was there for such a specific preventative procedure months before his annual physical examination. The doctor asked who scheduled the procedure. In a tone reflecting his expectation that it was common for patients to schedule proctosigmoidoscopies on their own volition, he replied "Well, your computer did."

No physician can be expected to remember the thousands of recommended interventions for each patient. The preventive health screening software queried the patient for the appropriate items based on his sex, age, and risk factors and compared them to the preventive guidelines of the U.S. Preventive Services Task Force. In the case of Mr. Gould, a flexible sigmoidoscopy was scheduled and a resectable severely dysplasic polyp was removed easily from his colon.

The large precancerous polyp that was discovered might have gone completely undetected without the intelligent prompting of the Instant Medical History program. Mr. Gould knew the importance of his decision to take the interview after his physician explained that he wouldn't have thought to do this test until his routine annual complete medical examination. The polyps were removed without complication before they could develop into colon cancer.

He was totally unaware of his risk for other conditions until he took the preventive interview. Now he strongly believes that Instant Medical History saved his life.

---

[5]Courtesy of Primetime Medical Software and Instant Medical History, used by permission.

Because interview software records subjective information from the patient, the data represents a more complete and accurate reflection of a patient's complaints than a physician's dictation after the visit. After asking a few confirmatory questions, physicians can complete the medical history in the examination room while the patient is still present.

The physician can add additional information as necessary and the exam note can be completed by the physician at the point of care. Finally, as the patient leaves, the patient can be given a copy of the exam note in addition to patient education materials and prescriptions.

Alternative Workflow

Patients can alternatively complete the symptom and history interview before the visit using the Internet at medical offices that imbed Instant Medical History in the practice Web site. In that case, the data will already be available to the clinician when the patient arrives at the office. In the case of E-visits, the clinician can make medical treatment decisions without a face-to-face visit in many instances. You will learn more about E-visits and the Internet in Chapter 9.

Improved Patient Information

Data from patient screening is useful for providing pertinent information that allows an immediate diagnosis. Not only does the physician have a reasonable idea of the patient's diagnosis before any examination begins but also the data are instantly ready to become part of the medical record.

Eliminating the bulk of transcription and dictation and replacing it with detailed, patient-entered data has transformed the office encounter from a data-gathering session into an opportunity to concentrate on the most important task at hand: caring for the patient.

The increased efficiency that computer screening allows makes office visits more enjoyable because the physician has more time to explain the diagnosis and educate the patient.

Preventive Health Screening

Another way that patient–computer interviews can help improve patient care is through preventive health screening. Because most patients wait 15 minutes to see a physician, it is medically appropriate to screen patients for compliance with health maintenance guidelines while they wait.

In the course of a year-long study, patients were invited to answer a few questions on the computer when they spoke to the triage nurse, but screening was completely voluntary. Over time, the software revealed the need for hundreds of tetanus shots, varicella vaccinations, papanicolaou smears, and other preventive measures by asking patients simple questions about the duration since their last assessment. (Preventive Health will be covered further in Chapter 7.)

Systems Integration for Better Patient Care

Beginning in 2002, leading manufacturers of electronic medical record systems started to embed Instant Medical History into their systems. For the first time, patients entering their own medical symptoms and history into automated interview software became an integral part of the EHR. Patients accepted a new role in their health care.

Because patient-entered information is in a codified, structured format, it can be searched, retrieved, and studied from within a comprehensive electronic health record. Instant Medical History is currently being mapped to the Medcin and SNOMed nomenclatures as well. Ultimately, the combination of computer screening and an electronic medical record can provide the most valuable patient data for determination of best practices and improved outcomes. Finally, enough reproducible data will be available for physicians to begin practicing evidenced-based medicine instead of medicine based on opinion and tradition.

Chapter Six Summary

This chapter described several additional methods to speed up documentation of the visit, manage the patient's health, and populate key portions of the patient chart using external sources. The external sources included electronic instruments and patient-entered data.

Patient Management

The patient management feature demonstrates the way an EHR can organize information from past encounters. Because most doctors see patients for multiple visits, the ability to view data from previous visits and to cite these data during a follow-up exam can significantly speed up documentation of the current visit.

Patient management has the following tabs:

◆ **Problems**—Clinicians use problem lists and problem-oriented views of the chart to help them during the examination. Problem-oriented views organize the data by problem and encounter date.

Problem lists provide an up-to-date list of the diagnoses and conditions that affect that particular patient's care. Problem lists track both acute and chronic conditions. Problems are removed from the list or set inactive once the patient is "cured" or the problem is "resolved." Problems that normally resolve themselves over a short period of time are called Acute Self-Limiting. The status of the problem is updated at each visit.

The following are typical of the types of status assigned to active problems:

Resolved

Resolving

Improving

Well controlled

Unchanged

Inadequately controlled

Mildly exacerbated

Failing to change as expected

Expanding

Worsening

Severely exacerbated

- **Care Plan**—provides a quick review of the plan from each previous encounter in a problem-oriented view. It is organized by problem and encounter date for which the patient was seen for that problem. Clicking on the encounter reveals the findings recorded in the plan for that visit.

- **Medications**—Keeps track of what medications the patient is currently taking. The Medications list is always reviewed before writing new prescriptions.

- **Vaccines**—provides a list of the patient's immunizations that have been administered at the clinic.

- **Allergies**—provides a list of food, drug, and other allergies the patient may have. This information is reviewed before writing a prescription.

- **Past Medical/Surgical History**—provides list of past history items recorded in the EHR during all previous encounters.

- **Family History**—provides list of family history items recorded in the EHR during all previous encounters.

- **Social History**—provides list of social and behavioral history items recorded in the EHR during all previous encounters.

- **Vitals**—displays key vital signs taken on previous visits in a column format.

Clicking the mouse on the label of a column within any tab of Patient Management will sort the rows in the tab by the values in the column that was clicked.

The patient management feature allows information from previous encounters to be updated and cited in the current encounter. In an EHR, citing from a previous exam note means to bring a finding into the current encounter. Tests can be ordered, reordered, or the results can be viewed. Prescriptions can be renewed or discontinued as well. All of this saves the clinician time and helps to ensure that each outstanding issue in the patient's care is followed up during the visit.

External Sources

A significant contribution of data into an EHR can come from sources other than direct entry by the clinic staff. These include vital signs directly from medical instruments as well as the results from test equipment used in the office such as ECG, spirometer, ultrasound, and in-house LIS systems.

National and regional reference laboratories offer medical practices the ability to send orders and receive lab results electronically in a format that allows them to be merged into the EHR. This codified lab result data allows the clinician to compare the change of certain test components over a period of time (trending). Lab results that have numerical results can be graphed so that the trending becomes visual.

Electronic ordering systems allow a provider to create and use quick pick-lists of frequently used orders for both prescriptions and lab orders. This is an important time-saving feature because there are thousands of tests that could be ordered and thousands of drugs to choose from, yet most clinicians find that they order a fairly narrow range of tests and write prescriptions for only a small group of medications.

Electronic ordering also allows the system to track tests that have been ordered but do not yet have results. The ability to see pending orders helps prevent duplicate orders, as a clinician can see what is already on order for a patient.

Because lab tests involve the collection of a specimen as well as additional information required by the lab, the efforts of multiple people must be organized. The workflow of the office is improved with an electronic orders/results system. When a clinician orders a lab test electronically, a sequence of steps automatically will be set in motion.

Electronic orders are transmitted to the lab either in batches throughout the day or in real time as each order is written. When an outside lab is used for blood tests, the patient is sometimes sent to the reference lab to have the blood drawn there. If the order has been sent electronically, it is already waiting in the lab system when the patient arrives. If the specimen is taken at the office, the order automatically initiates a "task" for a phlebotomist or nurse, who will obtain a specimen from the patient.

All lab orders have a status; these include:

Pending—sent but have no results

Preliminary—results provide an early indication of the test but awaiting verification

Final—results have been verified and are ready for review

Corrected—a change occurred as a result of repeat verification

As soon as any results are transmitted from the lab and merged into the EHR, the clinician is notified. A task list allows the clinician to review results for many patients without retrieving and opening each patient's chart individually. While reviewing lab results, the clinician can "sign" off on the order, order follow-up tests or a follow-up visit, send a "task" to have the patient called, add comments or annotations to the test, and compare the test to previous similar tests.

Triage

Nurses "triage" patients to determine the urgency of their condition, including the history and duration of present illness and a simplified, organ-specific review of system determined by the presenting complaint. In a primary care office, this often is done when the nurse records the vital signs.

Patient-Entered Data

Numerous studies have shown that patient data also can become a significant contributor to the EHR, for some of the following reasons:

◆ only the patient has the information about what symptoms were present at the outset of the illness;

◆ only the patient knows the outcome of medical treatment of those symptoms;

◆ the patient is also the source of past medical, family, and social history;

◆ patient-entered data is a more accurate reflection of a patient's complaints; and

◆ patients who can review their histories are better prepared for the visit.

Up to 67% of the nurse or clinician's time with the patient is spent entering the patient's symptom into the visit documentation. A computer can be used by the patient in the waiting room or exam room to enter the same symptom and history information that the nurse or clinician would have entered. This saves time and allows the triage nurse to focus on the review of the information with the patient rather than on the keying of data.

Patient-entered data is organized by the computer for the provider in a succinct and easy-to-read format that becomes the starting point for the encounter. Having a complete history in advance of the visit allows the clinician to ask fewer questions about the diagnosis and concentrate more on the effects of the illness on the patient. It also allows the clinician more time to discuss the treatment plan with the patient.

Testing Your Knowledge of Chapter 6

1. What is a problem list?
2. What is the idea of a problem list?
3. Name at least two reasons why clinicians use a problem list.
4. What is a reason that a "wellness" condition would appear on a problem list?
5. Where does the data that appears in the Patient Management tab come from?
6. What does it mean to cite a finding?
7. Name at least three external sources of data for populating the EHR.
8. Define trending of lab values.
9. What type of lab results can be graphed?
10. Describe the workflow of an office using an electronic lab interface.
11. What is a pending order?
12. Name at least two benefits of having patients entering their own symptoms and history.
13. What is triage (as used in this chapter)?
14. What percentage of a clinician's time is spent entering patient symptoms and history into the chart?
15. List the steps you would take to graph a lab value.

7 Using the EHR to Improve Patient Care

Learning Outcomes

After completing this chapter, you should be able to:

◆ Describe flow sheets

◆ Work with a flow sheet

◆ Create a graph of vital signs in the chart

◆ Document a well-baby check-up using a wellness form

◆ Explain the relationship between vitals signs and growth charts

◆ Create a pediatric growth chart

◆ Understand immunization schedules

◆ Order immunizations for a child

◆ Describe preventative care screening

Note

Important Information about the Student Edition Patient History Program

The classroom environment provides a challenge for computer programs because the exercises require multiple students to simultaneously retrieve patient charts and enter findings for the same patient, without disturbing the sample data for the next class.

To accommodate this, a special software program loads previous patient history into the computer's memory just for these exercises. The program must be running during the time you are performing the exercises in this chapter.

Warnings at key steps in the exercises will explain how to detect if the History Program needs to be restarted before you can continue. Instructions for starting this special software is provided in Appendix B.

If your classroom is part of a school network, the program probably is already running. If you reach a point in an exercise when you believe the History Program is not running, alert your instructor and refer to Appendix B in the back of this book.

Disease Management and Prevention

The value of an EHR increases as a practice uses it. As more of the patient's health record is stored in a codified EHR, more can be done with it. Thus far, you have learned how to use an EHR to document patient visits. In this chapter, we will discuss various ways in which data from past visits can be used to improve patient care through disease management, graphic analysis, preventative screening, and interactive alerts.

Flow Sheets

Flow sheets present data from multiple encounters in column form. This format allows for a side-by-side comparison of findings over a period of time. Some clinicians prefer to view a patient chart this way because it is easier to spot trends in the patient's health conditions. It is ideal for chronic disease management such as diabetes or long-term conditions such as pregnancy. OB offices use flow sheets to monitor pregnancy because it affords them a view of the previous visits when documenting the current one. Paper flow sheets have been in use long before they were used in EHR systems. EHR systems just create them without manual labor.

Not all EHR systems implement flow sheets in the same manner, so flow sheets in your medical office may vary from these exercises. Some EHR systems limit flow sheets to lab results or vital signs. However, by using a codified nomenclature, it is possible to create clinical flow sheets that present findings from entire encounters in columns by encounter date. Additionally, there are several different ways for an EHR to create a flow sheet based on a list, a problem, or a form.

Hands-On Exercise 41: Working with a Flow Sheet

In previous exercises, you worked with multiple diagnoses for a single patient. You also have learned that creating and using forms for specific diseases, conditions, or types of visits can speed up data entry because the form presents all of the findings likely to be needed by the clinician for a particular type of exam. This exercise will combine those two concepts and add a third concept, the flow sheet.

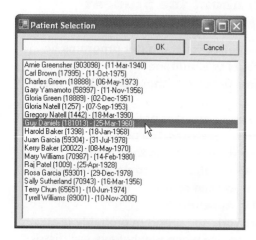

▶ **Figure 7-1 Selecting Guy Daniels from the Patient Selection Window.**

Patients with chronic diseases such as diabetes often develop additional chronic diseases, for example, hypertension, cardiovascular disease, macular degeneration, and a number of other diseases. Rather than try to develop complicated forms that cover different combinations of diseases, a practice can simply develop one form for each. As you will see in this exercise, you can switch forms throughout the exam without reentering findings. Because the forms share the same nomenclature, a finding that is used on both forms automatically displays the entered data when either form is loaded.

In this exercise, a patient with hypertension and borderline diabetes who has been seen quarterly to better manage his health returns for a 3-month check-up. Lab tests have been ordered and performed before his visit. The results were reviewed by the clinician when they arrived electronically earlier today.

Step 1

If you have not already done so, start the Student Edition software.

Click Select on the Menu bar, and then click Patient.

In the Patient Selection window, locate and click on **Guy Daniels**.

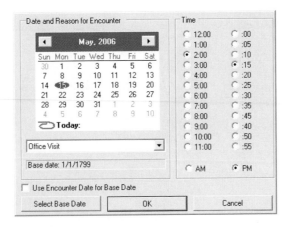

► **Figure 7-2 New Encounter for an Office Visit, May 15, 2006 2:15 PM.**

Step 2

Click Select on the Menu bar, and then click New Encounter.

Select the date **May 15, 2006**, the time **2:15 PM**, and the reason **Office Visit**.

Make certain that you set the date, time, and reason correctly. Compare your screen to Figure 7-2 before clicking on the OK button.

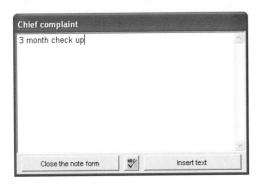

Step 3

Enter the Chief Complaint by locating the button in the toolbar labeled "Chief" and clicking on it.

In the dialog window that will open, type "3 month check up."

Compare your screen to Figure 7-3 and then click on the button labeled "Close the note form."

► **Figure 7-3 Chief Complaint Dialog for 3-Month Check-Up.**

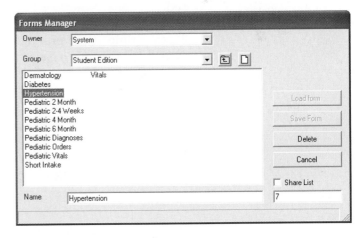

► **Figure 7-4 Active Forms Tab—Select Hypertension Form.**

Step 4

Locate and click on the tab labeled "Active Forms" at the bottom of your screen.

Locate and click on the Forms button in the toolbar at the top of your screen, as you have done in previous exercises.

Select the form labeled "Hypertension;" if it does not load automatically, click on the button labeled "Load Form".

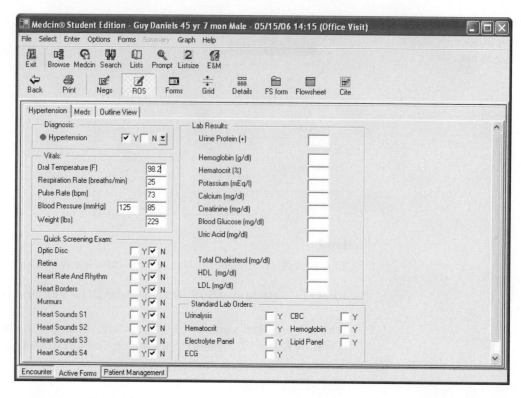

▶ Figure 7-5 Hypertension Form.

Step 5

Locate the Diagnosis Hypertension at the top of the form.

Click the **Y** check box for Hypertension. A circle next to the finding will turn red.

To save time at the practice, the form designer has incorporated the vital signs fields into the first page of the form. Enter the following vital signs for Guy Daniels:

Temperature: **98.2**

Respiration: **25**

Pulse: **73**

BP: **125/85**

Weight: **229**

Step 6

Locate and click on ROS button in the toolbar near the top of your screen. The button should appear depressed.

The clinician performs the Quick Screening exam.

Locate and click the Negs (auto negative) button to quickly document the clinician's physical findings.

Compare your screen to Figure 7-5.

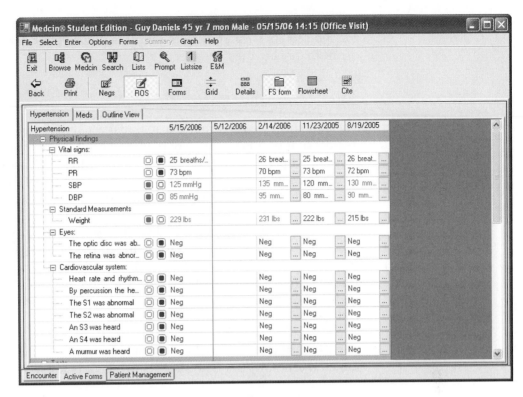

► Figure 7-6 Flow Sheet Based on Hypertension Form.

Step 7

You may have noticed previously that the toolbar near the top of your screen has additional buttons when you are on the Active Forms tab. Two of the buttons are used for invoking the flow sheet view. One button creates a flow sheet based on a form and the other creates a flow sheet based on a problem or list. In this exercise, you will learn to create a flow sheet based on the form.

To invoke the flow sheet view of Guy Daniels's chart, follow these steps:

Click on the button labeled List Size until the list size is set to **1**.

Locate and click on the button labeled "FS Form" in the toolbar near the top of your screen. (The icon resembles a file folder with a grid pattern.)

This button is used to view a flow sheet when you are in the Active Forms tab.

The screen will change to the flow sheet view and the button will appear depressed.

Compare your screen to Figure 7-6 as you read the following information.

! Alert

Important!

If the dated columns on the right of the flow sheet are empty, the Student Edition Patient History program is not running. *Stop the exercise* and notify your instructor. Refer to Appendix B at the end of this book.

If you click on the button again, the form will redisplay. Try it, click on the button labeled FS Form, notice the form is displayed. Click the FS Form button again to display the flow sheet.

About the Flow Sheet View

The flow sheet view resembles a spreadsheet similar to Microsoft Excel® or Lotus 1-2-3®; that is, it is made up of rows and columns of "cells." The first column displays descriptions as well as red and blue buttons for findings on the current form. The date of the current encounter is at the top of the column. The remaining columns to the right display encounter data from previous visits.

The flow sheet rows are grouped vertically into logical sections that match the sections you are accustomed to seeing in the exam note. The title of each section is printed in blue on a teal background. For example, sections in Guy Daniels's flow sheet are titled "Physical Findings" and "Tests," "Assessment," and "Plan." A small plus or minus sign next to the section title allows you to collapse or expand the findings below it.

The list of findings in the first column and how they are displayed is determined by the way the flow sheet is invoked as follows:

FS Form—When a flow sheet is invoked from a form, the software uses the data elements on the form to populate the first column.

Problem—If the flow sheet were invoked instead from the problem list on the Patient Management tab, the first column would be populated with findings pertinent to the selected problem in the problem list.

List—A third type of flow sheet view can be created from a list. When a list is used, the first column of the flow sheet is populated with findings in the list, findings that are within the tree view of the list, and findings of similar body systems.

Step 8

The columns on the right display the dates of previous visits. The cells within the column display the words POS (in red) or NEG (in blue), or a numerical value for the finding. A blank cell indicates no finding was recorded on that encounter date.

Each cell that has a finding recorded can display only one field of data. Where there is more than one type of data (for example, if entry detail fields have been used for a finding) the cell will contain a button with an ellipsis (three dots). Clicking on the ellipsis button will invoke a small window allowing you to view the additional details.

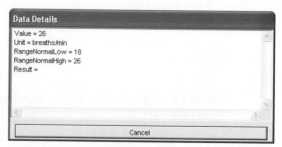

▶ Figure 7-7 Data Details Window Invoked from Ellipsis Button for 02/14/2006 RR.

Try this yourself. Locate the row under vital signs labeled RR (respiration rate); next, locate the column dated 02/14/2006; now position your mouse on the gray ellipsis button in the cell containing the value "26 breaths." Click on the ellipsis button.

A data details window will be invoked, as shown in Figure 7-7.

When you have finished looking at the data details, click on the button labeled cancel to close the data details window.

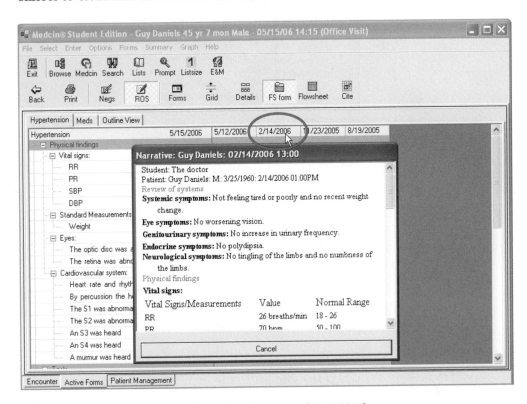

▶ Figure 7-8 Narrative Window of Previous Encounter (02/14/2006).

Step 9

The full exam note for any previous encounter can be viewed by positioning the mouse over the date at the top of any of the columns on the right and clicking the mouse on the date.

Locate and click on the column header date **02/14/2006**.

(Note that you must click on the date itself, not on the row or spaces adjoining it.)

A window displaying the full exam note will be invoked. Compare your screen to Figure 7-8.

Click on the cancel button to close the Narrative window for 2/14/2006.

Step 10

Locate and click on the button labeled "Cite" in the toolbar at the top of your screen. The button icon resembles a teal check mark over a grid. Whenever cite mode is enabled, the Cite button will appear as though it is depressed. (The cite button is circled in red in Figure 7-9.)

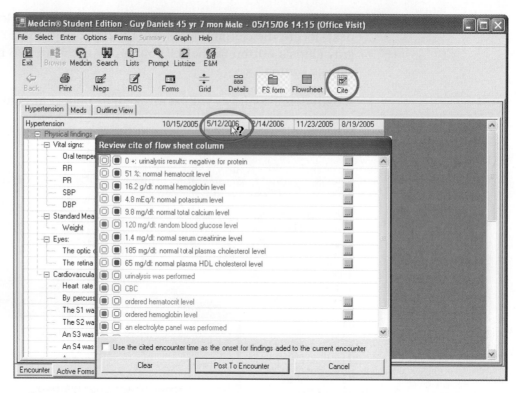

▶ **Figure 7-9 Window Used to Cite Items from Previous Encounter into Current Encounter.**

Cite is used to bring information forward from previous encounters into the current one. The information can be updated as it is brought forward. The findings also could be edited after they are in the current encounter, but the cite feature allows you to bring the finding into the current note and edit it in one step.

Step 11

When the cite button is depressed, clicking on the date of a column header will invoke a different window. The "Review cite" window will list findings from that encounter instead of the encounter narrative. The cite button changes which window is invoked. When the cite button is on, a window of findings is invoked; when it is off, the narrative window is invoked.

When the cite button is **on**, the mouse pointer will change to resemble a large question mark whenever you move over the cells of the flow sheet. If it does not, cite is not on; try clicking on the cite button in the toolbar again.

With the cite button on, position the mouse pointer on the column header date **05/12/2006**, as shown in Figure 7-9, and click the mouse.

(Note that you must click on the date itself, not on the row or spaces adjoining it.)

A window of findings from the May 12, 2006, encounter will be invoked. Compare your screen to Figure 7-9.

The red and blue buttons for each finding are used to select the finding just as they are elsewhere in the software. The description of the finding will include any numerical values entered in the previous encounter. Two additional buttons appear on the right of each finding.

The first is the ellipsis button, which you used in step 7 to view results. However, when cite mode is on, instead of displaying results, the ellipsis button allows you to modify any numerical data when citing the finding. The second button (whose icon resembles a red push-pin in a note pad) is used to add a free text comment to a finding when citing it.

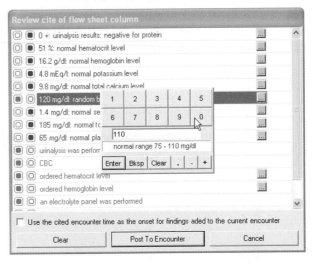

▶ Figure 7-10 Modify Numeric Values of Finding in Cite Window with Ellipsis Button.

Step 12

A new glucose test has been performed.

In the review cite of flow sheet column window, locate and highlight the finding for the "random blood glucose test" result.

Click on the ellipsis button for that finding. A small window resembling a calculator will appear.

Use your mouse to point to the numeric buttons and click on each number to change the previous test result from 120 to the current test result 110.

(Note that you must use the mouse, you cannot type the numbers on a keyboard.)

Click the number buttons **1 1** and **0**, then click on the button labeled "**Enter.**" This will record your modification and close the number pad.

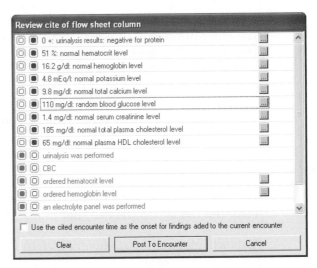

▶ Figure 7-11 Random Blood Glucose Level after Modification.

Step 13

From the cite window you can also select or deselect the red or blue buttons for any of the findings listed. Although it may appear that you are editing a past encounter, you are not. You are simply selecting and editing the findings that will copy to the current encounter. Do not be concerned that this will change any of the findings in a previous encounter.

Compare your screen to Figure 7-11.

Click on the button labeled "Post To Encounter" to cite the findings.

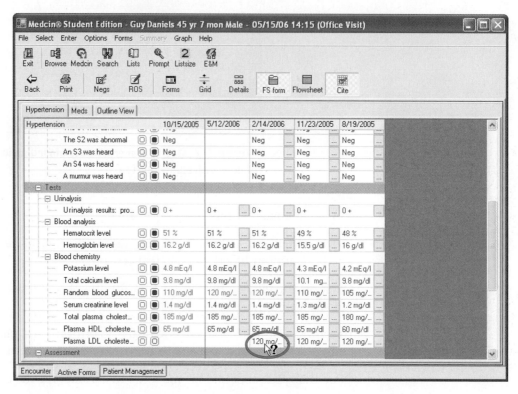

▶ Figure 7-12 Cite the Individual Finding Plasma LDL from the 02/14/2006 Column.

Step 14

Individual findings can be cited without invoking the cite review window. When the cite button is on, instead of positioning the mouse pointer on the date in the column header to invoke a window, you can position the mouse pointer on an individual cell of the flow sheet and click the mouse button. The data from that specific cell will be copied into the current encounter.

Scroll the flow sheet downward until you can see all the rows of the section labeled "Tests."

Locate the finding "Plasma LDL cholesterol" in the last row of that section.

Position your mouse pointer in that row, under the column dated 02/14/2006; click the mouse on the cell that reads "120 mg/dl," as shown in Figure 7-12.

This will cite a normal Plasma LDL in the column for the current encounter.

Locate and click on the button labeled "Cite" in the toolbar at the top of your screen. This will turn cite off.

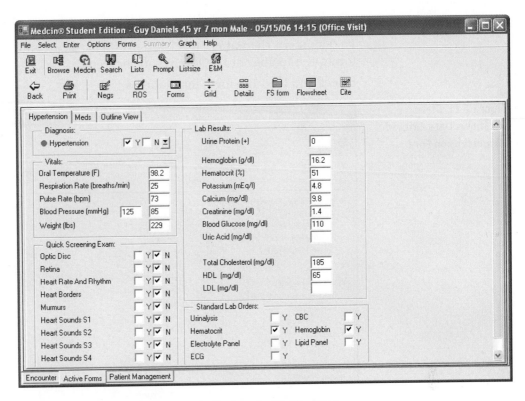

▶ **Figure 7-13 Hypertension Form Redisplayed with Cited Data.**

Step 15

As you learned earlier in this exercise, this FS form button acts like a toggle, shifting the screen between the flow sheet view and the form view.

Locate and click on the button labeled "FS Form" in the toolbar at the top of your screen. The form will redisplay. Compare your screen to Figure 7-13; notice the lab results in the center of the screen now have values that have been filled by using cite.

Here is a brief review of the buttons FS flow and cite:

◆ **FS Flow Off** (button normal) displays the form.

◆ **FS Flow On** (button depressed) displays the flow sheet view.

When the flow sheet is displayed:

◆ **Cite Off** (button normal)—Clicking on a column header date invokes the narrative of that encounter.

◆ **Cite On** (button depressed)—Clicking on a column header date invokes the findings from that encounter, which will be copied forward into today's encounter.

◆ **Cite On** (button depressed)—Clicking on an individual cell will copy only the specific finding forward into today's encounter.

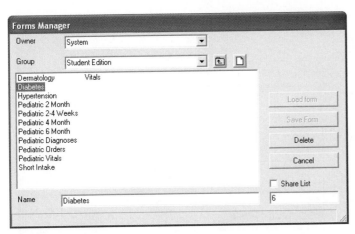

▶ **Figure 7-14 Selecting the Diabetes Form from the Form Manager Window.**

Step 16

To document the patient's second problem, locate and click on the forms button in the toolbar at the top of your screen.

Select and load the form for diabetes.

▶ **Figure 7-15 Diabetes Form Shows Data Entered on Hypertension Form.**

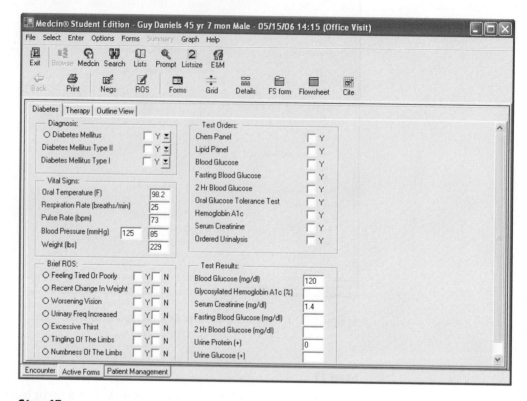

Step 17

Compare your screen to Figure 7-15. Notice that vital signs and several of the fields on the diabetes form already contain data, because these findings were

▶ **Figure 7-16 Setting the Diagnosis Diabetes Mellitus Well Controlled.**

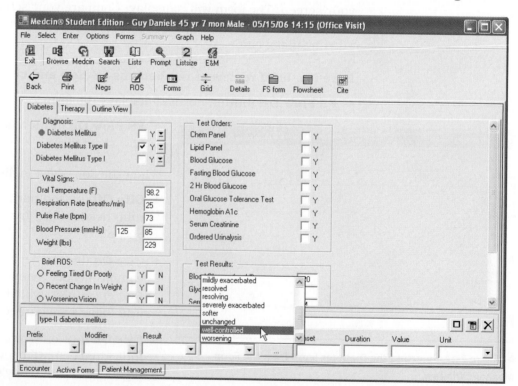

entered on the hypertension form. As mentioned earlier, any findings already in the current encounter will appear automatically as you change forms.

Step 18

Record the second diagnosis.

Locate the diagnosis Diabetes Mellitus Type II at the top of the form. Click on the check box next to the **Y**. A circle next to the finding will turn red.

Locate and click on the button labeled "Details" in the toolbar at the top of your screen. This will open the entry details section over the bottom of the form.

In previous exercises, you have used the details button to hide the details entry fields. In this step, we will display the fields so the status of the disease can be updated.

Locate the status field in the entry details section and click on the down arrow button in the field. Select the status "well controlled" from the drop-down list as shown in Figure 7-16.

Click on the button labeled "Details" in the toolbar at the top of your screen again, to hide the entry details section and to restore the full view of the form.

Step 19

Verify that the ROS button is still depressed, then click on the button labeled negs (auto negative) in the toolbar near the top of your screen.

Compare your screen to Figure 7-17.

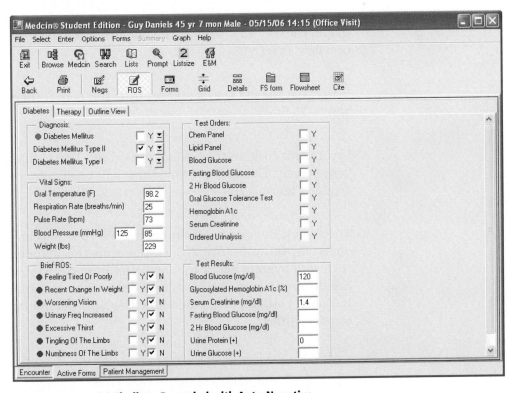

▶ **Figure 7-17 ROS Findings Recorded with Auto-Negative.**

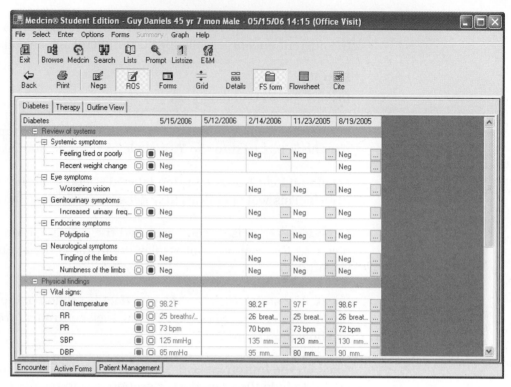

► Figure 7-18 Flow Sheet View Based on Diabetic Form.

Step 20

Not all findings from previous encounters are displayed in a form-based flow sheet. Only those findings that match the items in the form design are listed in the columns. Similarly, flow sheets based on a list only display findings that match the list. This step will demonstrate the difference a form design makes in a flow sheet.

Verify that the list size is still set to **1**; if it is not, then click on it until the list size is 1.

Locate and click on the button labeled "FS Form" in the toolbar at the top of your screen. The diabetes flow sheet will be displayed. Your screen should resemble Figure 7-18.

Turn back in your book and compare your screen with the earlier flow sheet shown in Figure 7-6. Notice that the diabetes flow sheet has a review of system section, which the hypertension does not. There also are differences in the tests ordered for the two diseases. From this comparison, you can easily see how the flow sheets for diabetes and hypertension differ.

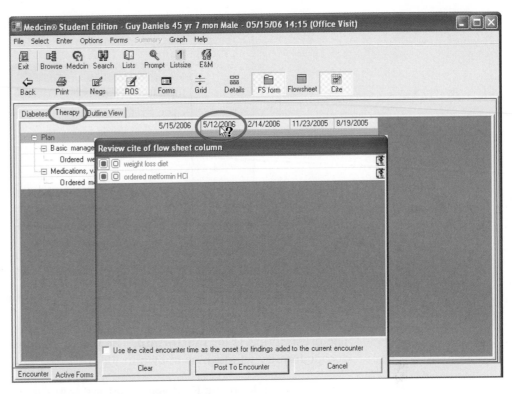

▶ **Figure 7-19 Cite of Therapy Tab Items.**

Step 21

Locate and click on the tab at the top of the diabetes form labeled "Therapy" (circled in red in Figure 7-19).

Locate and click the cite button on as you did early in this chapter (the button will appear depressed).

Locate and click on the column header date **05/12/2006** as you did in a previous step.

A small window of findings from that encounter will appear. Compare your screen to the review cite findings window in Figure 7-19. Notice that because these findings do not have numerical values, the gray ellipsis button is not present.

There also are fewer findings to cite. This is partly because of the items on the form but also because the cite feature is intelligent. It omits items already recorded in the current encounter during previous steps of the exercise.

After you have looked at the findings that are displayed, click the button labeled "Post To Encounter" to cite the findings.

Because one of the items in the list is a prescription, the prescription writer window will be invoked automatically.

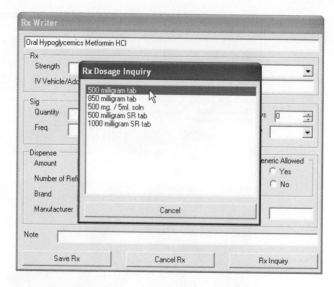

► Figure 7-20 Writing Guy Daniels's Prescription for Metformin HCL.

The prescription is for **metformin**. The prescription writer will display the Rx dosage inquiry window, as shown in Figure 7-20.

Locate and click on the Rx dosage **500 mg tab**; the window will next display a list of manufacturers.

Click on the default manufacturer when that window is displayed.

Locate the section labeled generic allowed and click on the circle next to **Yes**.

Click the button labeled "Save Rx."

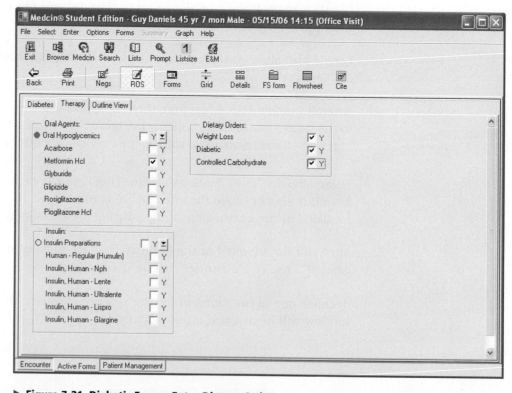

► Figure 7-21 Diabetic Form—Enter Dietary Orders.

Step 22

Locate and click on the button labeled "FS Form" in the toolbar at the top of your screen to return to the view of the form. If the form is not on the therapy tab, locate and click on the tab labeled therapy (at the top of the form).

Locate the section labeled "Dietary Orders" in the upper right corner of the form. Click the check box next to **Y** for the following findings:

✓ **Y** Weight Loss

✓ **Y** Diabetic (diet)

✓ **Y** Controlled Carbohydrate

Compare your screen to Figure 7-21.

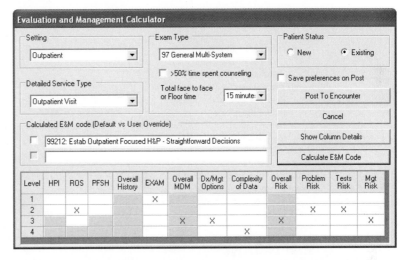

▶ **Figure 7-22 Evaluation and Management Code Calculator for Guy Daniels's Office Visit.**

Step 23

Locate and click on the encounter tab at the bottom of your screen.

Click on the E&M button in the toolbar at the top of your screen.

When the E&M Calculator window is invoked:

Set face-to-face time at **15 Minutes**.

Locate patient status and click on the circle next to existing.

Click the button labeled "Calculate E&M Code."

Compare your screen to Figure 7-22.

Click the button labeled "Post To Encounter."

Guy Daniels   Page 1 of 1

Student: Terry Jones
Patient: Guy Daniels: M: 3/25/1960: 10/15/2005 02:15PM
Chief complaint
The Chief Complaint is: 3 month check up.
Review of systems
Systemic symptoms: Not feeling tired or poorly and no recent weight change.
Eye symptoms: No worsening vision.
Genitourinary symptoms: No increase in urinary frequency.
Endocrine symptoms: No polydipsia.
Neurological symptoms: No tingling of the limbs and no numbness of the limbs.
Physical findings
Vital signs:

Vital Signs/Measurements	Value	Normal Range
Oral temperature	98.2 F	97.6 - 99.6
RR	25 breaths/min	18 - 26
PR	73 bpm	50 - 100
Blood pressure	125/85 mmHg	100-120/60-80
Weight	229 lbs	125 - 225

Eyes:
    General/bilateral:
      Optic Disc: ° Normal.
      Retina: ° Normal.
Cardiovascular system:
    Heart Rate And Rhythm: ° Normal.
    Heart Borders: ° By percussion the heart size and position were normal.
    Heart Sounds: ° S1 was normal. ° S2 was normal. ° No S3 was heard. ° No S4 was heard.
    Murmurs: ° No murmurs were heard.
Tests
Urinalysis Results: Value Normal Range
Urinalysis results: protein   0 + 0 - 0
Hematology:

Hematology:	Value	Normal Range
Hematocrit level	51%	42 - 52
Hemoglobin level	16.2 g/dl	14 - 18

Blood Chemistry:
    An electrolyte panel was performed and a lipid profile was performed.

Blood Chemistry:	Value	Normal Range
Potassium level	4.8 mEq/l	3.5 - 5.5
Total calcium level	9.8 mg/dl	8.5 - 10.5
Random blood glucose level	110 mg/dl	75 - 110
Serum creatinine level	1.4 mg/dl	0.7 - 1.5
Total plasma cholesterol level	185 mg/dl	140 - 200
Plasma HDL cholesterol level	65 mg/dl	30 - 70

    Normal plasma LDL cholesterol level.
Assessment
    • Hypertension
    • Type-II diabetes mellitus which is well-controlled
Counseling/Education

    • Weight loss diet
Plan
    • Hematocrit level
    • Hemoglobin level
    • Random blood glucose level
    • Weight loss diet
    • Diabetic diet
    • Controlled carbohydrate diet
    • Metformin HCl
500 mg tab Generic:Y Using:Glucophage Mfg: Bristol
Practice Management
 Estab outpatient focused h&p - straightforward decisions; Total face to face time 15 min

Step 24

Click File on the Menu bar, and then click Print Encounter or Print To HTML (as directed by your instructor).

If you are printing your work, you may alternatively click the Print button on the toolbar at the top of your screen.

Compare your printout or file output to Figure 7-23. If it is correct, hand it in to your instructor. If there are any differences, review the previous steps in the exercise and find your error.

You may stop at this point or, if time permits, you may continue with the next exercise without exiting.

Hands-On Exercise 42: Creating a Problem-Oriented Flow Sheet

In this exercise, you are going to view a flow sheet that is focused on a particular problem, rather than a form. You will not enter any new data.

Step 1

If you are continuing from the previous exercise, proceed to step 3.

Otherwise, start the Student Edition software.

Click Select on the Menu bar, and then click Patient.

In the Patient Selection window, locate and click on **Guy Daniels**.

Step 2

Click Select on the Menu bar, and then click New Encounter.

Select the date **May 15, 2006**, the time **2:15 PM**, and the reason **Office Visit**.

Make certain you set the date, time, and reason correctly. If necessary, refer to Figure 7-2.

▶ **Figure 7-24 Problem List for Guy Daniels.**

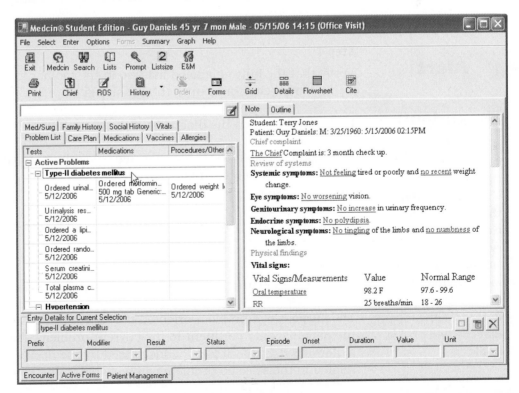

Step 3

Locate and click on the Patient Management tab at the bottom of your screen.

If the information pane on the left of your screen is not already displaying the problem list, click on the tab labeled "Problem List."

(Note that the right pane of Figure 7-24 is showing the exam note as if you were continuing from the previous exercise. If you are not, the right pane will contain less information; that is acceptable for this exercise.)

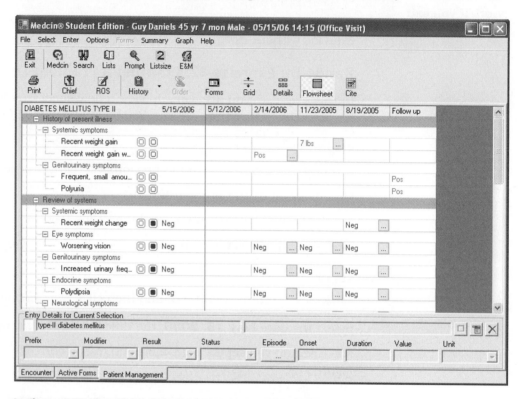

▶ Figure 7-25 Flow Sheet from Problem List for Guy Daniels.

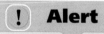 **Alert**

Important!

If the dated columns on the right of the flow sheet are empty, the Student Edition Patient History program is not running. Stop the exercise and notify your instructor. Refer to Appendix B at the end of this book.

Step 4

Verify that the button labeled list size in the toolbar at the top of your screen is 1. If it is not, click on it until the list size is **1**.

Locate and click on the diagnosis diabetes mellitus II in the problem list.

Locate and click on the button labeled "Flowsheet" in the toolbar at the top of your screen. (Note that this is *not* the FS form button that you used in the previous exercise.)

A flow sheet similar to that in Figure 7-25 will be displayed.

Step 5

Turn back to Figure 7-16. Compare your screen to the flow sheet in that figure.

The purpose of a problem-oriented flow sheet is to provide a historical view of the patient's data pertinent to the current problem. The difference in this type of flow sheet is that it is not constrained by the design of the form. Any finding related to the selected problem will be listed in the flow sheet.

The function of the cite button is the same in either flow sheet. That is, cite can be used to copy relevant findings into the current encounter.

As you learned in the previous chapter, most clinicians use a problem list at some point during the examination. The ability to quickly view and cite from a flow sheet specific to the problem not only can speed up the documentation process but also can ensure that the clinician recalls significant findings from previous visits.

The comparison of the problem-oriented flow sheet with the flow sheets base on the diabetes form concludes this exercise. You may exit the software, or if time permits, continue with the next exercise.

Patient Involvement in Their Own Health Care

Patients must become involved in their own health care to effectively manage and prevent diseases. In this exercise, a chart of the patient's weight measurements will be created and used for patient education; this might stimulate the patient to keep his own chart at home.

Hands-On Exercise 43: Graphing Vital Signs in the Chart

As discussed in Chapter 6, the ability to graph numeric findings is one advantage gained from a codified EHR. Not only are graphs useful to the clinician, but also they provide an excellent means of clarification when counseling patients.

In Exercise 40, you learned to graph a specific finding by locating it using the search tool. The graph menu allows the clinician to instantly create graphs of several key measurements without having to locate a specific finding. In Exercise 41, several of the doctor's orders concerned Mr. Daniels's weight. In this exercise, you will create a graph of the patient's weight for Mr. Daniels to take home with him. You will not enter any new data.

Step 1

If you are continuing from the previous exercise, proceed to step 2.

Otherwise, start the Student Edition software.

Click Select on the Menu bar, and then click Patient.

In the Patient Selection window, locate and click on **Guy Daniels**.

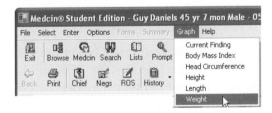

▶ Figure 7-26 Select Weight from the Graph Menu.

Step 2

Click the word "Graph" on the Menu bar, and then click "Weight" on the list of menu options.

A graph of the patient's weight measurements from previous visits is instantly displayed. You do not have to select a finding or even load an existing encounter.

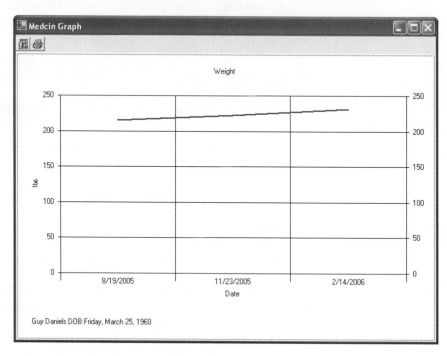

▶ **Figure 7-27 Graph of Change in Guy Daniels's Weight.**

Step 3

Compare your screen to Figure 7-27.

Locate and click on the print button in the upper left corner of the graph window to print the graph. When you have printed a copy, write your name on it and hand it in to your instructor.

Click on the exit button in the window displaying the weight graph.

You may also Exit the Student Edition software at this point.

Patient-Entered Data Graphs

Other vital signs such as blood pressure readings from quarterly office visits also can be graphed by the EHR software. However, it is not unusual for hypertensive patients to monitor their blood pressure at home and keep a log of daily readings that they bring to the doctor's office when they have a check-up.

Dr. Allen Wenner provides a spreadsheet template to patients who have Microsoft Excel on their home computers. The template is available on his Web site or on a diskette. He encourages them to record their daily blood pressure in an Excel workbook instead of on paper, and to bring or e-mail a copy of the workbook file when they come to his office.

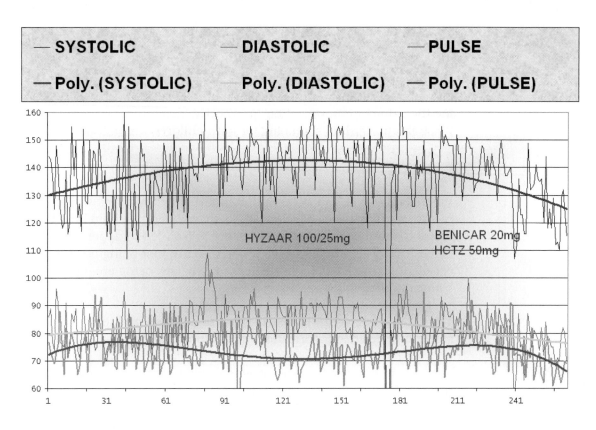

▶ **Figure 7-28 Graph of Blood Pressure Readings from February to May.**

During the patient's office visit, the clinician and the patient discuss the graph of the daily blood pressure readings compared with the regimen of blood pressure medicine. The physician tells the patient what are the parameters of control, for example, 140/90 for most patients and 130/80 for diabetics. The patient also can view the graph at home as he builds it with his own data. Following the graph on his home computer, the patient knows whether the therapy is working.

Figure 7-28 shows a graph created in Excel by Dr. Wenner and his patient. Notice during the Hyzaar treatment that the patient's blood pressure is tending higher than 140 over 90. The graph indicates the medication needs to be changed. After the doctor shows the patient how to read the graph during the office visit, the patient understands the normal and abnormal range. The patient knows when to call the physician for advice rather than wait until the next appointment. This shared information results in shared decision making. The interaction is transformed from one of gathering information to one of managing the patient's problem. Patients can now look actively at issues of the illness, the treatment regime, and the desired outcome.

This is an example of patients using technology to improve blood pressure management. Research has shown that controlling blood pressure will reduce stroke, heart attack, and vascular disease. Nearly 200 medications are approved for use. There is a combination of drugs that will work for most patients without side effects. Currently in the United States, only about one-third of hypertensive patients have their illness under good control. A number of reasons contribute to this, but increased patient involvement can improve their health.

Prevention and Early Detection

As we have seen in the previous section, patient participation in their health care, education, and counseling can help them to live healthier lives. Still, it is always better to prevent a disease than to treat it. In this section, we will examine the value of immunization, preventive measures, and early detection through appropriate screening for both children and adults.

Pediatric Wellness Visits

Whereas those of us who are adults may someday have an electronic health record, we may never have a completely codified personal health record, because too much of our medical history is isolated in paper records at medical offices that we no longer visit. Those who are just being born, however, have an excellent chance that their medical records are being created and stored electronically even today.

The care we receive in the early years is fundamental to lifelong health. Early screening, detection, education, and immunizations have all contributed to increased life spans of the population as a whole. Nowhere does this have more support than in the pediatric practice, where regular examinations are recommended for wellness visits, not just illness visits.

In the next exercises, you will use the Student Edition software to enter a pediatric visit, create a different kind of graph called a growth chart, and learn about childhood immunizations. This is a lot of material to cover and for that reason the pediatric visit will span several exercises.

Hands-On Exercise 44: A Well-Baby Check-Up

Step 1

If you have not already done so, start the Student Edition software.

Click Select on the Menu bar, and then click Patient.

In the Patient Selection window, locate and click on **Tyrell Williams**.

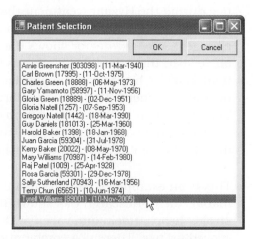

▶ **Figure 7-29 Selecting Tyrell Williams from the Patient Selection Window.**

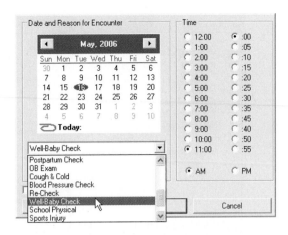

▶ **Figure 7-30 New Encounter for a Well-Baby Check, May 16, 2006 11:00 AM.**

Step 2

Click Select on the Menu bar, and then click New Encounter.

Use the date **May 16, 2006**, the time **11:00 AM**, and the reason **Well-Baby Check**.

Make certain you set the date, time, and reason correctly. (You will need to scroll the drop-down list of reasons to find Well-Baby Check.)

Compare your screen to Figure 7-30 before clicking on the OK button.

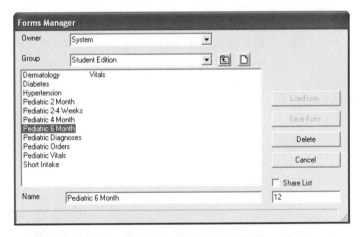

▶ **Figure 7-31 Selecting the Pediatric 6-Month from the Form Manager Window.**

Step 3

Locate and click on the tab labeled "Active Forms" at the bottom of your screen.

Locate and click on the forms button in the toolbar at the top of your screen, as you have done in previous exercises.

Notice that there are several pediatric forms. Because there are different developmental milestones and, therefore, different questions appropriate to different ages, pediatric practices typically have a form for each age-appropriate visit. In an actual pediatric practice, there would be more forms than are shown in the Student Edition.

Locate and click on the form labeled "Pediatric 6 Month." If it does not load automatically, click on the button labeled "Load Form."

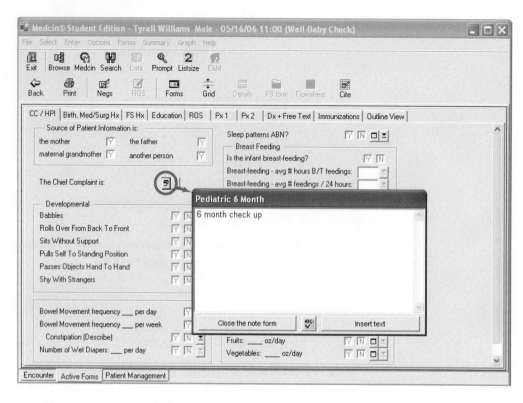

▶ Figure 7-32 Pediatric Form—CC/HPI Tab with Chief Complaint Dialogue Invoked.

Step 4

The pediatric form will be displayed. Take a moment to orient yourself. You will notice that there are quite a few tabs on the form.

Well-Baby check-ups are usually quite extensive, and involve the social history of the parents as well as of the baby. This form contains the items a practice might cover during a check-up for a 6-month-old baby. In the interest of time, you will not enter data for every question, although you would in an actual medical office.

Whereas practices seeing patients with chronic illnesses might use several different forms for a patient visit, the designer of this pediatric form has tried to combine in one form all the elements required for a well-baby visit. For example, the form has a button for the chief complaint imbedded in the form, and the vital signs also are imbedded in the form. This type of design allows the nurses and pediatricians to move right through the exam, ensuring that nothing is forgotten or overlooked.

Step 5

Locate the finding in the form labeled "The Chief Complaint is:"

Click on the note button to the right of the finding (circled in red in Figure 7-32). The chief complaint dialog window will be invoked.

In the dialog window, type "6 month check up."

Compare your screen to Figure 7-32, then click on the button labeled "Close the note form."

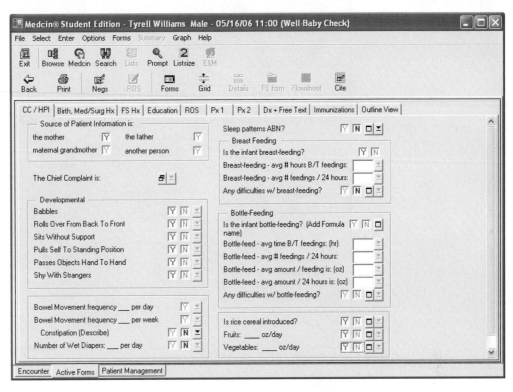

▶ **Figure 7-33 Pediatric Form—HPI Findings Recorded with Auto-Negative.**

Step 6

The first question asks for the source of information. Tyrell is accompanied by his mother. Click your mouse in the check box:

✓ **Y** "the mother"

Locate and click the button labeled "Negs" (auto negative) in the toolbar at the top of your screen.

Locate and click on the check box for sleep patterns on the top right of the form:

✓ **N** Sleep Patterns ABN

Step 7

Complete the HPI by clicking the indicated check boxes for the following findings about the patient's feeding:

✓ **Y** Breastfeeding

✓ **N** Difficulties breastfeeding

✓ **Y** Rice cereal introduced

✓ **Y** Fruits

✓ **Y** Vegetables

Compare your screen to Figure 7-33.

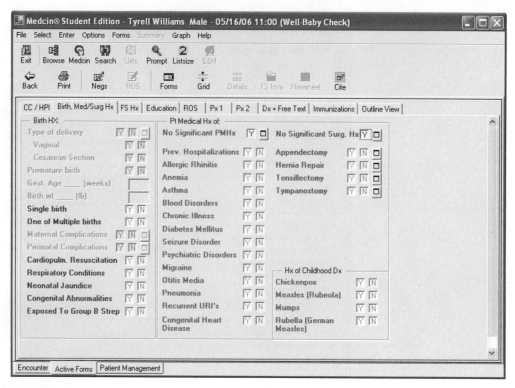

Step 8

Locate and click on the tab labeled "Birth, Med/Surg Hx" at the top of the form.

Tyrell has no pervious medical or surgical history. This is indicated by findings at the top of the middle and right columns, as shown in Figure 7-34. Locate and click on the following check boxes:

✓ **Y** No significant PM Hx

✓ **Y** No significant Surg Hx

Compare your screen to Figure 7-34.

► Figure 7-35 Family and
Social History Tab.

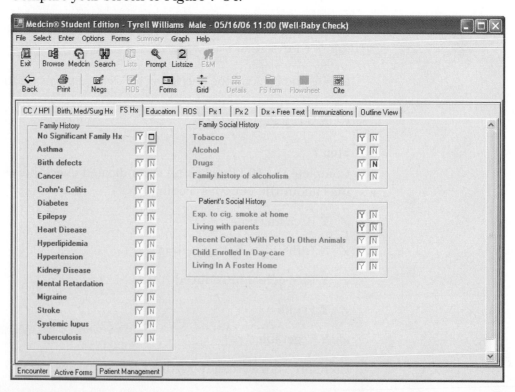

Step 9

Locate and click on the tab labeled "FS Hx" at the top of the form.

FS Hx stands for Family and Social History. In pediatric visits, the parent's social habits and environment are seen as influences that can affect the child. This page of the form is used to record findings about the family history, the child's environment, and the parents' behavioral habits. The Family Social history section is not asking if the baby uses tobacco, alcohol, or drugs, but if the parents do.

Locate and click on the check boxes as indicated for the following findings:

Family History:

✓ **Y** No significant Family Hx

Family Social History:

✓ **Y** Tobacco

✓ **Y** Alcohol

✓ **N** Drugs

Patient's Social History:

✓ **Y** Exposure to cig. smoke at home

✓ **Y** Living with parents

Compare your screen to Figure 7-35.

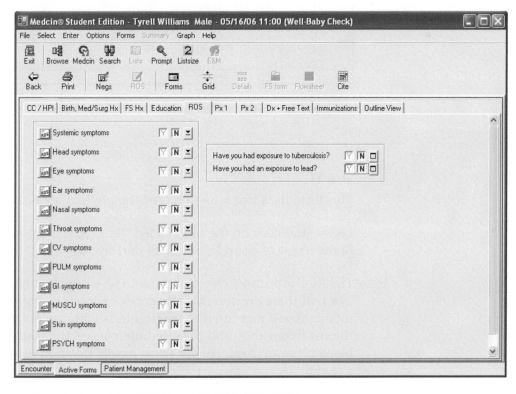

▶ **Figure 7-36 ROS Finding Recorded with Auto-Negative.**

Step 10

Locate and click on the tab labeled "ROS" at the top of the form.

Locate and click the button labeled "Negs" (auto negative) in the toolbar at the top of your screen.

Complete the ROS by clicking the check boxes for the following findings:

✓ **N** "Have you had exposure to tuberculosis"

✓ **N** "Have you had exposure to lead"

Compare your screen to Figure 7-36.

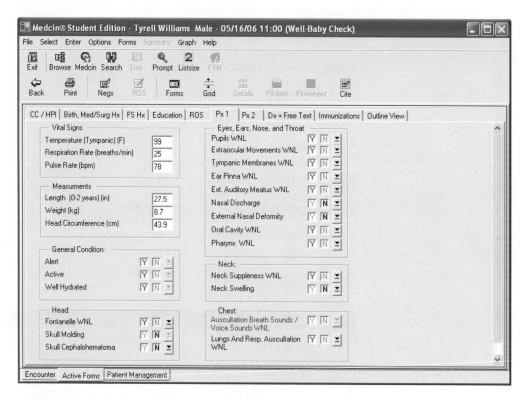

▶ **Figure 7-37 The First of Two Px Tabs Includes Vital Signs.**

Step 11

This form uses two tabs to record the physical exam.

Locate and click on the tab labeled "Px 1" at the top of the form. The first page of the physical exam form will be displayed.

The Px 1 tab allows the vital signs to be entered without leaving the form. Notice that there are several differences between pediatric and adult vital signs: infant growth measured in length not height, the temperature is measured in the ear (tympanic), and the circumference of the head is also recorded. Also, blood pressure readings are not typically taken in healthy children under the age of 3.

Enter the following measurements for Tyrell in the corresponding vital signs:

Temperature: **99**

Respiration Rate: **25**

Pulse: **78**

Length (in.): **27.5**

Weight (kg.): **8.7**

Head circumference (cm.): **43.9**

Click the button labeled "Negs" (auto negative) in the toolbar at the top of your screen to record the rest of the physical exam findings for this page.

Compare your screen with Figure 7-37.

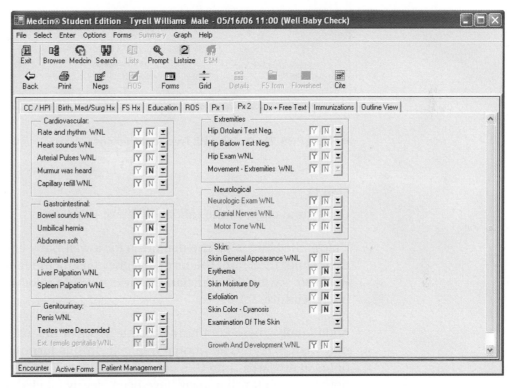

▶ **Figure 7-38 The Second Px Tab Completes the Physical Exam.**

Step 12

Record the remainder of the physical exam.

Locate and click on the tab labeled "Px 2" at the top of the form. The second page of the physical exam form will be displayed.

Click the button labeled "Negs" (auto negative) in the toolbar at the top of your screen to record the rest of the physical exam findings that are on this page.

Compare your screen with Figure 7-38.

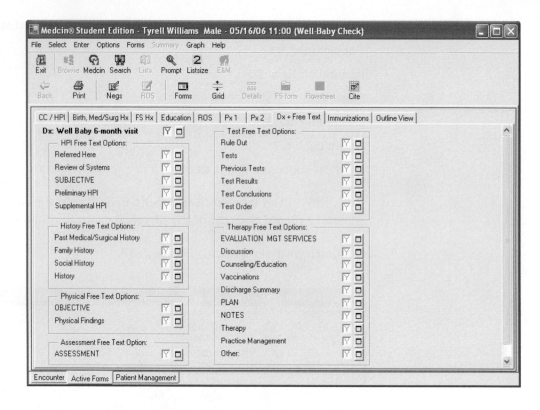

► **Figure 7-39 The Dx Tab with Free-Text Findings**

Step 13

Locate and click on the tab labeled "Dx + Free Text" at the top of the form.

Unless the child is ill, the diagnosis for a well-baby check-up is the same for each child; therefore, the form designer has included an option to record it via the form, saving the clinician the time it would take to search the nomenclature.

Additionally, there are many possible areas of the exam in which the pediatrian may wish to record additional free text. In this form, the clinician can add notes to any area from this one tab. The type of finding and the section of the note in which it will appear have been clearly labeled for the clinician.

Locate and click on the check box for the diagnosis:

✓ **Y** Dx Well Baby 6-Month Visit

Compare your screen to Figure 7-39.

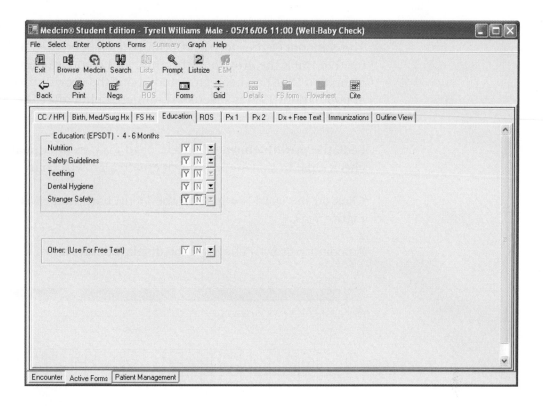

Step 14

During well-baby visits, the pediatrician provides educational information to the mother about the child's development, nutrition, immunizations, and safety.

Locate and click on the tab labeled "Education" at the top of the form.

Enter Y for each of the following to indicate that these points were covered during the visit:

✓ **Y** for Nutrition

✓ **Y** for Safety Guidelines

✓ **Y** for Teething

✓ **Y** for Dental Hygiene

✓ **Y** for Stranger Safety

Compare your screen to Figure 7-40.

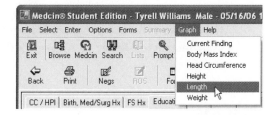

► Figure 7-41 Select Length from Graph Menu to Generate a Growth Chart.

Step 15

The National Center for Health Statistics has created a set of graphs that are used to track the growth of the child and compare him or her to statistical information that has been gathered about the growth rate of babies in the general population. This is discussed in more detail after the conclusion of this exercise.

Pediatric growth charts often are used for parent education during well-baby check-ups. In this step, you will create a growth chart for Tyrell Williams.

Click on the word "Graph" on the Menu bar, then click "Length" as shown in Figure 7-41.

A pediatric growth chart will be displayed, as shown in Figure 7-42.

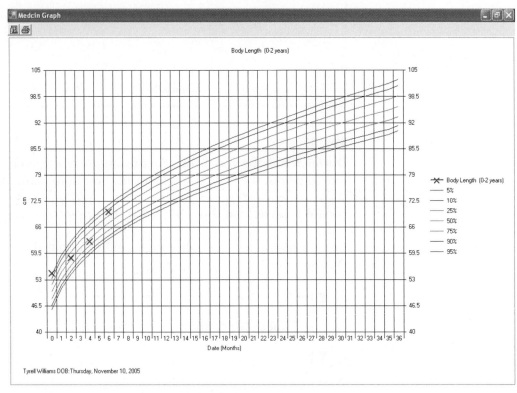

▶ Figure 7-42 Growth Chart for Tyrell Williams.

> **Alert**
>
> ## Important!
>
> **If you receive a message that there are no results to graph, the Student Edition Patient History program is not running. *Stop the exercise* and notify your instructor. Refer to Appendix B at the end of this book.**

Step 16

Review the growth chart for Tyrell Williams displayed on your screen. The blue X marks the patient's length at the various months, listed across the bottom of the graph. The curved lines represent the comparable growth rate as a percentage of the general population. This is called the percentile, which will be defined later. Similar growth charts also can be generated for a child's weight and head circumference.

Click on the Print button in the upper left corner of the graph window to print the growth chart. When you have printed a copy, write your name on it and give it into your instructor.

Click on the Exit button in the window displaying the growth chart.

This concludes Exercise 44. You may print the patient exam note, or you may exit the Student Edition software without printing (as directed by your instructor). Read the following information about Pediatric Growth Charts.

The Relation Between Vitals and Growth Charts

A patient's vital signs can be compared against statistical information of the general population. Comparing the height and weight measurements from the EHR to a series of growth charts is useful in two areas: measuring the growth rate of children, and fighting obesity in our society by determining if a person's weight is appropriate for their height.

Pediatric growth charts have been used by pediatricians, nurses, and parents to track the growth of infants, children, and adolescents in the United States since 1977. The 1977 growth charts were developed by the National Center for Health Statistics (NCHS) as a clinical tool for health professionals to determine if the growth of a child is adequate. The 1977 charts also were adopted by the World Health Organization (WHO) for international use.

Today, 16 pediatric growth charts are maintained and distributed by the CDC (eight for boys and eight for girls). The charts were revised in 2000, when two new charts were added. The new charts are body mass index-for-age for boys and girls ages 2 to 20 years. Body mass index is explained later.

What Is a Percentile?

Figure 7-43 shows one of the CDC growth charts; this actually combines two graphs on one page. The age of the child is indicated horizontally across the top of the graph and the height and weight measurements are listed vertically down the sides of the graph. The curved blue lines printed across the face of the graph are called percentiles. The curved lines represent what percent of the reference population the individual would equal or exceed. This graph includes the 5th through 95th percentiles; the CDC also has a version available that widens the spectrum by showing a 3rd and 97th percentile.

The patient's weight and height measurements can be marked on the chart under each age for which readings are available. By finding the percentile line closest to the patient's vitals, the clinician can assess the size and growth patterns of the individual as compared to other children in the United States.

For example, a 2-year-old boy whose weight is at the 25th percentile weighs the same or more than 25 percent of the reference population of 2-year-old boys but weighs less than 75 percent of the 2-year-old boys.

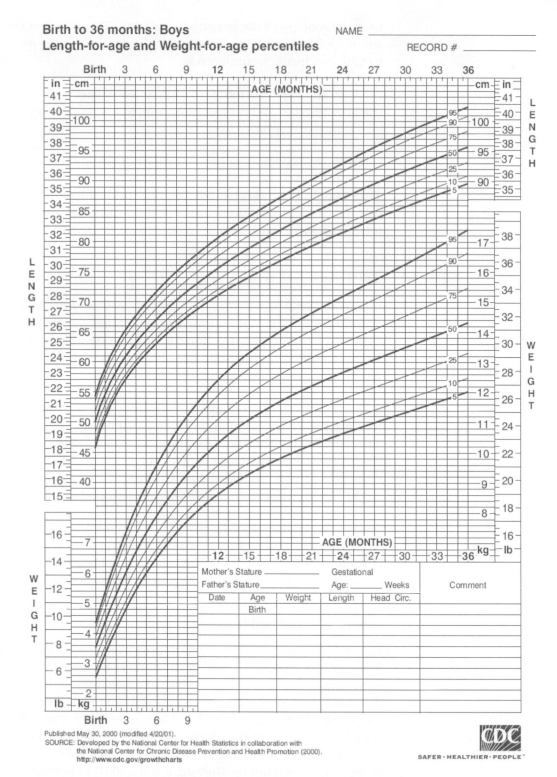

Birth to 36 months: Boys
Length-for-age and Weight-for-age percentiles

NAME _____

RECORD # _____

Published May 30, 2000 (modified 4/20/01).
SOURCE: Developed by the National Center for Health Statistics in collaboration with
the National Center for Chronic Disease Prevention and Health Promotion (2000).
http://www.cdc.gov/growthcharts

▶ **Figure 7-43 Boys Birth–36 Months Length-for-Age/Weight-for-Age Growth Chart.**

When vital signs are routinely entered in an EHR, those measurements can be used to create graphs and, in the case of children, to compare them to a reference population of other children. Most EHR systems have the ability to graph those measurements over an image of the CDC percentiles, as you have done in the previous exercise. Using the age of the patient, the EHR software determines if the graph should include the CDC growth chart. Because the growth charts are gender-specific, the software also uses the child's sex to determine which growth chart to display.

Body Mass Index

BMI stands for Body Mass Index. It is a number that shows body weight adjusted for height. BMI can be calculated with simple math (wt/ht2) using inches and pounds or meters and kilograms. BMI is gender-specific and age-specific for children. BMI-for-age is the measure used for ages 2 to 20 years, as BMI changes substantially as children get older. The CDC encourages pediatricians to replace usage of the older weight-for-stature charts with the new BMI-for-age charts.

There are several advantages to using BMI-for-age as a screening tool for overweight and underweight children. BMI-for-age provides a reference for adolescents, which was not available previously. Another advantage is that BMI-for-age is the measure that is consistent with the adult index, so BMI can be used continuously from 2 years of age to adulthood. This is important, as BMI in childhood is a determinant of adult BMI.[1]

A single BMI chart is used for adults of both genders age 20 years or older. Adult BMI falls into one of four categories: underweight, normal, overweight, or obese.

Optional Exercise 45: Calculate Your Own BMI

Because BMI is a useful measurement for adults as well as children, you may have an interest in seeing how you measure up. This exercise is completely optional and will not affect your grade.

Step 1

If you have access to the Internet, go to this Web site:

http://www.cdc.gov/nccdphp/dnpa/bmi/calc-bmi.htm

Step 2

Follow the on-screen instructions.

The Importance of Childhood Immunizations[2]

Immunization slows down or stops disease outbreaks. Vaccines prevent disease in the people who receive them and protect those who come into contact with unvaccinated individuals.

Although it is true that newborn babies are immune to many diseases because they have antibodies they obtained from their mothers, the duration of this immunity may last only a month to about a year. If a child is not vaccinated and is exposed to a disease germ, the child's body may not be strong enough to fight the disease. Before vaccines, many children died from diseases that vaccines now prevent.

Through childhood immunization, we are now able to control many infectious diseases that were once common in this country, including polio, measles, diphtheria, pertussis (whooping cough), rubella (German measles), mumps, tetanus, and Haemophilus influenzae type b (Hib).

---

[1]http://www.cdc.gov; U.S. Department of Health and Human Services, Centers for Disease Control Web site.
[2]Ibid.

Hands-On Exercise 46: Immunizations

One of the things a pediatrician does during the first two years of well-baby check-ups is to compare the child's immunization history against a recommended schedule of immunizations. At regular intervals, the well baby will receive one or more vaccines. By the age of 2 years, the child is then protected against a vast array of diseases that once the caused the death of many children.

When the pediatrician uses an EHR system, the information from all previous immunizations is readily at hand. The clinician can then easily order the next scheduled vaccines appropriate to the patient's age and vaccine history.

In commercial EHR systems, the next recommended immunizations can be calculated and displayed automatically. The Student Edition software does not have the ability to calculate this for you, but the EHR system you will use in a medical office quite likely will be able to do so.

In this exercise, you will use the patient management tab to verify what immunizations the child has had, and in the next step you will order vaccines that are required.

Step 1

If you have not already done so, start the Student Edition software.

Click Select on the Menu bar, and then click Patient.

In the Patient Selection window, locate and click on **Tyrell Williams** as you have previously (see Figure 7-29).

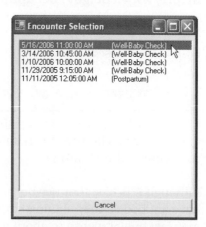

▶ Figure 7-44 Select Existing Encounter for May 16, 2006 11:00 AM.

Step 2

In this exercise, you are going to retrieve and work with an encounter for the well-baby check-up that began in Exercise 44.

Click Select on the Menu bar, and then click Existing Encounter.

Position your mouse pointer on the first encounter in the list, dated **May 16, 2006 11:00 AM** and click on it (as shown in Figure 7-44.)

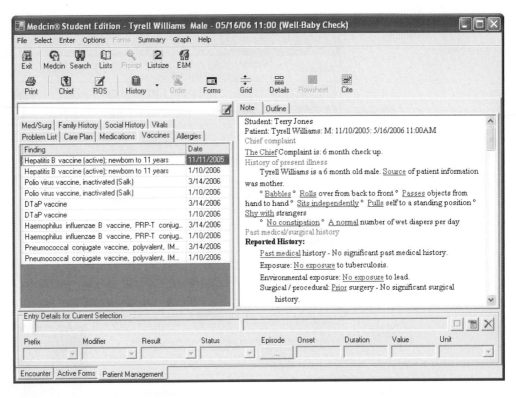

▶ **Figure 7-45** Patient Management Vaccines Tab History for Tyrell Williams.

Step 3

The right pane will display the encounter from Exercise 44.

Locate and click on the tab labeled "Patient Management" at the bottom of your screen. Click on the tab labeled vaccines.

The vaccine list can be sorted in two ways. If you click the mouse on the column header labeled "finding," the vaccines are sorted into groups, allowing you to see easily how many doses have been given of each vaccine. If you click the mouse on the column header for date, the list will be reordered so that you can see exactly which vaccines were administered during each well-baby check-up.

Click the mouse on the column header labeled "finding" so that the vaccines are sorted by type. Compare your screen to Figure 7-45.

(!) Alert

Important!

If the vaccine tab does not have data, the Student Edition Patient History program is not running. *Stop the exercise* and notify your instructor. Refer to Appendix B at the end of this book.

Immunization Schedules from the CDC

Immunizations must be acquired over time. Vaccines cannot be given all at once. Several require repeated applications over a period of time, and some such as the measles vaccine cannot be given to children under the age of 1 year. Therefore, the CDC and state health departments have designed a schedule to immunize children and adolescents from birth through 18 years.

Recommended Childhood and Adolescent Immunization Schedule UNITED STATES • 2005

Vaccine ▼ Age ▶	Birth	1 month	2 months	4 months	6 months	12 months	15 months	18 months	24 months	4–6 years	11–12 years	13–18 years
Hepatitis B	HepB#1	HepB #2			HepB #3					HepB Series		
Diphtheria, Tetanus, Pertussis			DTaP	DTaP	DTaP		DTaP			DTaP	Td	Td
Haemophilus influenzae type b			Hib	Hib	Hib	Hib						
Inactivated Poliovirus			IPV	IPV	IPV					IPV		
Measles, Mumps, Rubella						MMR #1				MMR#2	MMR #2	
Varicella						Varicella					Varicella	
Pneumococcal Conjugate			PCV	PCV	PCV	PCV				PCV / PPV		
Influenza					Influenza (Yearly)					Influenza (Yearly)		
Hepatitis A										Hepatitis A Series		

Vaccines below red line are for selected populations

This schedule indicates the recommended ages for routine administration of currently licensed childhood vaccines, as of December 1, 2004, for children through age 18 years. Any dose not given at the recommended age should be given at any subsequent visit when indicated and feasible.

Indicates age groups that warrant special effort to administer those vaccines not previously given. Additional vaccines may be licensed and recommended during the year. Licensed combination vaccines may be used whenever any components of the combination are indicated and the vaccine's other components are not contraindicated. Providers should consult the manufacturers' package inserts for detailed recommendations. Clinically significant adverse events that follow immunization should be reported to the Vaccine Adverse Event Reporting System (VAERS). Guidance about how to obtain and complete a VAERS form can be found on the Internet: www.vaers.org or by calling 800-822-7967.

Range of recommended ages
Preadolescent assessment
Only if mother HBsAg(–)
Catch-up immunization

DEPARTMENT OF HEALTH AND HUMAN SERVICES
CENTERS FOR DISEASE CONTROL AND PREVENTION
The Childhood and Adolescent Immunization Schedule is approved by:
Advisory Committee on Immunization Practices www.cdc.gov/nip/acip
American Academy of Pediatrics www.aap.org
American Academy of Family Physicians www.aafp.org

More information regarding vaccine administration can be obtained from the websites above or by calling
800-CDC-INFO
ENGLISH & ESPAÑOL
[800-232-4636]

Keep track of your child's immunizations with the
CDC Childhood Immunization Scheduler
www.cdc.gov/nip/kidstuff/scheduler.htm

▶ **Figure 7-46 Immunization Schedule from the CDC.**

Figure 7-46 shows the immunization schedule recommended by the CDC for children and adolescents. Age categories are shown across the top of the schedule. The full names of recommended vaccine combinations are shown down the left column. An abbreviation for the vaccine name is shown within the grid under the ideal age at which it should be administered.

Yellow bars within the grid indicate the ideal interval at which a particular series should be completed. Green bars indicate the ages that should be given special attention if the series has not been completed. The fact that colored bars extend over multiple age categories indicates the flexibility that is built into the recommended schedule.

For example, the chart shows that the CDC recommends that infants should receive the first dose of Hepatitis B vaccine (HepB) soon after birth and ideally before hospital discharge. The second dose would be administered at least 4 weeks after the first dose. The third dose should be given at least 16 weeks after the first dose and at least 8 weeks after the second dose. The last dose in the vaccination series (third or fourth dose) should not be administered before the age of 24 weeks.

Step 4

Compare the vaccine list on your screen to the CDC schedule, as shown in Figure 7-46. Notice the following:

Tyrell was born November 10, 2005.

He had his first dose of Hepatitis B (HepB) before leaving the hospital on 11/11/2005.

He had his second dose during his 2-month check-up on 01/10/2006.
He could receive his third dose during this visit or at his 12-month visit.

Compare his DTaP (Diphtheria, Tetanus, Pertussis) vaccines to the CDC schedule.
He had his first dose of DTaP during his 2-month check-up on 01/10/2006.
He had his second dose during his 4-month check-up on 03/14/2006.
He is due for his third dose during this visit.

Compare his Haemophilus Influenza Type B (Hib) doses to the CDC schedule.
He had his first dose of Hib during his 2-month check-up on 01/10/2006.
He had his second dose during his 4-month check-up on 03/14/2006.
He is due for his third dose during this visit.

Compare his IPV (Inactivated Polio Virus) doses to the CDC schedule.
He had his first dose IPV during his 2-month check-up on 01/10/2006.
He had his second dose during his 4-month check-up on 03/14/2006.
He is due for his third dose during this visit.

Compare his Pneumococcal Conjugate (PCV) doses to the CDC schedule.
He had his first dose of PCV during his 2-month check-up on 01/10/2006.
He had his second dose during his 4-month check-up on 03/14/2006.
He is due for his third dose during this visit.

Of the vaccines remaining on the CDC schedule, he is too young for the Varicella vaccine as well as the Measles, Mumps, Rubella (MMR) vaccine, which is not administered before 12 months.

He is old enough for a flu shot, but the office visit occurs in May and annual flu shots are not available until fall.

Step 5

Now that the clinician has a clear picture of the patient's immunization needs, they can be ordered and administered.

Locate and click on the tab labeled "Active Forms" at the bottom of your screen.

Locate and click on the forms button in the toolbar at the top of your screen as you have done in Exercise 44.

Locate and click on the form labeled "Pediatric 6 Month." If it does not load automatically, click on the button labeled "Load Form" (see Figure 7-31).

Step 6

Locate and click on the tab labeled "Immunizations" at the top of the form.

Locate the section labeled "Vaccines at 6 Months" and click the check box for each of the following:

✓ **Y** DTaP (dose 3)

✓ **Y** Haemophilus influenzae B (dose 3)

✓ **Y** IPV (dose 3)

✓ **Y** Pneumococcal conjugate (dose 3)

Compare your screen to Figure 7-47.

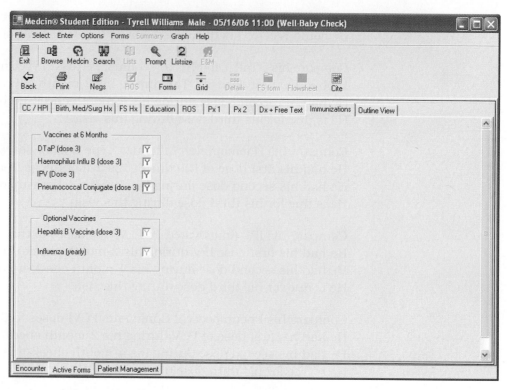

▶ Figure 7-47 Pediatric 6-Month Form—Immunization Tab.

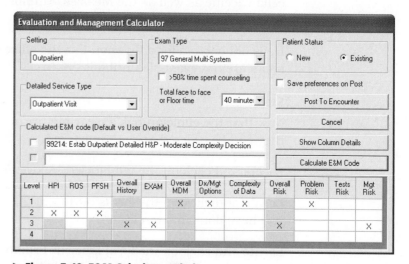

▶ Figure 7-48 E&M Calculator Window.

Step 7

Locate and click on the tab labeled "Encounter" at the bottom of your screen.

Locate and click on the button labeled "E&M" in the toolbar at the top of your screen. The E&M Calculator window will be invoked.

In the E&M Calculator window, set Face-to-face time at **40 Minutes**.

For Patient Status, click Existing.

Click the button labeled "Calculate E&M Code."

Compare your screen to Figure 7-48 and then click the button labeled "Post To Encounter."

Student: Terry Jones
Patient: Tyrell Williams: M: 11/10/2005: 5/16/2006 11:00AM
Chief complaint
The Chief Complaint is: 6 month check up.
History of present illness
    Tyrell Williams is a 6 month old male. Source of patient information was mother.
    ° Babbles ° Rolls over from back to front ° Passes objects from hand to hand
    ° Sits independently ° Pulls self to a standing position ° Shy with strangers
    ° No constipation ° A normal number of wet diapers per day
Past medical/surgical history
Reported History:
    Past medical history - No significant past medical history.
    Exposure: No exposure to tuberculosis.
    Environmental exposure: No exposure to lead.
    Surgical / procedural: Prior surgery - No significant surgical history.
    Dietary: Infant is breast-feeding.
    Pediatric history: No difficulty breast-feeding, rice cereal introduced, with pureed
       fruit introduced, and with pureed vegetables introduced.
Personal history
Habits: An abnormal sleep pattern.
Home environment: Lives with parents and the living environment has secondhand tobacco
smoke.
Family history
    Family medical history - No significant family history
    Tobacco use
    Alcohol
    Not using drugs.
Review of systems
Systemic symptoms: No systemic symptoms.
Head symptoms: No head symptoms.
Eye symptoms: No eye symptoms.
Otolaryngeal symptoms: No ear symptoms, no nasal symptoms, and no throat symptoms.
Cardiovascular symptoms: No cardiovascular symptoms.
Pulmonary symptoms: No pulmonary symptoms.
Skin symptoms: No skin symptoms.
Musculoskeletal symptoms: No musculoskeletal symptoms.
Psychological symptoms: No psychological symptoms.
Physical findings
Vital signs:

Vital Signs/Measurements	Value	Normal Range
Tympanic membrane temperature	99 F	99 - 101
RR	25 breaths/min	36 - 44
PR	78 bpm	110 - 175
Weight	8.7 kg	6.1 - 10
Body length	27.5 in	25.6 - 29.1
Head circumference	43.9 cm	42 - 47

General appearance:
    ° Alert. ° Well hydrated. ° Active.
Head:
    ° Showed no evidence of cephalohematoma. ° No skull molding was seen.
    ° Fontanelle was normal.

Eyes:
    General/bilateral:
        Extraocular Movements: ° Normal.
        Pupils: ° Normal.

▶ **Figure 7-49a Printed Exam Note for Tyrell Williams 6-Month Check-Up (page 1 of 2).**

Ears:
    General/bilateral:
      Outer Ear: ° Auricle was normal.
      External Auditory Canal: ° External auditory meatus showed no abnormalities.
      Tympanic Membrane: ° Normal.
Nose:
    ° External nose showed no deformities. ° No nasal discharge was seen.
Oral cavity:
    ° Normal.
Pharynx:
    ° Normal.
Neck:
    ° Not swollen. ° Demonstrated no decrease in suppleness.
Lungs:
    ° Clear to auscultation.
Cardiovascular system:
    Heart Rate And Rhythm: ° Normal.
    Heart Sounds: ° Normal.
    Murmurs: ° No murmurs were heard.
    Venous Filling Time: ° Normal.
    Arterial Pulses: ° Equal bilaterally and normal.
Abdomen:
    Auscultation: ° Bowel sounds were normal.
    Palpation: ° Abdomen was soft. ° No mass was palpated in the abdomen.
    Hepatic Findings: ° Liver was normal to palpation.
    Splenic Findings: ° Spleen was normal to palpation.
    Hernia: ° No umbilical hernia was discovered.
Genitalia:
    Penis: ° Normal.
    Testes: ° No cryptorchism was observed.
Skin:
    ° General appearance was normal. ° Showed no erythema. ° No cyanosis. ° Not dry.
    ° No exfoliation was seen.
Musculoskeletal system:
    General/bilateral: ° Normal movement of all extremities.
    Hips:
      General/bilateral: ° Hips showed no abnormalities.
Neurological:
    ° System: normal.
Growth and development:
    ° Normal.
Assessment
    • Normal routine history and physical well-baby (birth - 2 yr)
Vaccinations
    • Received dose of polio virus vaccine, inactivated (Salk)
    • Received dose of DTaP vaccine
    • Received dose of haemophilus influenzae B vaccine, PRP-T conjugate (4 dose schedule),
      for intramuscular use
    • Received dose of pneumococcal conjugate vaccine, polyvalent, IM use
Counseling/Education
    • Discussed safety practices
    • Discussed stranger safety
    • Discussed nutritional needs
    • Discussed concerns about teething
    • Discussed concerns about dental hygiene
Practice Management
    Estab outpatient detailed h&p - moderate complexity decision; Total face to face
      time 40 min

▶ **Figure 7-49b Printed Exam Note for Tyrell Williams 6-Month Check-Up (page 2 of 2).**

Step 8

Click File on the Menu bar, and then click Print Encounter or Print To HTML (as directed by your instructor).

If you are printing your work, you may alternatively click the Print button on the toolbar at the top of your screen.

Compare your printout or file output to Figure 7-49. If it is correct, hand it in to your instructor. If there are any differences, review the previous steps in the exercise and find your error.

You may stop at this point or, if time permits, you may continue with the next exercise without exiting.

Optional Exercise 47: Determine Your Adult Immunizations

The CDC also publishes a recommended immunization schedule for adults. Because adult immunizations are different from those you had as a child, you may have an interest in seeing what you need as an adult. This exercise is completely optional and will not affect your grade.

Step 1

If you have access to the Internet, go to the following Web site:

http://www2.cdc.gov/nip/adultImmSched/

Step 2

Follow the on-screen instructions.

Step 3

Print out your own immunization schedule.

Preventative Care Screening[3]

The U.S. Preventive Services Task Force, sponsored by Agency for Healthcare Research and Quality (AHRQ), is an independent panel of experts in primary care and prevention that systematically reviews the evidence of effectiveness and develops recommendations for clinical preventive services.

Established in 1984, the task force has helped establish the importance of including prevention in primary health care. It also influenced insurance companies to cover the cost of preventive tests and annual examinations.

The task force makes recommendations about preventive services based on age, sex, and risk factors for disease. These recommendations are published by the AHRQ and also are incorporated in EHR systems from several vendors. Figure 7-50 shows the Health Maintenance screen from EHR vendor NextGen.

---

[3]The Guide to Clinical Preventive Services 2005, by U.S. Preventive Services Task Force, published by the Agency for Healthcare Research and Quality, Rockville, MD.

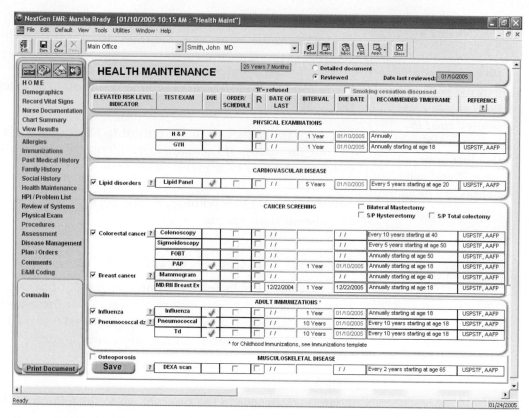

Courtesy of NextGen.

▶ **Figure 7-50 Health Maintenance Screen.**

Research has shown that the best way to ensure that preventive services are delivered appropriately is to make evidence-based information readily available at the point of care. As far back as 1990 EHR systems were developed to compare patient information in a medical office computer with age, sex, and risk factors. The system generated a list of preventive care measures individualized to the patient based on the U.S. Preventive Services Task Force guidelines at the point of care.

"Evidence-based guidelines" means analyzing scientific evidence from current research and studies to determine the effectiveness of preventive services. The guidelines recommend both for and against certain measures, including screening, counseling, and preventive medications. However, the guidelines are not set in stone. They vary not only by age and sex but change recommended intervals based on the individual patient. For example, a blood test measuring total cholesterol and high-density lipoprotein HDL-C is recommended every 5 years for a male over 35, but the interval shortens to every 2 years if the patient has additional risk factors such as high blood pressure, abnormal lipid levels on previous tests, or a family history of cardiovascular disease before age 50.

Using data in the EHR the computer is able to find the appropriate guideline based on the patient's age and sex, add to it based on the patient's problem list and history findings, and then reduce the intervals based on abnormal values of previous test results. The system then generates a guideline unique to the patient and delivers it to the clinician's computer screen. Using this information, the clinician can order tests, discuss important health care options, and recommend lifestyle changes to the patient at the point of care.

A Real-Life Story

Quality Care for Pediatric and Adult Patients

By Alison Connelly, P.A.

Alison Connelly is a Physician Assistant in a large multispecialty group in New York City. She was instrumental in setting up the preventative screening guidelines and designing many of the forms used in the EHR at her practice. Her group has eight clinics and 350 employees.

Our practice has implemented Electronic Health Records and uses many of the options the system offers. These include the electronic prescription system, document imaging, a Medcin-based EHR called OmniDoc™, the referral system, and Quality Care Guidelines (the health maintenance, preventative screening component of our EHR).

The document imaging component is terrific! That was actually what got doctors who were resistant to adopting the EHR to start using the system, because they could access their results and reports instantly. Now that we are on the imaging system, any type of patient results that come in are immediately scanned in so that doctors don't have to wait. This is especially useful in the off-site clinics. We have eight locations. Previously, a document would come in and it could float around for a couple of weeks before it got to the proper clinician, but now as soon as it arrives it is scanned and the clinicians have immediate access to the results on the report on the computer.

A little more than half our total providers use OmniDoc to enter their own exam notes, but all of the pediatric clinicians use it. We created multiple forms for pediatrics based on age and what the milestones and programs for that visit are. We have forms for well-baby visits at 2 months, 4 months, 6 months, 1 year, 15 months, 2 years, and so on. We also created one comprehensive pediatric form for all types of sick visits.

The pediatricians use the growth charts to ensure the pattern of the child's growth is appropriate and follows a trend. The vitals are automatically plotted on the growth chart after they are entered.

We use the Quality Care Guidelines module for age, sex, and disease-specific clinical reminders, primarily in the adult population. I will explain more about that later. Although the guideline system can be used for child immunization scheduling, we weren't able to get rid of the manual immunization sheet in each chart.

I initially set up a system that would track immunizations from the encounters. We created multiple codes for each vaccine and every series, for example, MMR1, MMR2, HIB1, and HIB2. This allowed us to capture the right instance of the vaccine in the series. You also can set up OmniDoc to update the guidelines as vaccines are ordered, but I haven't done that.

Our providers are still using the immunization sheet in the chart. There are several reasons for that. First was immunization history. We see about 150,000 visits a year and we didn't have the manpower to go back and enter the old immunization records manually. With 380 employees I also was afraid that manual entry could introduce errors. I couldn't come up with a method to validate the data if we did it that way so we went forward entering only new immunizations.

The second reason was consistency. The pediatricians didn't want to use the guideline system for some patients and not all of them. If a new patient started here when they were born and had all the vaccines administered here, the computer had an accurate record. However, if the patient already had an immunization record in the chart, or if the patient received some of their shots elsewhere, the guideline system would not be up to date. So for vaccines it turned out that pediatric providers didn't use it that frequently.

The third reason we didn't use the guideline system for immunizations was because of CIR, the citywide immunization registry. In New York City, we have to use CIR to report every vaccine we give to children between birth and 18 years old. So, in addition to putting it on the encounter, we have to send it into the city. If that were computerized, it would be much better; we could eliminate double entry by recording it in the EHR and then transmitting it to the city registry.

From a practical standpoint, the guideline system worked much better for adults in our practice. An adult population has more things that have to be monitored and more of the patients have chronic diseases than do children. In addition to the preventive health measures recommended by age and sex, we have special guidelines for the following conditions:

▶ Diabetes

▶ HIV

▶ Hypertension

▶ Hyperlipidemia

▶ Renal Failure

▶ Ischemic Heart Disease

▶ Anemia

▶ Asthma

Using the guideline system, we are able to make sure, for example, that a diabetes patient has a Hemoglobin A1C done every 3 months.

The guideline system uses patient data that is updated either manually or automatically. Many of the items on the guidelines are tests and it is possible to have the electronic lab system update them with orders and results. However, the interface to our local lab company never worked consistently so most of our guideline data is updated via the encounter. I created a section of the encounter that is labeled "QC Guidelines," which contains the factors that are followed. These are marked by the clinician, then our system automatically updates the guideline when the encounter is processed.

The other update process we use is related to our document image system, which updates the patient data when we scan images. For instance, we actually capture the mammogram referral and the mammogram result. When a mammogram result comes in, it is scanned and we update our system. This does three things; it stores an image of the results, it updates the patient data for the guideline, and it updates the managed care referral portion of the EMR.

We also run reports off the EHR data using the guideline system. In the case of the mammogram, this allows us to reconcile patients that are referred out with results we received back. We can then follow up with patients that just never went for their appointment.

I work in the HIV clinic and use both the guideline system and custom forms I designed for the EHR. While I write my notes in OmniDoc I pull up the guidelines; it is a great monitor.

Because HIV has a lot of clinical guidelines to follow, clinicians can become very focused on HIV and overlook the normal orders you would do based on age and sex, such as a mammogram or a fecal occult blood test. From that standpoint, the guideline system is very helpful, because it produces a complete list of recommendations for the patient's age and sex as well as any diseases the patient may have. I use it almost like a checklist that I go down to make sure I don't forget anything.

I also created forms in our EHR system specific for the HIV clinic that monitors certain clinical guidelines we have to follow and information such as the percentage of pills taken per week and the number of hours slept a night. I used an option in the form designer to make those fields required. The clinician can't exit the form until those questions are answered.

The EHR system is great but if it becomes more sophisticated we could do so much more. I like the idea that it could automatically update guidelines when results are received or automatically send vaccine data to the immunization registry. Similarly, we have to report sexually transmitted diseases within a certain time frame. If we could do that electronically when we received the lab result as well, it would be great.

Using EHR Data for Alerts

Chapter 1 discussed that one of the important reasons for the widespread adoption of EHR is the potential to reduce medical errors. Paper charts and even electronic charts that are comprised of scanned or text documents are dependent on something catching the eye of a person to alert the clinician to a risk factor for the patient. However, when data is stored in an EHR using standard nomenclature codes, then rules can be set up that allow the computer to do the monitoring. If a condition occurs that matches the rule, then an alert can be presented to the person using the EHR.

Alerts could be created about anything in the EHR. Different systems have this implemented to differing degrees. The most widely used alert systems are those implemented with electronic prescription systems.

Interactions between multiple prescription drugs, allergic reactions to certain classes of drugs, and patient health conditions that contraindicate certain drugs can all contribute to suffering, additional illness, and in extreme cases even death. To prevent this, most physicians consult the patient medication list, allergy list, and the book *Physician Desk Reference* (for interactions) before writing a prescription. As a further precaution, the pharmacy checks for drug conflicts and provides the patient with warning materials about the drug.

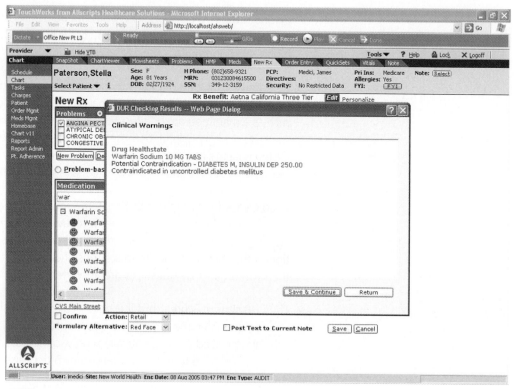

Courtesy of Allscripts, LLC

▶ **Figure 7-51 Electronic Prescription—DUR Alert.**

When prescriptions are written electronically, the computer can do a better job of checking, and present the clinician with warnings, alerts, and explanatory information about the risks. Figure 7-51 shows the clinical warning screen from the prescription writer of a popular EHR system, Allscripts.

Reactions to Drugs or Other Treatments

When the clinician writing an electronic prescription selects a drug and enters the Sig information, the EHR system scans the patient chart for allergy information, past and current diagnoses, and a list of current medications. This information is then passed to a Drug Utilization Review (DUR) program, which compares the prescription to a database of most known drugs. The database includes prescription drugs as well as over-the-counter drugs, and even nutritional herb and vitamin supplements. The DUR program performs the following functions:

◆ The drug about to be prescribed is checked against the patient medication list to determine if there is a conflict with any drug that the patient is already taking. Certain drugs remain in the system for a period of time after the patient has stopped taking them. This latency period is factored in as well.

◆ Ingredients that make up the drug are checked against the ingredients of current medications to see if they conflict or would hinder the effectiveness of the drug.

◆ Drugs are checked for duplicate therapy, where the patient is taking a different drug of the same class, which would have the effect of an overdose.

◆ Allergy records are checked for food and drug allergies, which would be aggravated by the new drug.

◆ Because some drugs cannot be given to patients with certain medical conditions, the patient diagnosis history is checked for to see if there is a problem.

◆ Patient education information is alerted when the drug might be affected by certain foods or alcohol interactions.

◆ If the Sig has been entered at the time of the DUR, then it is also checked to see if it matches recommended guidelines for the drug. Too much, too little, too many days, or too many refills could cause overdosing, underdosing (causing it to be ineffective), or abuse.

If the DUR finds any of these conditions, the clinician is given an alert message explaining exactly what the conflict is. The clinician can then alter the prescription or select a new drug and will not issue the incorrect one.

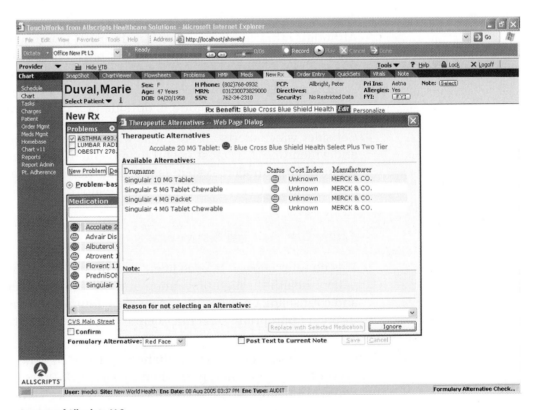

Courtesy of Allscripts, LLC.

▶ **Figure 7-52 Electronic Prescription Formulary Alert.**

Other Types of Alerts

Another type of alert that will be found in many EHR systems has to do with drug formularies, or lists of which drugs are covered by a patient's pharmacy benefit insurance. If the clinician prescribes a drug that is not on the list, then the pharmacy will call the physician to change it when the patient tries to have the prescription filled. This causes an inconvenience to the patient and wastes the doctor's time.

Electronic prescription writing systems offer formulary checking as an option. The option either presents the clinician with a selection of therapeutically equivalent drugs that are on the formulary of the patient's insurance plan, or waits to alert the clinician if a drug is selected that is not on the patient's insurance formulary. Figure 7-52 shows the Therapeutic Alternatives window of the Allscripts EHR system.

Electronic Lab order systems can have alerts as well. Certain tests will not be paid by Medicare. CMS requires that the patient sign a waiver that they were notified that the test is not covered. The waiver is called an "Advance Beneficiary Notice" (ABN). When certain tests are ordered the clinician is alerted if an ABN is required.

Alerts can be generated by nonactions as well. Task list systems can notify an administrator when medical items are not handled in a timely fashion. Order systems can generate alerts when results for a pending test order have not been received within the time that it would normally require for that type of test.

DUR is the most prevalent type of alert implemented in EHR systems today. Although other alerts exist within the EHR few medical practices use all of them. Some very useful alert systems have been designed, but they have been implemented only in large clinics or teaching hospitals. One example is an alert that monitors changes in values of certain blood tests and pages a doctor whenever the value is outside of a certain range.

Consider which alerts are available within your medical practice EHR system, and which would be most useful to implement. Once an EHR system contains codified data, an alert system is just a matter of programming a rule to detect for a finding with a certain event or threshold.

Chapter Seven Summary

This chapter showed how codified data in the EHR could be used to improve patient health through prevention and disease management. Patient education and counseling on preventive measures, immunizations, and early detection through appropriate screening help patients live healthier lives.

Immunization schedules published by the CDC and recommendations for preventative screening published by the U.S. Preventive Services Task Force are useful at the point of care. These are evidence-based guidelines.

"Evidence-based" means analyzing scientific evidence from current research and studies to determine the effectiveness of preventive or disease management services.

When clinicians treat patients with chronic diseases, they sometimes prefer to use flow sheets to view data from multiple encounters in column form. This format allows for a side-by-side comparison of findings over a period of time. There are three ways for a clinician to create a flow sheet based on a list, a problem, or a form.

Clinics also find that patients with diseases such as diabetes often develop additional chronic diseases as well. When regularly seeing patients with multiple diagnoses, it often is more practical to use several forms during a single exam than to create complex forms. As you have learned in this chapter, you can change forms as often as you like during an examination without losing any of the data.

A different approach to forms is taken by pediatricians. Because babies develop in several distinct stages, usually timed to their age in months, forms are designed for the type of information gathered at each age. Well-baby examinations are scheduled at 2-month intervals for the first 6 months, then at 3-month intervals from age 1–2 years, then annually thereafter.

Immunizations must be acquired over time. Vaccines cannot all be given at once. The CDC recommended immunizations are aligned with the well-baby visit intervals. A catch-up schedule also is published that specifies the minimum intervals for certain vaccines when the child has missed doses at an earlier age.

Using the data in the chart, the clinician compares the child's immunization history to the schedule recommended by the CDC (or state health department) to determine what is required each visit. Most EHR systems have a pediatric flow sheet that presents this data and highlights vaccines that are due, saving the clinician from calculating this manually.

The baby's length, weight, and head circumference are measured on each visit. These measurements can be plotted on a graph called a growth chart that compares the individual's growth to statistical information from the general population. Lines on the chart called percentiles represent the percentage of the population that was the same size at the same age. A child who is at the 50th percentile weighs the same or more than 50% of the reference population at that age.

The ability to graph weight, height, and BMI is also available for adult patients. These can provide an excellent means of clarification when counseling patients. The software decides rather to present the graph or the growth chart based on the age of the patient. Blood pressure readings also can be graphed in the EHR or at home from a daily log kept in a spreadsheet.

BMI stands for Body Mass Index. It is a number (wt/ht2) that represents body weight adjusted for height. BMI can be calculated with inches and pounds or meters and kilograms. BMI is gender-specific and age-specific for children, but a single BMI chart is used for adults of both genders. The CDC has replaced the older weight-for-stature charts with the new BMI charts.

Disease prevention through periodic screening and early detection also can save lives. Preventive guidelines, also known as health maintenance guidelines, can be generated by an EHR system. Tailored by the computer, these guidelines recommend tests and preventative measures based on the patient's age and sex, but then dynamically modify the recommendations due to past history and problems unique to the individual. Using this information, the clinician can order tests, discuss important health care options, and recommend lifestyle changes to the patient at the point of care.

Prescription drugs should be checked against the patient's medication list at the time that the prescription is written. Medical errors can be eliminated and time saved by electronic prescription ordering that automatically performs DUR checking and alerts the provider when conflicts are present.

When an EHR contains primarily codified findings many other types of alerts can be generated, helping to save the clinician time, and provide better care for the patient.

Testing Your Knowledge of Chapter 7

1. List at least three ways codified data in the EHR can be used to manage and prevent disease.
2. What is a flow sheet?
3. Describe how to create a flow sheet from a form.
4. Describe how to create a problem-oriented flow sheet.
5. Describe how to cite a finding from a flow sheet.
6. Describe how to graph a patient's weight.
7. Why are childhood immunizations important?
8. Describe how to change the order vaccines are displayed in patient management.

Give the full name for the following acronyms:

9. DTaP _____
10. HepB _____
11. BMI _____
12. DUR _____
13. What are "evidence-based" guidelines?
14. Name the organization that developed pediatric growth charts.
15. What is a growth chart percentile?

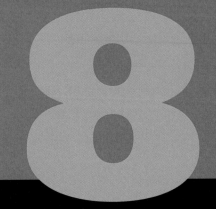

Chapter Eight

Privacy and Security of Health Records

Learning Outcomes

After completing this chapter, you should be able to:

◆ List HIPAA Transactions and Uniform Identifiers

◆ Apply HIPAA Privacy Policy in a medical office

◆ Discuss HIPAA Security Requirements

◆ Follow Security Policy guidelines in a medical office

◆ Explain Electronic Signatures

ACRONYMS USED IN CHAPTER 8	
Acronyms are used extensively in medicine, computers, the law, and government documents. The following are those that are used in this chapter.	
CDC	Centers for Disease Control
CMS	Centers for Medicare and Medicaid
COB	Coordination of Benefits
EDI	Electronic Data Interchange
EPHI	Protected Health Information in Electronic form
FDA	Food and Drug Administration
FEIN	Federal Employer Identification Number
HHS	U.S. Department of Health and Human Services
HIPAA	Health Insurance Portability and Accountability Act
JCAHO	Joint Commission on Accreditation of Healthcare Organizations
MOU	Memorandum of Understanding (between government entities)
NHII	National Health Information Infrastructure
NPI	National Provider Identifier
OCR	Office for Civil Rights
PHI	Protected Health Information
PIN	Personal Identification Number
PKI	Public Key Infrastructure

Understanding HIPAA

Chapter 2 briefly discussed the influence of HIPAA on the adoption of national standards. In this chapter, we will more thoroughly discuss HIPAA and its effect on medical practices. This chapter will make extensive use of documents prepared by the U.S. Department of Health and Human Services.

As someone who will work with patients' health records, it is especially important for you to understand the regulations regarding privacy and security. However, let us begin with a quick review of HIPAA, then study privacy and security portions in more depth.

In 1996 Congress passed legislation called the Health Insurance Portability and Accountability Act, or HIPAA. The law was intended to:

◆ Improve portability and continuity of health insurance coverage.

◆ Combat waste, fraud, and abuse in health insurance and health care delivery.

◆ Promote use of medical savings accounts.

◆ Improve access to long-term care.

◆ Simplify administration of health insurance.

HIPAA law regulates many things. However, a portion known as the Administrative Simplification Subsection of HIPAA (Title 2, f) covers entities such as health plans, clearinghouses, and health care providers. HIPAA refers to these as "covered entities" or a "covered entity." This means the medical practice or health plan and all of its employees. If you work in the health care field, these regulations likely govern your job and behavior. Therefore, it is not uncommon for medical offices to use the term HIPAA when they actually mean only the Administrative Simplification Subsection of HIPAA.

The Administrative Simplification Subsection has four distinct components:

1. Transactions and Code Sets.

2. Uniform Identifiers.

3. Privacy.

4. Security.

HIPAA Transactions and Code Sets

The first section of the regulations to be implemented governed the electronic transfer of medical information for business purposes such as insurance claims, payments, and eligibility. When information is exchanged electronically both sides of the transaction must agree to use the same format in order to make the information intelligible to the receiving system. Before HIPAA, transactions for nearly every insurance plan used a format that contained variations that made it different from another plan's format. This meant that plans could not easily exchange or forward claims to secondary payers and that most providers could only send to a few plans electronically.

HIPAA standardized these formats by requiring specific Transaction Standards for eight types of EDI or Electronic Data Interchange. Two additional EDI transactions are not yet finalized. The HIPAA transactions are:

1. Claims or Equivalent Encounters and Coordination of Benefits (COB)

2. Remittance and Payment Advice

3. Claims Status

4. Eligibility and Benefit Inquiry and Response

5. Referral Certification and Authorization

6. Premium Payments

7. Enrollment and Deenrollment in a Health Plan

8. Health Claims Attachments (Not Final)

9. First Report of Injury (Not Final)

10. Retail Drug Claims, Coordination of Drug Benefits and Eligibility Inquiry

In an EDI transaction, certain portions of the information are sent as codes. For the receiving entity to understand the content of the transaction both the sender and the receiver must use the same codes. For example, two of the code sets that you have worked with in this book that are required by HIPAA are:

◆ Diagnoses (ICD-9CM) Codes

◆ Procedure (CPT-4 and HCPCS) Codes

In an insurance claim, charges for patient visits are sent as CPT-4 or HCPCS procedure codes instead of their long descriptions. The medical reason for the procedure is sent in the claim as ICD-9CM diagnosis codes. Under HIPAA, any coded information within a transaction is also subject to standards. Examples include codes for sex, race, type of provider, relation of the policy holder to the patient, and hundreds of others.

HIPAA Uniform Identifiers

You can see the importance of both the sending and receiving system using the same formats and code sets to report exactly what was done to the patient. Similarly, it is necessary for multiple systems to identify the doctors, nurses, and health care businesses sending the claim or receiving the payment. ID numbers are used in a computer processing instead of names because there could be many providers named John Smith.

However, before HIPAA, each provider had multiple ID numbers assigned to them for use on insurance claims, prescriptions, and so on. A provider typically received a different ID from each plan and sometimes multiple numbers from the same plan. This created a problem for the office to get the right ID on the right claim and made electronic coordination of benefits all but impossible.

HIPAA established Uniform Identifier Standards, which will be used on all claims and other data transmissions. These will include:

◆ National Provider Identifier for doctors, nurses, and other health care providers. Providers began to obtain numbers May 23, 2005. All covered entities must use the NPI by the compliance date May 23, 2007.

◆ Employer Identifier will be used to identify employer sponsored health insurance. It is the same ID as the Federal Employer Identification Number (FEIN) already assigned today.

◆ National Health Plan Identifier will be a unique identification number that will be assigned to each insurance plan, and to the organizations that administer insurance plans, such as payers and third-party administrators.

HIPAA Privacy Rule

The HIPAA privacy standards are designed to protect a patient's identifiable health information from unauthorized disclosure or use in any form, while permitting the practice to deliver the best health care possible. When the HIPAA legislation was passed, "Congress recognized that advances in electronic technology could erode the privacy of health information. Consequently, Congress incorporated into HIPAA provisions that mandated the adoption of Federal privacy protections for individually identifiable health information."[1]

---

[1]*Guidance on HIPAA Standards for Privacy of Individually Identifiable Health Information*, U.S. Department of Health and Human Services Office for Civil Rights December 3, 2002, and revised April 3, 2003.

PHI

HIPAA privacy rules frequently refer to PHI or Protected Health Information; this is the patient's personally identifiable health information.

Health care providers have a strong tradition of safeguarding private health information and have established privacy practices already in effect for their offices. For instance:

◆ "By speaking quietly when discussing a patient's condition with family members in a waiting room or other public area;

◆ By avoiding using patients' names in public hallways and elevators, and posting signs to remind employees to protect patient confidentiality;

◆ By isolating or locking file cabinets or records rooms; or

◆ By providing additional security, such as passwords, on computers maintaining personal information.

"However, The Privacy Rule establishes, for the first time, a foundation of Federal protections for the privacy of protected health information. The Rule does not replace Federal, State, or other law that grants individuals even greater privacy protections, and covered entities are free to retain or adopt more protective policies or practices."[2]

To comply with the law that became effective April 14, 2003, privacy activities in the average medical office might include:

◆ Providing a copy of the office privacy policy informing patients about their privacy rights and how their information can be used.

◆ Asking the patient to acknowledge receiving a copy of the policy or signing a consent form.

◆ Obtaining signed authorization forms and in some cases tracking the disclosures of patient health information when it is to be given to a person or organization outside the practice for purposes other than treatment, billing, or payment purposes.

◆ Adopting clear privacy procedures for its practice.

◆ Training employees so that they understand the privacy procedures.

◆ Designating an individual to be responsible for seeing that the privacy procedures are adopted and followed.

◆ Securing patient records containing individually identifiable health information so that they are not readily available to those who do not need them.

Let us examine each of these points.

Privacy Policy

"The HIPAA Privacy Rule gives individuals a fundamental new right to be informed of the privacy practices of their health plans and of most of their health care providers, as well as to be informed of their privacy rights with respect to their personal health information. Health plans and covered health care providers are

---

[2]Ibid.

required to develop and distribute a notice that provides a clear explanation of these rights and practices. The notice is intended to focus individuals on privacy issues and concerns, and to prompt them to have discussions with their health plans and health care providers and exercise their rights.

"Covered entities are required to provide a notice in *plain language* that describes:

◆ How the covered entity may use and disclose protected health information about an individual.

◆ The individual's rights with respect to the information and how the individual may exercise these rights, including how the individual may complain to the covered entity.

◆ The covered entity's legal duties with respect to the information, including a statement that the covered entity is required by law to maintain the privacy of protected health information.

◆ Whom individuals can contact for further information about the covered entity's privacy policies.

Any use or disclosure of protected health information for treatment, payment, or health care operations must be consistent with the covered entity's notice of privacy practices."[3]

Consent

When the privacy rule was initially issued it required providers to obtain patient "consent" to use and disclose protected health information (PHI) for purposes of treatment, payment, and health care operations, except in emergencies. The rule was almost immediately revised to make consent optional.

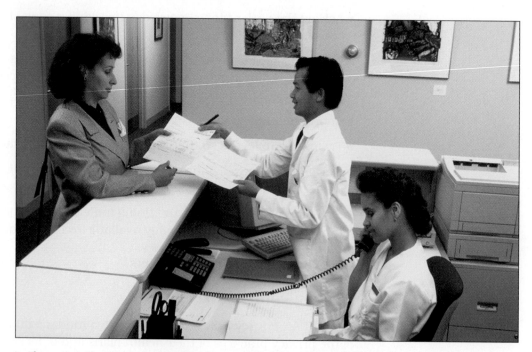

▶ **Figure 8-1 The Patient Acknowledges Receipt of the Medical Office Privacy Policy.**

---

[3]Ibid.

Under the revised privacy rule, the patient gives consent to the use of their PHI for purposes of treatment, payment, and operation of the health care practice. The patient does this by signing a consent form or signing an acknowledgment that they have received a copy of the office's privacy policy. Figure 8-1 shows a patient receiving a copy of the medical office privacy policy. The office has the patient sign a form acknowledging receipt of the privacy policy.

Although most health care providers who see patients obtain patient "consent" as part of the routine demographic and insurance forms patients sign, the rule states:

"A covered entity may, without the individual's authorization:

◆ Use or disclose protected health information for its own treatment, payment, and health care operations activities.

   For example: A hospital may use protected health information about an individual to provide health care to the individual and may consult with other health care providers about the individual's treatment.

◆ A health care provider may disclose protected health information about an individual as part of a claim for payment to a health plan.

◆ A covered entity may disclose protected health information for the treatment activities of any health care provider (including providers not covered by the Privacy Rule).

   For example: A primary care provider may send a copy of an individual's medical record to a specialist who needs the information to treat the individual. A hospital may send a patient's health care instructions to a nursing home to which the patient is transferred.

◆ A covered entity may disclose protected health information to another covered entity or a health care provider (including providers not covered by the Privacy Rule) for the payment activities of the entity that receives the information.

   For example: A physician may send an individual's health plan coverage information to a laboratory who needs the information to bill for services it provided to the physician with respect to the individual. A hospital emergency department may give a patient's payment information to an ambulance service provider that transported the patient to the hospital in order for the ambulance provider to bill for its treatment.

◆ A health plan may use protected health information to provide customer service to its enrollees."[4]

Others within the office also can use PHI; for example, doctors and nurses can share the patient's chart; discuss what the best course of care might be, and so on. The doctor's administrative staff, can access the patient's information to perform billing, transmit claims electronically, post payments, file the charts, type up the doctor's progress notes, and print and send out patient statements.

The office also can use PHI for operation of the medical practice, for example, to determine how many staff they will need on a certain day, whether they should invest in a particular piece of equipment, what types of patients they

---

[4]Ibid.

are seeing the most, where most of their patients live, and any other uses that will help make the office operate more efficiently.

The HHS Guidance document states: "A covered entity may voluntarily choose, but is not required, to obtain the individual's consent for it to use and disclose information about him or her for treatment, payment, and health care operations. A covered entity that chooses to have a consent process has complete discretion under the Privacy Rule to design a process that works best for its business and consumers.

"A 'consent' document is not a valid permission to use or disclose protected health information for a purpose that requires an 'authorization' under the Privacy Rule. . .

"Individuals have the right to request restrictions on how a covered entity will use and disclose protected health information about them for treatment, payment, and health care operations. A covered entity is not required to agree to an individual's request for a restriction, but is bound by any restrictions to which it agrees.

"Individuals also may request to receive confidential communications from the covered entity, either at alternative locations or by alternative means. For example, an individual may request that her health care provider call her at her office, rather than her home. A health care provider must accommodate an individual's reasonable request for such confidential communications."[5]

Authorization

Authorization differs from consent in that it *does* require the patient's permission to disclose PHI. Some examples of instances that would require an authorization would include sending the results of an employment physical to an employer, sending immunization records, or the results of an athletic physical to the school.

The appearance of an authorization form is up to the practice, but the Privacy Rule requires that it contain specific information. This includes a date signed, an expiration date, to whom the information may be disclosed, what is permitted to be disclosed, and for what purpose the information may be used. Unlike the privacy rule concept of consent, authorizations are not global. A new authorization is signed each time there is a different purpose or need for the patient's information to be disclosed.

Research Authorizations are usually required for researchers to use PHI. The authorization may be combined with consent to participate in a clinical trial study, for example. An exception is that research authorizations are not required to have an expiration date.

To protect the patient's information while at the same time ensuring that researchers continue to have access to medical information necessary to conduct vital research the privacy rule also allows some exceptions that permit researchers to access PHI without individual authorizations. Typically, these

---

[5]Ibid.

are cases in which the patients are deceased; the researcher is using PHI only to prepare a research protocol; or in which a waiver has been issued by an internal review board and none of the information will be removed or used for any other purpose.

Marketing The privacy rule specifically defines marketing and *requires* individual authorization for all uses or disclosures of PHI *for marketing* purposes with limited exceptions. These exceptions are generally when information from the provider is sent to all patients in the practice about improvements or additions to the practice; or when the information is sent to the patient about their own treatments. For example, a reminder about an annual check-up is not marketing.

Government Agencies

One area that permits the disclosure of PHI without a patient's authorization or consent is when it is requested by an authorized government agency. Generally such requests are for legal (law enforcement, subpoena, court orders, etc.) or public health purposes. A request by the FDA for information on patients who are having adverse reactions to a particular drug might be an example. Another example might be an audit of medical records by CMS to determine if sufficient documentation exists to justify Medicare claims.

The Privacy Rule also permits the disclosure of PHI, without authorization, to public health authorities for the purpose of preventing or controlling disease or injury as well as maintaining records of births and deaths. This would include, for example, the reporting of a contagious disease to the CDC or an adverse reaction to a regulated drug or product to the FDA.

One new authority for government involves enforcement of the protections in the Privacy Rule itself. To ensure that covered entities protect patients' privacy as required, the Rule requires that health plans, hospitals, and other covered entities cooperate with efforts by the HHS Office for Civil Rights (OCR) to investigate complaints or otherwise ensure compliance.

To comply with various states' Workers' Compensation laws, providers are permitted to disclose PHI concerning on-the-job injuries to Workers' Compensation insurers, state administrators, and other entities to the extent required by state law.

Minimum Necessary

The Privacy Rule includes a minimum necessary standard intended to limit unnecessary or inappropriate access to and disclosure of PHI beyond what is necessary. For example, if an insurance plan requests the result of a patient's hematocrit test to justify a claim for the drug Epogen, then the minimum necessary would be to send only the value of that particular test.

Note	**No Restrictions on PHI for Treatment of the Patient**
	The minimum necessary standard does not apply to disclosures to or requests by a health care provider for PHI used for treatment purposes.

"The Privacy Rule generally requires covered entities to take reasonable steps to limit the use or disclosure of, and requests for, protected health information to the minimum necessary to accomplish the intended purpose. The minimum necessary standard does not apply to the following:

♦ Disclosures to or requests by a health care provider for treatment purposes.

♦ Disclosures to the individual who is the subject of the information.

♦ Uses or disclosures made pursuant to an individual's authorization.

♦ Uses or disclosures required for compliance with the Health Insurance Portability and Accountability Act (HIPAA) Administrative Simplification Rules.

♦ Disclosures to the Department of Health and Human Services (HHS) when disclosure of information is required under the Privacy Rule for enforcement purposes.

♦ Uses or disclosures that are required by other law.

The implementation specifications for this provision require a covered entity to develop and implement policies and procedures appropriate for its own organization, reflecting the entity's business practices and workforce."[6]

A Patient's Right to Know about Disclosures

Whether the practice has disclosed PHI based on a signed authorization or to comply with a government agency, the patient is entitled to know about it. Therefore, in most cases the medical office must track the disclosure.

The privacy rule gives the individuals the right to receive a report of all disclosures made for purposes other than treatment, payment, or operations. The report must include the date of the disclosure, whom the information was provided to, a description of the information and the stated purpose for the disclosure. The patient can request the report at any time and the practice must keep the records for at least 6 years.

Patient Access to Medical Records

In addition to protecting privacy, the law generally allows patients to be able to see and obtain copies of their medical records and request corrections if they identify errors and mistakes. Health plans, doctors, hospitals, clinics, nursing homes, and other covered entities generally must provide access to these records within 30 days, but they may charge patients for the cost of copying and sending the records.

---

[6]Ibid.

Incidental Disclosures

"Many customary health care communications and practices play an important or even essential role in ensuring that individuals receive prompt and effective health care. Due to the nature of these communications and practices, as well as the various environments in which individuals receive health care or other services from covered entities, the potential exists for an individual's health information to be disclosed incidentally. For example, a hospital visitor may overhear a provider's confidential conversation with another provider or a patient, or may glimpse a patient's information on a sign-in sheet or nursing station whiteboard. The HIPAA Privacy Rule is not intended to impede these customary and essential communications and practices and, thus, does not require that all risk of incidental use or disclosure be eliminated to satisfy its standards. Rather, the Privacy Rule permits certain incidental uses and disclosures of protected health information to occur when the covered entity has in place reasonable safeguards and minimum necessary policies and procedures to protect an individual's privacy."[7]

Personal Representatives

"There may be times when individuals are legally or otherwise incapable of exercising their rights, or simply choose to designate another to act on their behalf with respect to these rights. Under the Rule, a person authorized to act on behalf of the individual in making health care related decisions is the individual's personal representative.

"The Privacy Rule requires covered entities to treat an individual's personal representative as the individual with respect to uses and disclosures of the individual's protected health information, as well as the individual's rights under the Rule.

"The personal representative stands in the shoes of the individual and has the ability to act for the individual and exercise the individual's rights. . . . In addition to exercising the individual's rights under the Rule, a personal representative may also authorize disclosures of the individual's protected health information."[8]

In general, the personal representative's authority over privacy matters parallels their authority to act on other health care decisions.

◆ Where the personal representative has broad authority in making health care decisions, the personal representative is treated as the individual for all purposes under the Privacy Rule.

Examples include a parent with respect to a minor child or a legal guardian of a mentally incompetent adult.

---

[7]Ibid.

[8]Ibid.

♦ Where the representative's authority is limited to particular health care decisions, their authority concerning PHI is limited to the same area.

For example, a person with limited health care power of attorney about artificial life support could not sign an authorization for the disclosure of protected health information for marketing purposes.

♦ When the patient is deceased, a person who has authority to act on the behalf of the deceased or their estate is the personal representative for all purposes under the Privacy Rule.

Figure 8-2 provides a chart of who must be recognized as the personal representative for a category of individuals.

If the Individual Is:	The Personal Representative Is:	Examples:
An Adult or an Emancipated Minor	A person with legal authority to make health care decisions on behalf of the individual	Health care power of attorney Court appointed legal guardian General power of attorney
A Minor (not emancipated)	A parent, guardian, or other person acting in loco parentis with legal authority to make health care decisions on behalf of the minor child	Parent, guardian, or other person (with exceptions in state law)
Deceased	A person with legal authority to act on behalf of the decedent or the estate (not restricted to health care decisions)	Executor of the estate Next of kin or other family member Durable power of attorney

▶ **Figure 8-2 Persons Automatically Recognized as Personal Representatives for Patients.**

Minor Children

"The Privacy Rule defers to State or other applicable laws that address the ability of a parent, guardian, or other person acting as parent to obtain health information about a minor child.

"In most cases under the Rule, the parent is the personal representative of the minor child and can exercise the minor's rights with respect to protected health information, because the parent usually has the authority to make health care decisions about his or her minor child. Regardless of whether a parent is the personal representative, the Privacy Rule permits a covered entity to disclose to a parent, or provide the parent with access to, a minor child's protected health information when and to the extent it is expressly permitted or required by State or other laws.

"Likewise, the Privacy Rule prohibits a covered entity from disclosing a minor child's protected health information to a parent, or providing a parent with access to, such information when and to the extent it is expressly prohibited under State or other laws.

"However, the Privacy Rule specifies three circumstances in which the parent is not the personal representative with respect to certain health information about his or her minor child. The three exceptional circumstances when a parent is not the minor's personal representative are:

♦ When State or other law does not require the consent of a parent or other person before a minor can obtain a particular health care service, and the minor consents to the health care service;

Example: A State law provides an adolescent the right to obtain mental health treatment without the consent of his or her parent, and the adolescent consents to such treatment without the parent's consent.

♦ When a court determines or other law authorizes someone other than the parent to make treatment decisions for a minor;

Example: A court may grant authority to make health care decisions for the minor to an adult other than the parent, to the minor, or the court may make the decision(s) itself.

♦ When a parent agrees to a confidential relationship between the minor and the physician.

Example: A physician asks the parent of a 16-year-old if the physician can talk with the child confidentially about a medical condition and the parent agrees.

"In these exceptional circumstances, where the parent is not the personal representative of the minor, if State or other law is silent or unclear concerning parental access to the minor's protected health information, a covered entity has discretion to provide or deny a parent with access to the minor's health information, provided the decision is made by a licensed health care professional in the exercise of professional judgment."[9]

Summary of Patient Privacy Rights

Figure 8-3 provides a summary of patient rights under the privacy rule. It is published by HHS Office of Civil Rights, which enforces the HIPAA Privacy Rule.

---

[9]Ibid.

► Figure 8-3 Patient Privacy Summary Published by the U.S. Department of Health and Human Services Office for Civil Rights.

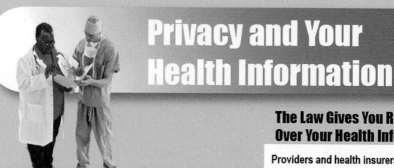

Privacy and Your Health Information

Your Privacy Is Important to All of Us

Most of us feel that our health and medical information is private and should be protected, and we want to know who has this information. Now, Federal law

► Gives you rights over your health information

► Sets rules and limits on who can look at and receive your health information

Your Health Information Is Protected By Federal Law

Who must follow this law?

► Most doctors, nurses, pharmacies, hospitals, clinics, nursing homes, and many other health care providers

► Health insurance companies, HMOs, most employer group health plans

► Certain government programs that pay for health care, such as Medicare and Medicaid

What information is protected?

► Information your doctors, nurses, and other health care providers put in your medical record

► Conversations your doctor has about your care or treatment with nurses and others

► Information about you in your health insurer's computer system

► Billing information about you at your clinic

► Most other health information about you held by those who must follow this law

The Law Gives You Rights Over Your Health Information

Providers and health insurers who are required to follow this law must comply with your right to

► Ask to see and get a copy of your health records

► Have corrections added to your health information

► Receive a notice that tells you how your health information may be used and shared

► Decide if you want to give your permission before your health information can be used or shared for certain purposes, such as for marketing

► Get a report on when and why your health information was shared for certain purposes

► If you believe your rights are being denied or your health information isn't being protected, you can

  ▷ File a complaint with your provider or health insurer

  ▷ File a complaint with the U.S. Government

You should get to know these important rights, which help you protect your health information. You can ask your provider or health insurer questions about your rights. You also can learn more about your rights, including how to file a complaint, from the website at www.hhs.gov/ocr/hipaa/ or by calling 1-866-627-7748; the phone call is free.

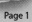

Page 1

Business Associates

"The HIPAA Privacy Rule applies only to covered entities—health care providers, plans, and clearinghouses. However, most health care providers and health plans do not carry out all of their health care activities and functions by themselves. Instead, they often use the services of a variety of other persons or businesses. The Privacy Rule allows covered providers and health plans to disclose protected health information to these business associates if the providers or plans obtain written satisfactory assurances that the business associate will use the informa-

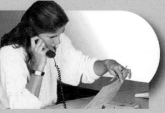

PRIVACY

The Law Sets Rules and Limits on Who Can Look At and Receive Your Information

To make sure that your information is protected in a way that does not interfere with your health care, your information can be used and shared

► For your treatment and care coordination

► To pay doctors and hospitals for your health care and help run their businesses

► With your family, relatives, friends or others you identify who are involved with your health care or your health care bills, unless you object

► To make sure doctors give good care and nursing homes are clean and safe

► To protect the public's health, such as by reporting when the flu is in your area

► To make required reports to the police, such as reporting gunshot wounds

Your health information cannot be used or shared without your written permission unless this law allows it. For example, without your authorization, your provider generally cannot

► Give your information to your employer

► Use or share your information for marketing or advertising purposes

► Share private notes about your mental health counseling sessions

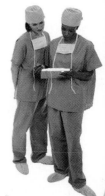

Published by:

U.S. Department of Health & Human Services Office for Civil Rights

The Law Protects the Privacy of Your Health Information

Providers and health insurers who are required to follow this law must keep your information private by

► Teaching the people who work for them how your information may and may not be used and shared

► Taking appropriate and reasonable steps to keep your health information secure

Page 2

tion only for the purposes for which it was engaged by the covered entity, will safeguard the information from misuse, and will help the covered entity comply with some of the covered entity's duties under the Privacy Rule.

"The covered entity's contract or other written arrangement with its business associate must contain the elements specified in the privacy rule. For example, the contract must:

◆ Describe the permitted and required uses of protected health information by the business associate;

◆ Provide that the business associate will not use or further disclose the protected health information other than as permitted or required by the contract or as required by law; and

◆ Require the business associate to use appropriate safeguards to prevent a use or disclosure of the protected health information other than as provided for by the contract."[10]

Civil and Criminal Penalties

"Congress provided civil and criminal penalties for covered entities that misuse personal health information. For civil violations of the standards, OCR may impose monetary penalties up to $100 per violation, up to $25,000 per year, for each requirement or prohibition violated. Criminal penalties apply for certain actions such as knowingly obtaining protected health information in violation of the law. Criminal penalties can range up to $50,000 and one year in prison for certain offenses; up to $100,000 and up to five years in prison if the offenses are committed under 'false pretenses'; and up to $250,000 and up to 10 years in prison if the offenses are committed with the intent to sell, transfer or use protected health information for commercial advantage, personal gain or malicious harm."[11]

HIPAA Security Rule

The final security rule for HIPAA was passed and became effective two years after the final privacy rule. The delay was caused by differences in the language of the two rules which had to be reconciled in the Security Rule. This delay could have created a difficult situation because in order to fully comply with the Privacy Rule covered entities needed to implement some of the same requirements listed in the Security Rule. Fortunately the final Security Rule became effective April 21, 2003, only a week after the compliance date for Privacy. This meant that although providers had until 2005 to comply with the Security Rule, careful implementation of certain safeguards required by the Privacy Rule would simplify compliance with the Security Rule.

There are clearly areas in which the two rules supplement each other as both the HIPAA Privacy and Security Rules are designed to protect identifiable health information. However, the privacy rule covers PHI in all forms of communications, whereas the security rule covers only electronic information. Because of this difference, security discussions are assumed to be about the protection of EHR, but the security rule actually covers all PHI that is stored electronically. This is called EPHI.

---

[10]Ibid.

[11]*Fact Sheet: Protecting the Privacy of Patients' Health Information,* HHS Press Office, April 14, 2003.

A Real-Life Story

The First HIPAA Privacy Case[12]

T he first legal case under the privacy rule concerned the theft of patient demographic information (name, address, date of birth, Social Security number) by an employee in a medical office.

The former employee of a cancer care facility pled guilty in federal court in Seattle, Washington, to wrongful disclosure of individually identifiable health information for economic gain. This is the first criminal conviction in the United States under the health information privacy provisions of the Health Insurance Portability and Accountability Act (HIPAA), which became effective in April 2003. Those provisions made it illegal to wrongfully disclose personally identifiable health information.

The ex-employee admitted that he obtained a cancer patient's name, date of birth, and Social Security number while employed at the medical facility, and that he disclosed that information to get four credit cards in the patient's name. He also admitted that he used several of those cards to rack up more than $9,000 in debt in the patient's name. He used the cards to purchase various items, including video games, home improvement supplies, apparel, jewelry, porcelain figurines, groceries, and gasoline for his personal use. He was fired shortly after the identity theft was discovered.

"Too many Americans have experienced identity theft and the nightmare of dealing with bills they never incurred. To be a vulnerable cancer patient, fighting for your life, and having to cope with identity theft is just unconscionable," stated United States Attorney John McKay. "This case should serve as a reminder that misuse of patient information may result in criminal prosecution."

The case was investigated by the Federal Bureau of Investigation (FBI) and prosecuted by the United States Attorney's Office. The man was sentenced to a term of 10 to 16 months. He also has agreed to pay restitution to the credit card companies, and to the patient for expenses he incurred as a result of the misuse of his identity.

Although identity theft is serious, the consequences are much greater in a medical setting than if the same information had been stolen from an ordinary business. Why? Because even the patient's name and date of birth are part of the PHI. Additionally, the disclosure of medical information for financial gain could have resulted in a sentence of 10 years for each violation. The case serves as a reminder for everyone in the health care field of the personal responsibility for protecting PHI.

Although the patient privacy rule under HIPAA does not restrict the internal use of health information by the staff for treatment, payment and office operations, you should make every effort to protect your patients' privacy and always follow the privacy policy of the practice.

---

[12]Press Release, August 19, 2004, United States Attorney's Office, Western District of Washington.

PHI—EPHI

The Security Rule applies only to EPHI, whereas the Privacy Rule applies to PHI which may be in electronic, oral, and paper form.

In order to comply fully with the Privacy Rule, it is necessary to understand and implement the requirements of the Security Rule. As an employee of a covered entity, it is important that you participate in the security training and follow the security policy and procedures of your health care organization.

In this section, you will learn about the Security Rule. As with the previous section, much of the information provided is drawn directly from HHS documents. HHS regulates and enforces HIPAA using two different divisions for enforcement. OCR or Office of Civil Rights enforces the Privacy Rule whereas CMS enforces the Security Rule.

Why Security?

"Prior to HIPAA, no generally accepted set of security standards or general requirements for protecting health information existed in the health care industry. At the same time, new technologies were evolving, and the health care industry began to move away from paper processes and rely more heavily on the use of computers to pay claims, answer eligibility questions, provide health information and conduct a host of other administrative and clinically based functions.

"In order to provide more efficient access to critical health information, covered entities are using web-based applications and other 'portals' that give physicians, nurses, medical staff as well as administrative employees more access to electronic health information. While this means that the medical workforce can be more mobile and efficient (i.e., physicians can check patient records and test results from wherever they are), the rise in the adoption rate of these technologies creates an increase in potential security risks. [Portals and remote access will be discussed in Chapter 9.]

"As the country moves towards its goal of a National Health Information Infrastructure (NHII), and greater use of electronic health records, protecting the confidentiality, integrity, and availability of EPHI becomes even more critical.

"The security standards in HIPAA were developed for two primary purposes. First, and foremost, the implementation of appropriate security safeguards protects certain electronic health care information that may be at risk. Second, protecting an individual's health information, while permitting the appropriate access and use of that information, ultimately promotes the use of electronic health information in the industry—an important goal of HIPAA.

The Privacy Rule and Security Rule Compared

"The Privacy Rule sets the standards for, among other things, who may have access to PHI, while the Security Rule sets the standards for ensuring that only those who should have access to EPHI will actually have access. The primary distinctions between the two rules follow:

◆ Electronic vs. oral and paper: The Privacy Rule applies to all forms of patients' protected health information, whether electronic, written, or oral. In contrast, the Security Rule covers only protected health information that is in electronic form. This includes EPHI that is created, received, maintained or transmitted.

◆ "Safeguard" requirement in Privacy Rule: While the Privacy Rule contains provisions that currently require covered entities to adopt certain safeguards for PHI, the Security Rule provides for far more comprehensive security requirements and includes a level of detail not provided in the Privacy Rule section.

Security Standards

"The security standards are divided into the categories of administrative, physical, and technical safeguards. Each category of the safeguards is comprised of a number of standards, which generally contain a number of implementation specifications.

◆ **Administrative safeguards:** In general, these are the administrative functions that should be implemented to meet the security standards. These include assignment or delegation of security responsibility to an individual and security training requirements.

◆ **Physical safeguards:** In general, these are the mechanisms required to protect electronic systems, equipment and the data they hold, from threats, environmental hazards and unauthorized intrusion. They include restricting access to EPHI and retaining off site computer backups.

◆ **Technical safeguards:** In general, these are primarily the automated processes used to protect data and control access to data. They include using authentication controls to verify that the person signing onto a computer is authorized to access that EPHI, or encrypting and decrypting data as it is being stored and/or transmitted.

"In addition to the safeguards (listed above), the Security Rule also contains several standards and implementation specifications that address organizational requirements, as well as policies and procedures and documentation requirements."[13]

Implementation Specifications

An implementation specification is an additional detailed instruction for implementing a particular standard. Implementation requirements and features within the categories were listed in the Security Rule by alphabetical order to convey that no one item was considered to be more important than another.

Implementation specifications in the Security Rule are either "Required" or "Addressable." Addressable does *not* mean optional.

To help you understand the organization of safeguards, security standards, and implementation specifications, a matrix of the HIPAA Security Rule is provided in Figure 8-4. The matrix is a part of the official rule and published as an appendix to the rule. You may wish to refer to Figure 8-4 as we discuss each of the following sections.

---

[13]Adapted from: Security 101 for Covered Entities, CMS HIPAA paper 1 of 7 on security.

Security Standards Matrix[14]

Administrative Safeguards

Standards	Section of Rule	Implementation Specifications	Required or Addressable
Security Management Process	§ 164.308Addressable(1)	Risk Analysis	Required
		Risk Management	Required
		Sanction Policy	Required
		Information System Activity Review	Required
Assigned Security Responsibility	§ 164.308Addressable(2)		Required
Workforce Security	§ 164.308Addressable(3)	Authorization and/or Supervision	Addressable
		Workforce Clearance Procedure	Addressable
		Termination Procedures	Addressable
Information Access Management	§ 164.308Addressable(4)	Isolating Health Care Clearinghouse Function	Required
		Access Authorization	Addressable
		Access Establishment and Modification	Addressable
Security Awareness and Training	§ 164.308Addressable(5)	Security Reminders	Addressable
		Protection from Malicious Software	Addressable
		Log-In Monitoring	Addressable
		Password Management	Addressable
Security Incident Procedures	§ 164.308Addressable(6)	Response and Reporting	Required
Contingency Plan	§ 164.308Addressable(7)	Data Backup Plan	Required
		Disaster Recovery Plan	Required
		Emergency Mode Operation Plan	Required
		Testing and Revision Procedure	Addressable
		Applications and Data Criticality Analysis	Addressable
Evaluation	§ 164.308Addressable(8)		Required
Business Associate Contracts and Other Arrangement	§ 164.308(b)(1)	Written Contract or Other Arrangement	Required

▶ Figure 8-4 HIPAA Security Standards Matrix.[14]

Administrative Safeguards[15]

The name "Security Rule" sounds like it might be very technical, but the largest category of the rule is Administrative Safeguards. The Administrative Safeguards comprise over half of the HIPAA Security requirements.

---

[14]Adapted from Appendix A to Subpart C of Part 164—Security Standards Matrix, Health Insurance Reform: Security Standards; Final Rule, Federal Register, February 20, 2003.

[15]Adapted from: Security Standards: Administrative Safeguards, CMS HIPAA paper 2 of 7 on security.

Physical Safeguards

Standards	Section of Rule	Implementation Specifications	Required or Addressable
Facility Access Controls	§ 164.310Addressable(1))	Contingency Operations	Addressable
		Facility Security Plan	Addressable
		Access Control and Validation Procedures	Addressable
		Maintenance Records	Addressable
Workstation Use	§ 164.310(b)Required		Required
Workstation Security	§ 164.310(c)Required		Required
Device and Media Controls	§ 164.310(d)(1)	Disposal	Required
		Media Re-use	Required
		Accountability	Addressable
		Data Backup and Storage	Addressable

Technical Safeguards

Standards	Section of Rule	Implementation Specifications	Required or Addressable
Access Control	§ 164.312Addressable(1)	Unique User Identification	Required
		Emergency Access Procedure	Required
		Automatic Logoff	Addressable
		Encryption and Decryption	Addressable
Audit Controls	§ 164.312(b)		Required
Integrity	§ 164.312(c)(1)	Mechanism to Authenticate Electronic Protected Health Information	Addressable
Person or Entity Authentication	§ 164.312(d)		Required
Transmission Security	164.312(e)(1)	Integrity Controls	Addressable
		Encryption	Addressable

Administrative Safeguards are the policies, procedures, and actions to manage the implementation and maintenance of security measures to protect EPHI. The Administrative Standards are as follows:

Security Management Process

The Security Management Process is the first step. It is used to establish the administrative processes and procedures. There are four implementation specifications in the Security Management Process standard.

1. **Risk Analysis** Identify potential security risks, and determine the probability of occurrence and magnitude of risks.

2. **Risk Management** Make decisions about how to address security risks and vulnerabilities.

Risk analysis and risk management serve as tools to assist in the development of a strategy to protect the confidentiality, integrity, and availability of EPHI.

3. **Sanction Policy** Appropriate sanctions must be in place so that workforce members understand the consequences of failing to comply with security policies and procedures, to deter noncompliance.

4. **Information System Activity Review** Information System Activity Review requires regular review records such as audit logs, access reports, and security incident tracking reports. The information system activity review helps to determine if any EPHI is used or disclosed in an inappropriate manner.

Assigned Security Responsibility

Security responsibility is assigned to one individual designated as having overall responsibility (the Security Official); however, specific security responsibilities may be assigned to other individuals (e.g., facility security or network security) as illustrated by Figure 8-5.

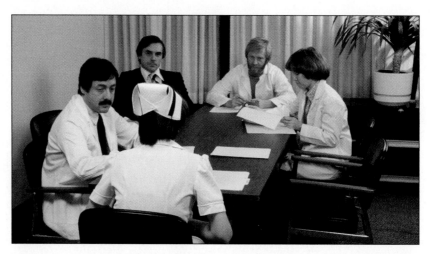

▶ **Figure 8-5 Medical Office Staff Review Security Policy and Appoint Security Officer.**

This standard corresponds to the Privacy Rule, which requires covered entities to designate a Privacy Official. The Security Official and Privacy Official can be the same person but does not have to be.

Workforce Security

Within Workforce Security there are three addressable implementation specifications:

1. **Authorization or Supervision** Authorization is the process of determining whether a particular user (or a computer system) has the right to carry out a certain activity, such as reading a file or running a program.

2. **Workforce Clearance Procedure** Ensures members of the workforce with authorized access to EPHI receive appropriate clearances.

3. **Termination Procedures** Whether the employee leaves the organization voluntarily or involuntarily, termination procedures must be in place to remove access privileges when an employee, contractor, or other individual previously entitled to access information no longer has these privileges.

Information Access Management

Restricting access to only those persons and entities with a need for access is a basic tenet of security. By managing information access, the risk of inappropriate disclosure, alteration, or destruction of EPHI is minimized. This safeguard supports the "minimum necessary standard" of the HIPAA Privacy Rule.

The Information Access Management standard has three implementation specifications.

1. **Access Authorization** In the Workforce Security standard (above) the practice determined who has access. This section requires policies and procedures to identify who has authority to grant those access privileges and the process for doing so.

2. **Access Establishment and Modification** Once a covered entity has clearly defined who should get access to what EPHI and under what circumstances, it must consider how access is established and modified.

3. **Isolating Health Care Clearinghouse Functions** This implementation specification only applies in the situation in which a health care clearinghouse is part of a larger organization.

Security Awareness and Training

Security awareness and training for all new and existing members of the workforce is required. Figure 8-6 illustrates training an employee. In addition, periodic retraining should be given whenever environmental or operational changes affect the security of EPHI.

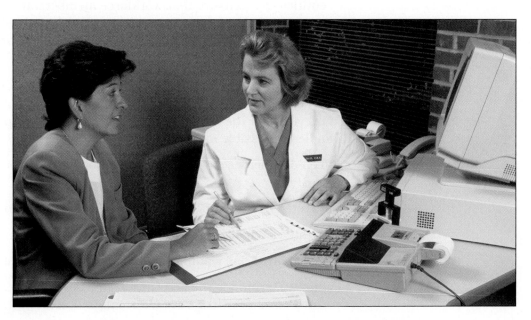

▶ **Figure 8-6 Training a Medical Assistant on Security Policy and Procedures.**

Regardless of the Administrative Safeguards a covered entity implements, those safeguards will not protect the EPHI if the workforce is unaware of its role in adhering to and enforcing them. Many security risks and vulnerabilities within covered entities are internal. This is why the Security Awareness and Training standard is so important.

The Security Awareness and Training standard has four implementation specifications.

1. **Security Reminders** Security reminders might include notices in printed or electronic form, agenda items and specific discussion topics at monthly meetings, focused reminders posted in affected areas, as well as formal re-training on security policies and procedures.

2. **Protection from Malicious Software** One important security measure that employees need to be reminded of is that malicious software is frequently brought into an organization through email attachments and programs that are downloaded from the Internet. As a result of an unauthorized infiltration, EPHI and other data can be damaged or destroyed or, at a minimum, can require expensive and time-consuming repairs.

3. **Log-In Monitoring** Security awareness and training also should address how users log onto systems and how they are supposed to manage their passwords.

   Typically, an inappropriate or attempted login is when someone enters multiple combinations of user names or passwords to attempt to access an information system. Fortunately, many information systems can be set to identify multiple unsuccessful attempts to log in. Other systems might record the attempts in a log or audit trail. Still other systems might disable a password after a specified number of unsuccessful log in attempts. Once capabilities are established the workforce must be made aware of how to use and monitor them.

4. **Password Management** In addition to providing a password for access, entities must ensure that workforce members are trained on how to safeguard the information. Train all users and establish guidelines for creating passwords and changing them during periodic change cycles.

Security Incident Procedures

Security incident procedures must address how to identify security incidents and provide that the incident be reported to the appropriate person or persons. Examples of possible incidents include:

◆ Stolen or otherwise inappropriately obtained passwords that are used to access EPHI.

◆ Corrupted backup tapes that do not allow restoration of EPHI.

◆ Virus attacks that interfere with the operations of information systems with EPHI.

◆ Physical break-ins leading to the theft of media with EPHI.

◆ Failure to terminate the account of a former employee that is then used by an unauthorized user to access information systems with EPHI.

◆ Providing media with EPHI, such as a PC hard drive or laptop, to another user who is not authorized to access the EPHI before removing the EPHI stored on the media.

There is one required implementation specification for this standard.

1. **Response and Reporting** Establish adequate response and reporting procedures for these and other types of events.

Contingency Plan

The contingency plan consists of strategies for recovering access to EPHI should the organization experience an emergency or other occurrence, such as a power outage or disruption of critical business operations. The goal is to ensure that EPHI is available when it is needed.

The Contingency Plan standard includes five implementation specifications:

1. **Data Backup Plan** Data Backup plans are an important safeguard and a required implementation specification. Most covered entities already have backup procedures as part of current business practices.

2. **Disaster Recovery Plan** These are procedures to restore any loss of data.

3. **Emergency Mode Operation Plan** When operating in emergency mode because of a technical failure or power outage, security processes to protect EPHI must be maintained.

4. **Testing and Revision Procedures** Periodically test and revise contingency plans.

5. **Application and Data Criticality Analysis** Analyze software applications that store, maintain, or transmit EPHI and determine how important each is to patient care or business needs. A prioritized list of specific applications and data will help determine which applications or information systems get restored first or that must be available at all times.

Evaluation

Periodically evaluate strategy and systems to ensure that the security requirements continue to meet the organization's operating environments. Ongoing evaluation of security measures is the best way to ensure all EPHI is adequately protected.

Business Associate Contracts and Other Arrangements

The Business Associate Contracts and Other Arrangements standard is comparable to the Business Associate Contract standard in the Privacy Rule, but is specific to business associates who create, receive, maintain, or transmit EPHI. The standard has one implementation specification.

1. **Written Contract or Other Arrangement**

Physical Safeguards[16]

The Security Rule defines physical safeguards as "*physical measures, policies, and procedures to protect a covered entity's electronic information systems and related buildings and equipment, from natural and environmental hazards, and unauthorized intrusion.*"

Facility Access Controls

Facility Access Controls are policies and procedures to limit physical access to electronic information systems and the facility or facilities in which they are

---

[16]Adapted from: Security Standards: Physical Safeguards, CMS HIPAA paper 3 of 7 on security.

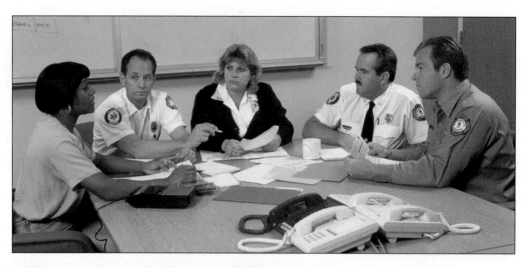

▶ **Figure 8-7 Review Facility Security and Emergency Contingency Plans Periodically.**

housed. Figure 8-7 illustrates a staff meeting on security. There are four implementation specifications.

1. **Access Control and Validation Procedures** Access Control and Validation are procedures to determine which persons should have access to certain locations within the facility based on their role or function.

2. **Contingency Operations** Contingency operations refer to physical security measures to be used in the event of the activation of contingency plans.

3. **Facility Security Plan** The Facility Security Plan defines and documents the safeguards used to protect the facility or facilities. Some examples include:

   ◆ Locked doors, signs warning of restricted areas, surveillance cameras, alarms.

   ◆ Property controls such as property control tags, engraving on equipment.

   ◆ Personnel controls such as identification badges, visitor badges, or escorts for large offices.

   ◆ Private security service or patrol for the facility.

   In addition, all staff or employees must know their roles in facility security.

4. **Maintenance Records** Document facility security repairs and modifications such as changing locks, making routine maintenance checks, or installing new security devices.

Workstation Use

Inappropriate use of computer workstations can expose a covered entity to risks, such as virus attacks, compromise of information systems, and breaches of confidentiality. Specify the proper functions to be performed by electronic computing devices.

Workstation use also applies to workforce members that who off-site using workstations that can access EPHI. This includes employees who work from home, in satellite offices, or in another facility.

Workstation Security

Although the Workstation Use standard addresses the policies and procedures for how workstations should be used and protected, the Workstation Security standard addresses how workstations are to be physically protected from unauthorized users.

Device and Media Controls

Device and Media Controls are policies and procedures that govern the receipt and removal of hardware and electronic media that contain EPHI, into and out of a facility, and the movement of these items within the facility.

The Device and Media Controls standard has four implementation specifications, two required and two addressable.

1. **Disposal** When disposing of any electronic media that contains EPHI make sure it is unusable or inaccessible.

2. **Media Reuse** Instead of disposing of electronic media, covered entities may want to reuse it. The EPHI must be removed before the media can be reused.

3. **Accountability** If a covered entity's hardware and media containing EPHI are moved from one location to another, a record should be maintained as documentation of the move.

   Portable workstations and media present a special accountability challenge. Portable technology is getting smaller, less expensive, and has an increased capacity to store large quantities of data. As a result, it is becoming more prevalent in the health care industry, making accountability even more important and challenging.

4. **Data Backup and Storage** This specification protects the availability of EPHI and is similar to the Data Backup Plan for the contingency plan.

Technical Safeguards[17]

The Security Rule defines technical safeguards as *"the technology and the policy and procedures for its use that protect electronic protected health information and control access to it."*

In the CMS guidance documents, some security measures and technical solutions are provided as examples to illustrate the standards and implementation specifications. These are only examples. The Security Rule is based on the fundamental concepts of flexibility, scalability, and technology neutrality. No specific technologies are required by the rule.

Access Control

Access Control consists of technical policies and procedures to allow access only to those persons or software programs that have been granted access rights (as specified in Information Access Management discussed earlier).

---

[17]Adapted from: Security Standards: Technical Safeguards, CMS HIPAA paper 4 of 7 on security.

Four implementation specifications are associated with the Access Controls standard.

1. **Unique User Identification** Unique User Identification provides a way to identify a specific user, typically by name or number. This allows an entity to track specific user activity and to hold users accountable for functions performed when logged into those systems. Figure 8-8 illustrates a login procedure.

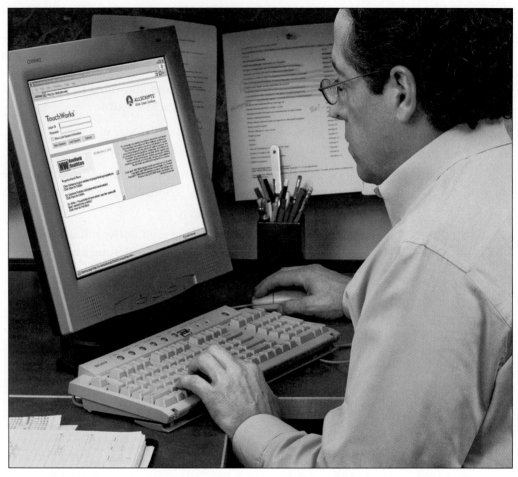

Courtesy of Allscripts, LLC.

▶ **Figure 8-8 A Clinician Logs on Touchworks Using a Unique User ID and Secure Password.**

2. **Emergency Access Procedure** Emergency Access procedures are documented instructions and operational practices for obtaining access to necessary EPHI during an emergency situation. Access Controls are necessary under emergency conditions, although they may be very different from those used in normal operational circumstances.

3. **Automatic Logoff** As a general practice, users should log off the system they are working on when their workstation is unattended. However, there will be times when workers may not have the time, or will not remember, to log off a workstation. Automatic logoff is an effective way to prevent unauthorized users from accessing EPHI on a workstation when it is left unattended for a period of time.

Many applications have configuration settings for automatic logoff. After a predetermined period of inactivity, the application will automatically log off the user. Some systems that may have more limited capabilities may activate an operating system screen saver that is password-protected after a period of system inactivity. In either case, the information that was displayed on the screen is no longer accessible to unauthorized users.

4. **Encryption and Decryption** Encryption is a method of converting an original message of regular text into encoded text. The text is encrypted by means of an algorithm (a mathematical formula). The receiving party who has the key to decrypt (i.e., translate) the text can convert it back into plain, comprehensible text. There are many different encryption methods and technologies to protect data from being accessed and viewed by unauthorized users.

Audit Controls

Audit Controls are *"hardware, software, and/or procedural mechanisms that record and examine activity in information systems."*

Most information systems provide some level of audit controls and audit reports. These are useful, especially when determining if a security violation occurred. This standard has no implementation specifications.

Integrity

Protecting the integrity of EPHI is a primary goal of the Security Rule. EPHI that is improperly altered or destroyed can result in clinical quality problems, including patient safety issues. The integrity of data can be compromised by both technical and nontechnical sources.

There is one addressable implementation specification in the Integrity standard.

1. **Mechanism to Authenticate Electronic Protected Health Information** Once risks to the integrity of EPHI data have been identified during the risk analysis, security measures are put in place to reduce the risks.

Person or Entity Authentication

The Person or Entity Authentication standard has no implementation specifications. This standard requires *"procedures to verify that a person or entity seeking access to electronic protected health information is the one claimed."*

There are several ways to provide proof of identity for authentication.

◆ Require something known only to that individual, such as a password or PIN.

◆ Require something that individuals possess, such as a smart card, a token, or a key.

◆ Require something unique to the individual such as a biometric. Examples of biometrics include fingerprints, voice patterns, facial patterns, or iris patterns.

Most covered entities use one of the first two methods of authentication. Many small provider offices rely on a password or PIN to authenticate the user.

Transmission Security

Transmission Security procedures are the "*measures used to guard against unauthorized access to electronic protected health information that is being transmitted.*"

The Security Rule allows for EPHI to be sent over an electronic open network as long as it is adequately protected. This standard has two implementation specifications.

1. **Integrity Controls** Protecting the integrity of EPHI maintained in information systems was discussed previously in the Integrity standard. Integrity in this context is focused on making sure the EPHI is not improperly modified during transmission.

   A primary method for protecting the integrity of EPHI being transmitted is through the use of network communications protocols. Using these protocols, the computer verifies that the data sent is the same as the data received.

2. **Encryption** As previously described in the Access Control standard, encryption is a method of converting an original message of regular text into encoded or unreadable text that is eventually decrypted into plain comprehensible text.

   Encryption is necessary for transmitting EPHI over the Internet. There are various types of encryption technology available, but for encryption technologies to work properly both the sender and receiver must be using the same or compatible technology. Currently no single interoperable encryption solution for communicating over open networks exists.

Organizational, Policies and Procedures and Documentation Requirements[18]

In addition to the standards in the Administrative, Physical, and Technical Safeguards categories of the Security Rule, there also are four other standards that must be implemented. These are not listed in the Security Standards Matrix (Figure 8-4), but they must not be overlooked.

Organizational Requirements

There are two implementation specifications of this standard.

1. **Business Associate Contracts** The Business Associate Contracts used if the business associate creates, receives, maintains, or transmits EPHI must meet the Security Rule requirements.

2. **Other Arrangements** The Other Arrangements implementation specifications apply when both parties are government entities. There are two alternative arrangements:

   1. A memorandum of understanding (MOU), which accomplishes the objectives of the Business Associate Contracts section of the Security Rule;

   2. A law or regulations applicable to the business associate that accomplishes the objectives of the Business Associate Contracts section of the Security Rule.

---

[18]Adapted from: Security Standards: Organizational, Policies and Procedures and Documentation Requirements, CMS HIPAA paper 5 of 7 on security.

Policies and Procedures

Although this standard requires covered entities to implement policies and procedures, the Security Rule does not define either "policy" or "procedure." Generally, policies define an organization's approach. Procedures describe how the organization carries out that approach, setting forth explicit, step-by-step instructions that implement the organization's policies. Policies and procedures may be modified as necessary.

Documentation

The Documentation standard has three implementation specifications.

1. **Time Limit** Retain the documentation required by [the rule] for 6 years from the date of its creation or the date when it last was in effect, whichever is later.

2. **Availability** Make documentation available to those persons responsible for implementing the procedures to which the documentation pertains.

3. **Updates** Review documentation periodically, and update as needed, in response to environmental or operational changes affecting the security of the electronic protected health information.

The Security Rule also requires that a covered entity document the rationale for all security decisions.

Electronic Signatures for Medical Records

The HIPAA Security Rule was originally titled "Security and Electronic Signature Standards." The original Security Rule also proposed a standard for electronic signatures. The final rule covered only security standards.

In 2000, President Clinton signed into federal law the Electronic Signatures in Global and National Commerce Act, which made digital signatures as binding as their paper-based counterparts. The law made digital signatures valid for commerce, but HIPAA does not require the use of electronic signatures, because HIPAA does not yet have a Rule for Electronic Signature standards. A Rule for Electronic Signature standards may be proposed at a later date.

Electronic Signature standards eventually will be necessary to achieve a completely paperless EHR. In this section, we will discuss Electronic Signatures and the criteria required for successful implementation.

What Is an Electronic Signature and What Is Not?

Compare Figure 8-9 and Figure 8-10. Which of these has an Electronic Signature? If you said Figure 8-10, you are correct. An Electronic Signature is not a scanned image of someone's paper signature. Valid Electronic Signatures must meet three criteria.

1. **Message Integrity** Message Integrity means the recipient must be able to confirm that the document has not been altered since it was signed.

2. **Nonrepudiation** The signer must not be able to deny signing the document.

3. **User Authentication** The recipient must be able to confirm that the signature was in fact "signed" by the real person.

► **Figure 8-9 Document with Digital Image of Signature.**

► **Figure 8-9 Document with Digital Image of Signature.**

4/28/2006 11:00AM

S. Rosa Garcia is a 27 year old female complaining of chronic/recurring headaches for more than 5 days. Headaches are occurring daily, recently worse, inadequately controlled, and lasting 2-4 hours.
Daily coffee consumption was 7-8 cups per day but she recently stopped all coffee consumption.

O. Physical exam showed no evidence of a head injury. A mental status exam was normal.
Vital Signs were WNL:

Vital Signs/Measurements	Value
Oral temperature	98.6 F
RR	25 breaths/min
PR	75 bpm
Blood pressure	117/75 mmHg
Weight	140 lbs
Height	64 in

A. Vasoconstrictor withdrawal headache from caffeine

P. Eat regular meals, get plenty of exercise, and limit intake of caffeine, and alcohol

Terry Jones, M.D

► **Figure 8-10 Electronically Signed Document with a PKI Signature.**

► **Figure 8-10 Electronically Signed Document with a PKI Signature.**

```
<Signed SigID=001>
```

4/28/2006 11:00AM

S. Rosa Garcia is a 27 year old female complaining of chronic/recurring headaches for more than 5 days. Headaches are occurring daily, recently worse, inadequately controlled, and lasting 2-4 hours.
Daily coffee consumption was 7-8 cups per day but she recently stopped all coffee consumption.

O. Physical exam showed no evidence of a head injury. A mental status exam was normal.
Vital Signs were WNL:

Vital Signs/Measurements	Value
Oral temperature	98.6 F
RR	25 breaths/min
PR	75 bpm
Blood pressure	117/75 mmHg
Weight	140 lbs
Height	64 in

A. Vasoconstrictor withdrawal headache from caffeine

P. Eat regular meals, get plenty of exercise, and limit intake of caffeine, and alcohol

// Electronically Signed by Terry Jones, M.D. 200604281114EST

```
</Signed>
<Signature SigID=001 PsnID=jones001>
2AB3764578CB212990BA5C18A29870F40198B240C330249C9461D20774C1622D
39D2302B2349802DE002342
</Signature>
```

The electronic signature process involves the successful identification and authentication of the signer at the time of the signature, binding of the signature to the document and non-alterability of the document after the signature has been affixed. Only "digital signatures" meet all three of these criteria.

How Digital Signatures Work

Digital signatures use a branch of mathematics called cryptography and PKI, which stands for Public Key Infrastructure. Each PKI user has two "keys," a private key for signing documents and a public key for verifying his or her signature. Only you know your private key, whereas your public key is available to all through a public directory.

Usually the directory for your public key is maintained by a certificate authority. The certificate authority is a trusted third party who has validated your identity and issued a certificate to that effect. A certificate is an electronic record of your public key, which has been digitally signed by the certificate authority. The certificate can be validated by its own key. This provides reasonable assurance that the signer and their public key are genuine.

Figure 8-11 illustrates the Electronic Signature and verification process of PKI. Compare Figure 8-11 with the following steps:

1. A computer software program performs a mathematical calculation on the entire contents of the electronic document to be signed.
2. The result is a unique code referred to as the "message digest."
3. This code is encrypted using your "private" key. Your private key might be similar to a password, which you must keep secret so that no one else can "forge" your signature.

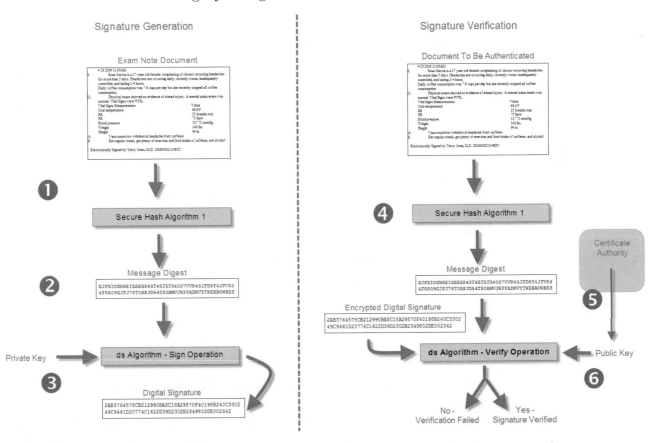

▶ **Figure 8-11 How a Digital Signature Works.**[19]

---

[19]Figure adapted from: Digital Signature Standard, published by U.S. Department of Commerce/National Institute of Standards and Technology, 2000.

The digital signature is then typically attached to or sent with the document.

When the recipient wishes to validate your signature they use a computer program that decodes the signature with your public key, and determines if the message digest is identical to that which was originally sent.

4. The validation process uses the same algorithm as the original program to produce a "message digest" of the text of the document.

5. The public key is retrieved from a public directory or certificate authority.

6. The signature verification process decodes the digital signature using your public key and compares it to the message digest. If the results of the algorithm match, the signature is verified.

PKI digital signatures not only confirm that you are the signer but also that the document has not been altered since you signed it.

Some Electronic Signatures Are Not Truly Signatures

Even though HIPAA has not adopted an official standard for Electronic Signatures, they are already necessary in the EHR. Prescriptions are sent to a pharmacy, dictation and electronic medical records are "signed," and orders are issued from EHR systems every day. However, most of the systems currently in use do not use the process described earlier to produce and store an electronic signature.

Many systems have a process to "sign" their records with a PIN, a password, or even a fingerprint, but the underlying software simply sets a field in the database indicating the provider "signed" the record. This is adequate to the particular EHR system, but it would not meet the criteria of an Electronic Signature if it were necessary to send a copy of the record to an outside entity. Partly this is the fault of HHS. Until there is a national infrastructure for issuing certificates and national standards for signing and validating digital signatures, EHR software cannot comply.

Whether electronic signatures in your office are true digital signatures or just mechanisms for locking and protecting EHR system records, it is important that you follow the policies and procedures of your facility. Most EHR systems have an internal audit trail detailing who has created each document and medical record.

◆ Always log on to the EHR as yourself.

◆ Always log off when you are through.

◆ Always keep your passwords or PIN numbers private.

This will prevent someone else from signing medical records under your ID.

The Future of Electronic Signatures

The Joint Commission on Accreditation of Healthcare Organizations (JCAHO) accepts the use of electronic signatures in hospital, ambulatory care, home care, long-term care, and mental health settings. The JCAHO requirement for electronic signatures and computer key signatures is simple: "The practitioner must sign a statement that he or she alone will use it."[20]

---

[20]*Comprehensive Accreditation Manual for Hospitals (CAMH)*, Standard IM. 6.10, Joint Commission on Accreditation of Healthcare Organizations, 2004.

Currently, CMS permits the authentication of medical records by computer key but does not specify methods. The President of the United States directed the U.S. Department of Commerce, National Institute of Standards and Technology to develop a set of standards for Digital Signatures. HHS will likely adopt the same cryptographically based digital signature for the HIPAA standard.

State laws vary on electronic signatures for medical records and some do not address it at all. States will likely come into alignment only after HHS publication of HIPAA standards for electronic signatures. If you have any question about regulations in your state, check with the medical licensing authority in your state.

HIPAA Privacy, Security, and You

As someone who will work with patients' health records, it is especially important for you to understand the regulations regarding privacy and security. Follow the privacy policy and security rules at your place of work. Know who the Privacy and Security Officials are. Ask them if you have any questions regarding policies at your practice or if you feel that you need additional training.

It is especially important not to give others your password and to always log out of a medical records computer when you are not using it. Remember to treat every medical record, paper or electronic, in a confidential manner.

Hands-On Exercise 48: Medical Office Privacy Policy

The purpose of this exercise is let you compare what you have learned in this chapter to an example from the real world. Visit a medical office and ask for a copy of their HIPAA Privacy Policy. Some offices provide their privacy policy on their Web site as well. You may print a copy of that as an acceptable alternative for the exercise.

Compare the contents of the privacy policy with the points in the sample CMS brochure shown in Figure 8-3. Write a brief paper comparing the points of the government document with the copy of the privacy policy you obtained. Give your instructor a copy of the privacy policy you obtained along with your paper.

Chapter Eight Summary

The Health Insurance Portability and Accountability Act, or HIPAA, was passed in 1996. The Administrative Simplification Subsection (Title 2, f) (hereafter just called HIPAA) has four distinct components:

1. Transactions and Code Sets
2. Uniform Identifiers
3. Privacy
4. Security

HIPAA regulates health plans, clearinghouses, and health care providers as "covered entities" or a "covered entity" with regard to these four areas.

HIPAA standardized formats for EDI or Electronic Data Interchange by requiring specific Transaction Standards. These currently are used for eight types of transactions between covered entities. This was the first of the Administrative Simplification Subsection to be implemented. This section also requires standardized code sets such as HCPCS, CPT-4, ICD-9CM, and others to be used.

HIPAA also established Uniform Identifier Standards, which will be used on all claims and other data transmissions. These will include:

◆ National Provider Identifier for doctors, nurses, and other health care providers.

◆ Federal Employer Identification Number used to identify employer-sponsored health insurance.

◆ National Health Plan Identifier, a unique identification number that will be assigned to each insurance plan, and to the organizations that administer insurance plans, such as payers and third-party administrators.

The privacy and security rules use two acronyms: PHI, which stands for Protected Health Information, and EPHI, which stands for Protected Health Information in an Electronic Format.

The HIPAA privacy standards are designed to protect a patient's identifiable health information from unauthorized disclosure or use in any form, while permitting the practice to deliver the best health care possible. To comply with the law that became effective April 14, 2003, privacy activities in the average medical office might include:

◆ Providing a copy of the office privacy policy informing patients about their privacy rights and how their information can be used.

◆ Asking the patient to acknowledge receiving a copy of the policy or signing a consent form.

◆ Obtaining signed authorization forms and in some cases tracking the disclosures of patient health information when it is to be given to a person or organization outside the practice for purposes other than treatment, billing, or payment.

◆ Adopting clear privacy procedures for its practice.

◆ Training employees so that they understand the privacy procedures.

◆ Designating an individual to be responsible for seeing that the privacy procedures are adopted and followed.

◆ Securing patient records containing individually identifiable health information so that they are not readily available to those who do not need them.

When the privacy rule initially was issued, it required providers to obtain patient "consent" to use and disclose protected health information (PHI) for purposes of treatment, payment, and health care operations, except in emergencies. The rule was almost immediately revised to make consent optional. In general, the practice can use PHI for almost anything related to treating the patient, running the medical practice, and getting paid for services. This means doctors, nurses, and other staff can share the patient's chart within the practice.

Authorization differs from consent in that it *does* require the patient's permission to disclose PHI. Some examples of instances that would require an authorization would include sending the results of an employment physical to an employer, sending immunization records, or the results of an athletic physical to the school.

The authorization form must include a date signed, an expiration date, to whom the information may be disclosed, what is permitted to be disclosed, and for what purpose the information may be used. The authorization must be signed by the patient or a representative appointed by the patient. Unlike the open concept of consent, authorizations are not global. A new authorization is signed each time there is a different purpose or need for the patient's information to be disclosed.

Practices are permitted to disclose PHI without a patient's authorization or consent when it is requested by an authorized government agency. Generally such requests are for legal (law enforcement, subpoena, court orders, etc.) public health purposes, or for enforcement of the Privacy Rule itself. Providers also are permitted to disclose PHI concerning on-the-job injuries to Workers' Compensation insurers, state administrators, and other entities to the extent required by state law.

Whether the practice has disclosed PHI based on a signed authorization or to comply with a government agency, the patient is entitled to know about it. The privacy rule gives the individuals the right to receive a report of all disclosures made for purposes *other than treatment, payment, or operations*. Therefore, in most cases the medical office must track the disclosure and keep the records for at least 6 years.

Most health care providers and health plans use the services of a variety of other persons or businesses. The Privacy Rule allows covered providers and health plans to disclose protected health information to these "business associates." The Privacy Rule requires that a covered entity obtain a written agreement from its business associate, which states the business associate will appropriately safeguard the protected health information it receives or creates on behalf of the covered entity.

Congress provided civil and criminal penalties for covered entities that misuse personal health information. The privacy rule is enforced by the HHS Office for Civil Rights (OCR).

The Privacy Rule sets the standards for, among other things, who may have access to PHI, whereas the Security Rule sets the standards for ensuring that only those who should have access to EPHI actually will have access. The Privacy Rule applies to all forms of patients' protected health information, whether electronic, written, or oral. In contrast, the Security Rule covers only protected health information that is in electronic form.

Security standards were designed to provide guidelines to all types of covered entities, while affording them flexibility regarding how to implement the standards. Covered entities may use appropriate security measures that enable them to reasonably implement a standard.

Security standards were designed to be "technology neutral." The rule does not prescribe the use of specific technologies, so that the health care community will not be bound by specific systems or software that may become obsolete.

The security standards are divided into the categories of administrative, physical, and technical safeguards.

◆ **Administrative safeguards.** In general, these are the administrative functions that should be implemented to meet the security standards. These include assignment or delegation of security responsibility to an individual and security training requirements.

◆ **Physical safeguards.** In general, these are the mechanisms required to protect electronic systems, equipment and the data they hold, from threats, environmental hazards, and unauthorized intrusion. They include restricting access to EPHI and retaining off-site computer backups.

◆ **Technical safeguards.** In general, these are primarily the automated processes used to protect data and control access to data. They include using authentication controls to verify that the person signing onto a computer is authorized to access that EPHI, or encrypting and decrypting data as it is being stored or transmitted.

The original Security Rule also proposed a standard for electronic signatures. The final rule covered only security standards.

In 2000, President Clinton signed into federal law the Electronic Signatures in Global and National Commerce Act, which made digital signatures as binding as their paper-based counterparts. Although the law made digital signatures valid for commerce, HIPAA does not require the use of electronic signatures. Electronic Signature standards will eventually be necessary to achieve a completely paperless EHR. A Rule for Electronic Signature standards may be proposed at a later date.

A valid Electronic Signature must meet three criteria.

1. **Message Integrity**—the recipient must be able to confirm that the document has not been altered since it was signed.

2. **Nonrepudiation**—the signer must not be able to deny signing the document.

3. **User Authentication**—the recipient must be able to confirm that the signature was in fact "signed" by the real person.

Digital signatures meet all three of these criteria. Digital signatures use a branch of mathematics called cryptography and PKI, which stands for Public Key Infrastructure.

Each PKI user has two "keys," a private key for signing documents and a public key for verifying his or her signature. A computer software program performs a mathematical calculation on the entire contents of the electronic document to be signed. The result is a unique "message digest," which is then encrypted using the "private" key.

The digital signature is then attached to or sent with the document. When the recipient wishes to validate the signature, a similar computer program regenerates the "message digest" and decodes the digital signature with the public key. Comparing the two, the program determines if the message digest is identical to that which was originally sent. In this way digital signatures not only confirm that you are the signer but also that the document has not been altered since it was signed.

Testing Your Knowledge of Chapter 8

Answer the following questions:

1. What do the acronyms PHI and EPHI stand for?
2. List the three criteria of an Electronic Signature.
3. Compare the difference between Consent and Authorization.
4. Does a provider need the patient's consent to share PHI with an authorized government agency?
5. List the four components of the HIPAA Administrative Simplification Subsection.
6. Which part of the regulation went into effect first?
7. Which part of the regulation went into effect last?
8. Business Associate Agreements apply to which components of the Administrative Simplification Subsection?
9. What department of the U.S. government enforces HIPAA?
10. List the three categories of the Security Rule.
11. Name the covered entities under HIPAA.
12. Which components of the Administrative Simplification Subsection require employee training?
13. List the requirements for the medical office privacy policy.
14. Name three of the Technical Safeguards.
15. Who may sign an authorization to release PHI?

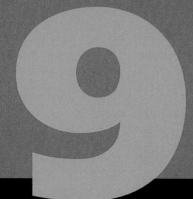

EHR and Technology

Learning Outcomes

After completing this chapter, you should be able to:

◆ Explain how technology impacts implementation of EHR

◆ Compare the use of workstations, laptop computers, Tablet PCs, and PDA devices

◆ Understand how the clinician's style and mobility affect the choice of EHR devices

◆ Understand how wireless networks work

◆ Understand how speech recognition works

◆ Use an EHR drawing tool to annotate drawings in an exam note

◆ Discuss the effect of the Internet on the future of the EHR

◆ Describe the differences between provider-to-patient e-mail, secure messaging, and e-visits

◆ Discuss patient access to electronic health records

Acronyms are used extensively in both medicine and computers. The following are those that are used in this chapter.

CAT	Computerized Axial Tomography
ECG	Electrocardiogram
EPHI	Protected Health Information in Electronic Form
IOM	Institute of Medicine
LAN	Local Area Network
OB	Obstetrics
PC	Personal Computer
PDA	Personal Digital Assistant
SSL	Secure Socket Layer
RAM	Random Access Memory (computer memory)
VPN	Virtual Private Network
WEP	Wired Equivalent Privacy
Wi-Fi	Wireless Fidelity (wireless computer networking)

How Technology Impacts Implementation of EHR

In the book *The Electronic Physician*, the authors compare the adoption of the EHR to the automobile. Let us begin this chapter by expanding on that useful analogy.[1]

A hundred years ago, the most common means of transportation was the horse and carriage. As the first automobiles began to appear, people referred to them as "horseless carriages." The people of that era conceptualized this new invention in terms of the existing technology. Even the inventors of the technology were not immune to this viewpoint. Isn't the engine in the front of a car today because that's where the horse was yesteryear?

As the automobile began to appear across the country, many people did not rush to adopt it or understand the full potential of the change that society was about to undergo. The new vehicles seemed to some to be fancy toys, inferior to the horse and carriage in many ways. The supply chain of the period was built to feed and water the horse, not gas up the car. The state of the roads, which were passable by horse, often led cars to being stuck. Viewed within the existing infrastructure of their time, the critics were right; driving an automobile instead of a carriage seemed like a lot of work for very little gain.

People of our era use the term Electronic Medical Records because we are thinking in terms of paper Medical Records. However, the opinion in a report by the IOM is that "Merely automating the form, content, and procedures of current patient records will perpetuate their deficiencies and will be insufficient to meet emerging user needs."[2]

---

[1]Analogy paraphrased from *The Electronic Physician*, ed. Todd Stein, Allscripts Healthcare Solutions, Chicago, IL. © 2005.

[2]R. S. Dick and E. B. Steen, *The Computer-based Patient Record: An Essential Technology for Health Care*, Institute of Medicine, Washington, DC: National Academy Press 1991, revised 1997, 2000.

Using the horseless carriage analogy, you can see that the office workflow has been designed around the infrastructure of a paper chart. Adapting the electronic chart to fit the old technology provides a level of comfort during the transition to the new system, but it also prevents us from seeing the full potential of the EHR. Similar to driving early automobiles on inadequate roads, implementing an EHR without considering the landscape can make it seem like a lot of work for very little gain.

In this chapter, we are going to examine how the office environment and the choice of computers, devices, and technology can affect the successful adoption of an EHR. To quote Peter Gerloffs, Medical Director of Allscripts, LLC, a leading EHR vendor, "If physicians don't use it, nothing else matters." This means, of course, that the EHR has to be designed and deployed in a way that enables clinicians to make it a part of their workflow that is as natural as driving their car to the office. We also are going to look at the impact of the Internet on the medical office, the patient, and the physician.

Style of Practice

The first consideration is not just the physical layout of your office but the style of clinician–patient interaction with which you are comfortable. In some ways, this will determine how and where you want to use computers to achieve point-of-care EHR.

Allen R. Wenner M.D. and John W. Bachman M.D. describe three types of patient–physician relationships:[3]

1. The doctor is paternalistic telling the patient what to do;

2. The doctor gives the patient information and the patient decides what to do;

3. Patients and doctors share information to determine the best plan for given conditions.

Wenner and Bachman believe patients will help the physician when they are given some degree of control, as reflected in points 2 and 3. Doctors also have found that patients react favorably to the use of a computer during the exam, especially when they are part of the process, able to see the screen, and able to participate in the review of their information.

▶ **Figure 9-1 Stages of Change in EHR Adoption**

Stages of Change in EHR Technology Adoption			
Stage	Technology Adoption	Medical Records	Medical Practice
Stage I	Do it the old way	The paper chart used and viewed as an historical document by physicians	Health care providers are the center of health care
Stage II	Adopt technology but continue to do it the old way	Transcribing dictation onto paper, using the EHR for data storage only managed by staff	Providers continue to dominate medical decisions and maintain all health care data
Stage III	Change the workflow to leverage the technology Paperless medical office	Use EHR at the point-of-care with providers and patients participating to allow real-time continuity of care	Patients and providers will share decision making as health care information is available to both

---

[3]Allen R. Wenner and John W. Bachman, *Transforming the Physician Practice: Interview with a Computer*, Healthcare Information Management Systems, 3rd Edition, Copyright © 2003.

Figure 9-1, provided by Dr. Wenner, lists the stages of change resulting from adoption of an EHR.

The Physical Clinic and Clinician Mobility

Another consideration is how mobile the providers are when they are in the office.

1. Does a clinician have a preassigned set of exam rooms they always use for their patients or does the office have a number of rooms which are shared randomly by several providers throughout the day?

2. Is the clinician likely to complete the note and all orders when in the exam room, or do so on the way to the next room?

3. Where/when will the clinician review lab results, radiology reports, e-mail messages, prescription renewals, and so on; on the move throughout the day, at a desk in his or her office, or from home over the Internet?

The following discussion of various technology and devices used in EHR solutions today will provide you with an idea of how these installations work in a medical office.

EHR on Computer Workstations

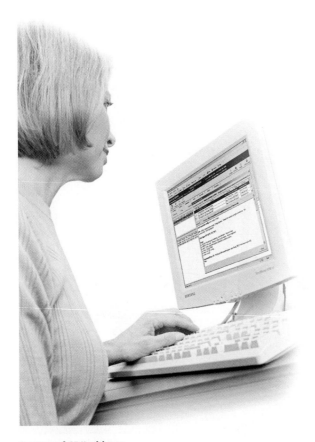

Courtesy of GE Healthcare.

▶ **Figure 9-2 Computer Workstation Connected to the Wired LAN.**

In most offices, you will find computer workstations in the billing, nursing, and lab areas, as shown in Figure 9-2. In some offices, you will find them in the exam room, and in a comparatively few offices you will find them in the waiting room or a subwaiting area for patients to use.

Computer workstations are cheap, reliable, dependable, and usually fixed in one location. You are probably working on one right now. They take up more space, requiring extra room for the keyboard and mouse. They are, however, easier for the IT department to manage and usually easier to upgrade when necessary.

Certainly workstations at fixed positions will be the right choice for some of the personnel who input data in your EHR. Whether they make sense at the point of care depends on how much free space you have in your exam rooms and if your providers want to finish up their exam notes before or after leaving the room. Most medical facilities were built long before anyone thought of putting computers in the exam rooms. Many exam rooms are already filled with supplies and equipment used for the exams and have only a small counter or writing area.

Although workstations can pose a security risk in the exam room when left unattended, that is easily handled through any number of biometric, or smart card, and auto sign-off solutions. With these solutions, the screen blanks or the EHR is logged off whenever an authorized user is not present. An ID badge or other device has a computer chip imbedded in it that can be detected by the workstation. Biometric solutions usually involve a pad on the keyboard or mouse that reads and authenticates a user's fingerprint.

One final advantage of the workstation is that it can support a substantially higher screen resolution (finer picture) than any other device. This makes it the only viable choice for radiologists and others who "read" diagnostic quality images of x-rays, CAT scans, and so on.

Of course, the medical office EHR is actually on a network server somewhere else. Workstations and other devices are connected to the network. This can be done with cables that have been wired in the building walls or through "wireless" access points that connect to the network through high-frequency radio signals. One advantage of a workstation is that it is ideally suited to a wired network connection. These are usually much faster and less subject to failure.

EHR on Laptop Computers

A laptop computer, as shown in Figure 9-3, packages the screen, keyboard, mouse, and computer in one unit, about the size of an 8″ × 11″ notebook. In a medical office, these provide mobility for clinicians who want to stay connected and take their work from room to room.

Although laptops can be connected to a wired network fairly easily, it is usually bothersome to have to plug the computer in and log on to the network each time you enter a room. For this reason, most laptops use a wireless standard

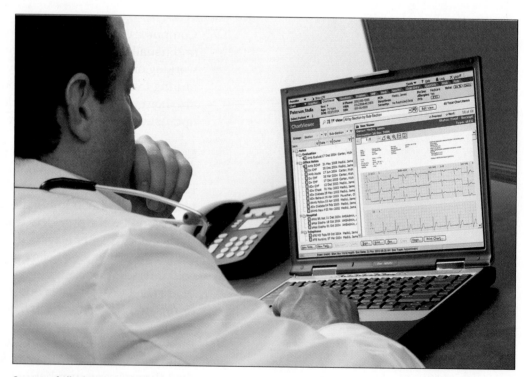

Courtesy of Allscripts, LLC.

▶ **Figure 9-3 Laptop Computers with Wi-Fi Connectivity Provide Portability.**

called "Wi-Fi," which stands for "wireless fidelity," to connect to the network. Wi-Fi capability is standard on many higher-end laptop computers.

Wireless networking, however, works only for very short distances; therefore, it requires infrastructure in the medical facility. Transmitters and receivers called "access points" must be installed throughout the building in close enough proximity that the laptop (or other wireless device) can always find the radio signal. Wireless networks will be discussed in more detail later in this chapter.

There are some concerns that wireless access points can be used by unauthorized computers to enter the network, or that wireless transmissions containing EPHI can be intercepted. However, medical systems installed by qualified installers use secure authentication and encryption techniques (discussed in technical safeguards in Chapter 8), which effectively protect the EHR and patient data.

The real risk with laptop computers is that providers and clinical users will save PHI data to the laptop computer's hard drive. That data may then not be protected by the same safeguards used on the office network or built into the EHR system. Laptops also are more troublesome for the IT department to manage and update, and laptops eventually become obsolete because they have only limited capability for hardware upgrades.

Laptops have other issues as well. Typically they run on batteries. This means after 2 to 4 hours of use, the batteries need to be recharged. Although laptop computers have A/C adapters, most users don't like having to plug them in every time they come into a room. The small appearance of a laptop is deceptive. They typically weigh from 3.5 to 9 pounds; after carrying it all day, that weight feels quite heavy.

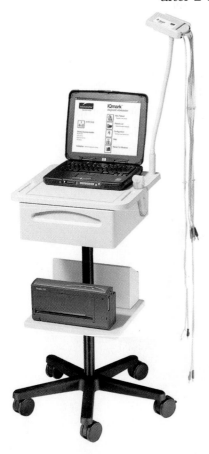

Being mobile, laptops also are more susceptible to being dropped, lost, or damaged. The keyboards are smaller and the built-in pointing devices that replace the mouse take some getting use to. However, laptops typically have high-resolution screens and will run almost any program that will run on a workstation.

One choice for offices with limited counter space in the exam rooms is to combine the laptop with a portable cart, as shown in Figure 9-4. The cart can easily be rolled from room to room and provides a stable and comfortable work area for the clinician. If the laptop has Wi-Fi connectivity, there is nothing to plug in. Also, if the batteries begin to run low, the A/C adapter-battery charger is usually right on the back of the cart. You also may have seen computer carts used on hospital floors. Carts are especially useful when there are extra cords or devices to carry such as the IQ-Mark™ Digital ECG, attached to the cart as shown in Figure 9-4.

EHR on a Tablet PC

The Tablet PC offers the size and portability (and drawbacks) of a laptop computer. However, it offers one feature that many providers really like. Users can move and click the mouse by just touching the screen with a special stylus supplied with the Tablet PC.

Courtesy of Midmark Diagnostics Group.

▶ **Figure 9-4 Laptop on Computer Cart.**

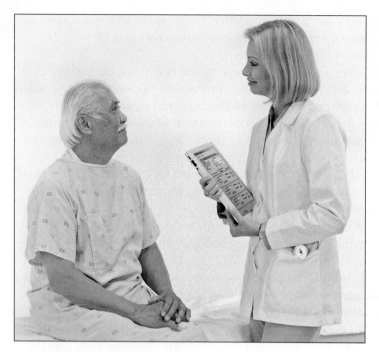

Courtesy of GE Healthcare.

▶ **Figure 9-5 Tablet PC Uses a Stylus Instead of a Mouse.**

EHR systems that involve primarily opening lists and clicking findings with a mouse (similar to the Student Edition software) work well on a Tablet PC.

If 95% of the charting is done with a mouse, then a Tablet PC is ideal. However, a Tablet PC typically does not have a keyboard for touch typing. Most have a small keyboard that can appear on the screen. Typing is done by clicking the mouse over each letter of the alphabet. This technique is serviceable for a word or two but painful for a clinician who uses a lot of free-text.

To compensate for the lack of a keyboard, the Tablet PC has two other features. One is handwriting recognition, which allows you to hand print characters on the screen, and then a few seconds later it will convert them into typed characters. The other is speech recognition, which is built into the Tablet PC operating system. Spoken words are recorded and then processed with special software to produce a text note. Both of these features require you to train the computer to recognize your handwriting or speech patterns. For some providers, these features work relatively well; others find that the error rate is too high.

Like laptops, a Tablet PC uses wireless networking and runs on batteries. Some models have a screen that flips over to become a laptop computer when a keyboard is needed for more extensive typing (see Figure 9-6).

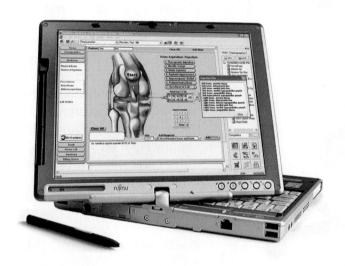

Courtesy of NextGen.

▶ **Figure 9-6 Annotate Drawings or Enter Findings with an Image on a Tablet PC.**

Most applications that run on a workstation will run on a Tablet PC. Some EHR applications are even enhanced to detect the Tablet PC and more fully take advantage of the Tablet PC features.

A Tablet PC is also an excellent choice for providers who annotate medical illustrations of body systems for either the medical record or for patient education. With a drawing application invoked, the stylus can be used on the screen just like an ink pen on paper. The experience is very similar. Ophthalmologists and dermatologists are two examples of medical specialists who tend to annotate illustrations in the medical record to record their observations. Later in this chapter, you will be able to experiment with annotated drawings, but you will not need a Tablet PC for the exercise.

EHR on Handheld PDA Devices

PDA or Personal Digital Assistants are ubiquitous today. Look around your class and you will probably find any number of fellow students who have a Palm Pilot™ or similar device. However, most of these don't qualify for an EHR. Remember, with all the devices we have discussed so far, the real EHR is somewhere else, on the network server.

A PDA that is to be used for an EHR requires the same wireless connectivity as the laptop and Tablet PC. It also usually requires a special piece of software that can act as a "client" to the EHR application. Because a PDA screen is significantly smaller than a computer screen, applications that run on a workstation, laptop, and Tablet PC will almost never run "as is" on a PDA. A PDA also has less memory and a much smaller microprocessor. Therefore, most EHR systems that offer PDA capability have a special component that communicates with and sends limited information to the PDA.

A PDA that can be used as an EHR device costs significantly more than the PDA devices you see around school, but they are about half the price of a laptop. For some providers, they are ideal. They are slightly heavier but not much larger than a prescription pad. In fact, the first widespread adoption of the PDA in medical offices was as an electronic prescription writer.

Except for the smaller screen, a PDA functions similarly to the Tablet PC. A special stylus is supplied with the device, which can be used as a mouse to write or draw directly on the screen. Handwriting recognition software is built in as well.

A number of documents and reference guides are available for download into the PDA. Some examples include The Guide to

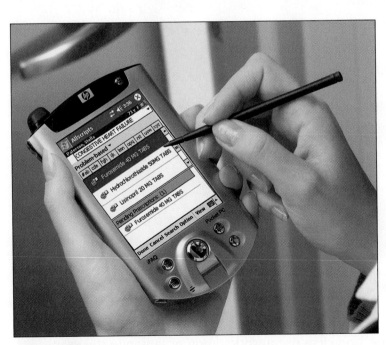

▶ **Figure 9-7 A Handheld PDA Is Light and Portable but Has a Small Screen.**

Preventive Services, the *Physicians Desk Reference*, CDC Immunization Schedules, and contact listings for doctors and facilities in the local area. Although these documents may not be integrated into the EHR, having them available at the point of care is considered a significant benefit by many clinicians.

Most EHR PDA devices also include a digital voice recorder that can be used by clinicians who still dictate. The advantage over other methods of recording dictation is that the clinician can see a list of patients, appointments, and other useful information on the PDA, and then select the patient and dictate. The digital dictation file is sent electronically through the wireless network to the transcription department; it is already associated with the correct patient, expediting the merge of the finished document with the patient's chart when the doctor approves it.

The real limitation for the PDA is the small screen size. The screen resolution is very good. Text is surprisingly readable, even the lengthy exam notes that you have created in recent exercises can be easily reviewed on a PDA. It is also easy to write orders, write prescriptions, and review lab results. It is not, however, easy to create a miniature version of an EHR such as you have been using in the Student Edition software. The screen just doesn't have enough space for comfortable data entry. As a result, some providers use multiple devices.

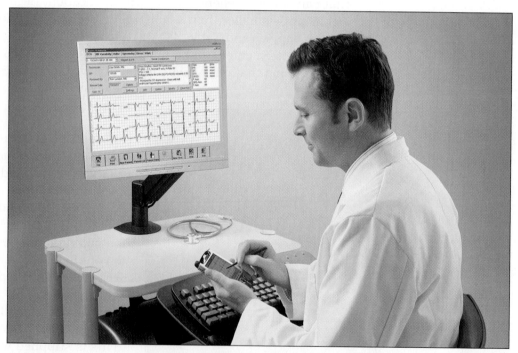

Courtesy of Midmark Diagnostics Group.

▶ **Figure 9-8 Providers Often Use Both a PDA and a Workstation or Laptop.**

In some medical offices, providers use a workstation or laptop in the exam room during the patient visit, whereas they carry a PDA to use for prescriptions, chart review, and scheduling. The most popular EHR systems can handle a mix of all these devices on the network and keep the patient record as perfect as if it were all maintained from a single type of device.

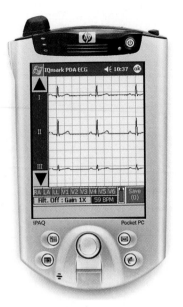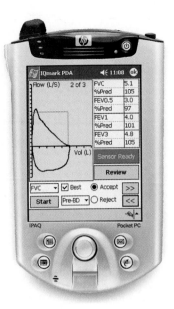

Courtesy of Midmark Diagnostics Group.

▶ Figure 9-9 IQmark™ Diagnostic PDA ECG and Spirometer.

Because the PDA has real microprocessing power, it has been adapted for several custom applications where its small size offers unparalleled portability. One example of that is IQmark™ Diagnostic PDA Software, which allows a provider to use a PDA to perform ECG (electrocardiogram) and spirometery tests. The PDA provides a pocket-sized test apparatus that, when connected to Midmark devices, captures and stores the test data. The test results can be saved into the EHR.

Note

How Wireless Networks Work

The Wi-Fi feature of many of the devices discussed in this chapter allows the clinician to move freely throughout the clinic yet stay connected to the EHR system. To make use of this feature, the medical office will need to have a "wireless" network.

Workstations in a medical office are usually connected to the main computer or "server" via cables wired throughout the building. This is called the local area network or LAN. Information between the workstation and the server is exchanged in small packets of data. A wireless network works exactly the same except that the data packets are exchanged using radio signals.

Each Wi-Fi device is equipped with a radio transceiver. This may be built in the device by the manufacturer or a wireless LAN adapter card that is added later. The "wired" LAN is connected to similar radio transceivers, called "access points," which are usually mounted in the ceiling throughout the building.

Each access point has a 150- to 300-foot range in which a quality wireless connection can be maintained. The actual distance varies depending on the construction of the building. To ensure complete coverage, multiple access points may be installed. A clinician can "roam" from one access point to another. The wireless network hardware automatically changes to the access point with the best signal, transparent to the user.

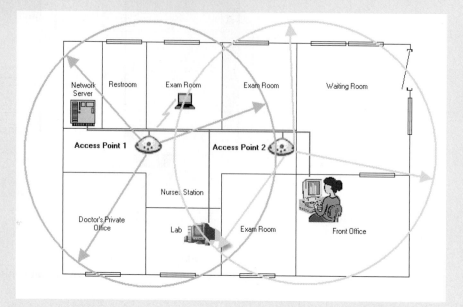

Network Server Restroom Exam Room Exam Room Waiting Room

Access Point 1 Access Point 2

Nurse Station

Doctor's Private Office Lab Exam Room Front Office

▶ Figure 9-10 Multiple Access Points Connected to the LAN Provide Overlapping Coverage.

Figure 9-10 illustrates the coverage area of an office with multiple access points. The red lines indicate the wired LAN cables connecting the computers and access points. The overlapping teal and lavender circles represent the range of radio signals from each access point. The laptop computer in the exam room is communicating with access point 1 because of its proximity.

There are potential security issues with wireless networks because the physical access controls that protect the wired network do not apply. The existence of the wireless network can be detected by any other wireless computer within its range. That does not mean, however, that wireless communications cannot be protected. Wireless networks use a standard called 802.11, which operates at 2.4GHz and cannot be received by a scanner or ordinary radio.

There are several methods that can be used individually or together to ensure that the wireless network stays private. 802.11 wireless communications use WEP (which stands for Wired Equivalent Privacy), to encrypt data sent over the network using 128-bit encryption. In secure systems, a foreign device won't even reach the network without the correct 128-bit WEP key.

A measure of security is also provided by a technique called "frequency hopping spread spectrum," which divides each data packet and sends parts of it across several adjacent radio frequencies. The interval in which the hopping signals change the radio frequency is too fast for most radios to follow.

Finally, a wireless network can use a Virtual Private Network or VPN just like a wired network. However, wireless networks today are slower than a wired network. A VPN adds additional data to packets, which may further slow down the rate of exchange.

EHR Devices and the Patient

Earlier in this chapter, you learned that the size of the exam rooms and the philosophy of clinician–patient relationship to some extent determine the type of EHR computers in your office. The photos in Figures 9-11 to 9-18 illustrate how these choices work in the doctor–patient relationship.

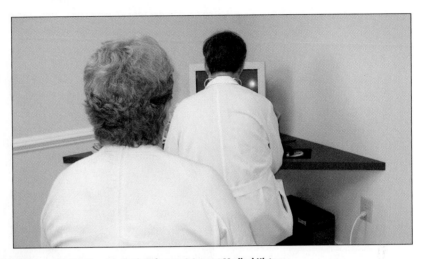

Courtesy of Primetime Medical Software & Instant Medical History.

▶ **Figure 9-11 Doctor Turns His Back on Patient When Using the Computer.**

In Figure 9-11, the doctor has installed computers in the exam room, allowing for point-of-care documentation. However, in this configuration, his back is turned away from his patient any time he wants to check something, review the history and symptoms, or enter findings himself.

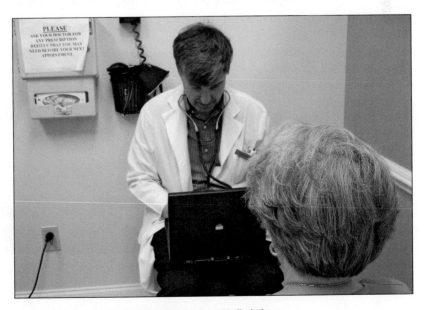

Courtesy of Primetime Medical Software & Instant Medical History.

▶ **Figure 9-12 Physician Using a Laptop During a Patient Visit.**

In Figure 9-12, you see a better approach to EHR input. At least the doctor can look up periodically and make eye contact when typing. Even though the computer is called a "laptop," actually holding it on your lap when using the mouse is uncomfortable and makes it difficult to type. Notice that the doctor is focused on using the computer and not on the patient. Doesn't the computer feel like an obstacle between them?

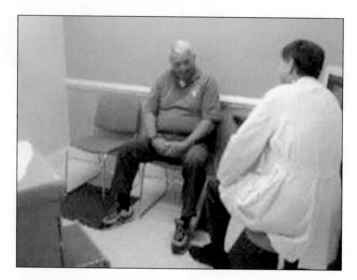

Courtesy of Primetime Medical Software & Instant Medical History.

▶ Figure 9-13 Doctor and Patient Converse with Computer at Doctor's Side.

In Figure 9-13, the doctor is focused on the patient. The computer is in the exam room and the doctor is positioned so that he can glance at it during any salient point in the discussion. Notice, however, that in this position the doctor still maintains the control over anything from the chart.

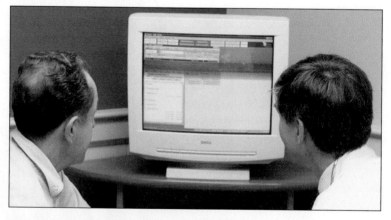

Courtesy of Primetime Medical Software & Instant Medical History.

▶ Figure 9-14 Patient and Doctor Share Computer.

Figure 9-14 illustrates a configuration recommended by Dr. Wenner. The patient, doctor, and computer form a triangle, which allows both of them to see the screen at once. This has been found useful for reviewing history and symptoms that have been entered by the patient (using Instant Medical History).

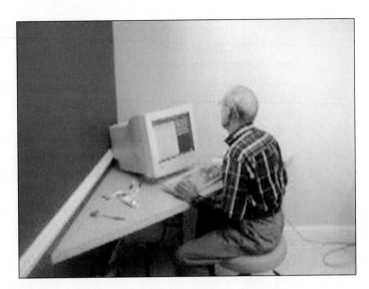

Courtesy of Primetime Medical Software & Instant Medical History.
▶ **Figure 9-15 Patient Entering Their Own History and Symptoms.**

As you learned in Chapter 6, one of the ways that a practice can more fully document patient medical history is to let the patient participate in the process. Dr. Wenner and his peers have found most patients willing and eager to answer a computer interview about their reason for the visit. Figure 9-15 shows a patient using a computer to do this in the privacy of the exam room. Alternatively, some offices using this technique have a private area of the waiting room or a subwaiting area for the computer interview.

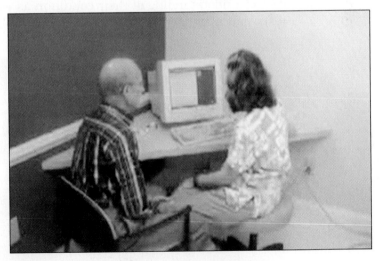

Courtesy of Primetime Medical Software & Instant Medical History.
▶ **Figure 9-16 Nurse Reviews with the Patient Data from the Computer Interview.**

Once the patient has completed their portion of the history and symptom information, a nurse is alerted. In Figure 9-16, the nurse reviews the patient entered information, asks further questions, and edits the note if there is additional information.

After the nurse has completed the review and taken and recorded the patient's vital signs, the patient is ready to see the doctor. The doctor enters the room, greets the patient, reviews the portions of the medical record already completed, and is able to focus on the patient. If the exam room is configured as shown earlier in Figure 9-14, the patient is able to engage in the mutual process of documenting the visit.

The patient benefits from this arrangement because when the patient and physician share information the patient feels a part of the decisions and has a vested interest in following the plan of care. The patient also benefits because the time the doctor has saved from having to input the symptoms and history can be focused fully on the patient and used for counseling and education.

John Mayne at the Mayo Clinic observed, "If the time physicians spend collecting, organizing, recording, and retrieving data could be reduced, at least in part, by information technology, more time would be available for actual delivery of medical care (and, thus, in effect increase the number of physicians) and at the same time the physician's capabilities for collecting information from patients would be extended."[4]

Using a point-of-care EHR, when the exam is complete, the note is complete. The clinician can then provide not only patient education materials for the patient to take home but also can actually print a copy of the finished note. Giving the patient a copy of the notes from that day's visit ensures that they will remember the key elements of their plan of treatment. They also will have a clearer understanding of their condition as well as any information on any tests that may have been ordered or performed.

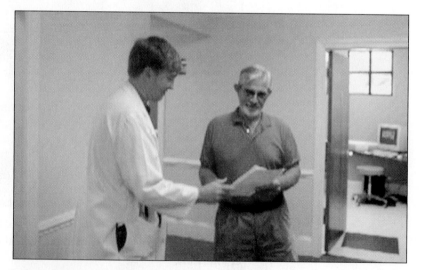

Courtesy of Primetime Medical Software & Instant Medical History.

▶ **Figure 9-17 Doctor Provides Patient with a Copy of Exam Notes from Visit.**

---

[4]Mayne JG, Weksel W, Sholtz PN. Toward automating the medical history. *Mayo Clin Proc* 1968; 43:1–25.

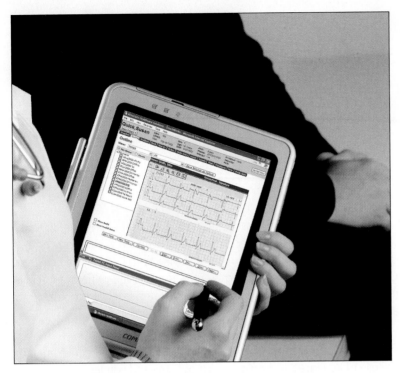

Courtesy of Allscripts, LLC.

▶ **Figure 9-18 Using a Tablet PC Doctor Discusses ECG Results with Patient.**

Dr. John Bachman M.D., a professor of Family Medicine at the Mayo Medical School in Rochester, Minnesota, has stated this in what he refers to as Bachman's rule and law:

Bachman's Rule: "A patient who has a copy of a note is impressed by the fact that all the information they provided and were given is included for them to review. It also is useful in that it has immunizations prevention information and instructions. Outcome studies have shown it to be helpful in compliance and improvement of health; crossing the Quality Chasm."

Bachman's Law: "A clinician who gives a patient a copy of their note has all their work complete. Consequently there is no dictation, rework, signing, or any activity of maintaining the administrative workflow. This saves a great deal of money and means the workflow systems are extremely efficient."

The availability of information from the EHR during the patient visit is an invaluable tool in counseling and patient education. The clinician has access to graphs, medical images, test results, and anatomical drawings, all of which are useful in explaining something related to the patient's condition or to illustrate an upcoming procedure. Using a Tablet PC, the doctor in Figure 9-18 is able to access the results of the patient's most recent electrocardiogram wirelessly and explain them to the patient.

Remote EHR Access for the Provider

The end of the scheduled day for most physicians really just means that the patients have left. Many physicians then turn to the task of "paperwork," reviewing test results, transcribed dictation, radiology reports, and patient charts.

Increasingly, medical office networks are configured to allow providers to access their patients' medical records away from the office. This often is called "remote access." The benefits to the provider and the patient are tremendous. Instead of staying late, the provider can go home, have dinner with the family, relax for a few hours, then sign on to the office computer system and complete any chart reviews or other work that would have previously meant staying late. Additionally, if the clinician receives an emergency call from or about a patient, the patient's records can be accessed from home, helping the clinician to make better decisions.

Networks can be enabled to allow remote sign-on. Clinicians connect to their office network and sign on just as they would in the office. There are several means by which remote access can be accomplished. However this is accomplished, it must be done securely, to protect the patient's EPHI (as you learned in Chapter 8).

The most secure method of connecting is through direct dial. Small offices with only one or two doctors can set up phone lines with special modems that receive a call from the doctor's home, disconnect, and redial the number for the

A Real-Life Story

Enhancing Process Efficiency Through Remote Access[5]

By Julie DeSantis

Hinsdale Hematology Oncology Associates, Ltd. (HHOA) of Hinsdale, Illinois, switched from traditional paper records to the advanced technology of wireless, mobile electronic medical records (EMR) from IMPAC Medical Systems. At HHOA, the result of implementing an EMR is improved patient and clinician satisfaction, an increased patient load, and an elevated level of process efficiency that has paid for itself within 2 years of implementation.

Michele White, practice administrator at HHOA, said that patient confidence improved with the use of advanced technology, such as PDAs and wireless laptop systems. "Our patients have noticed that our medical documentation is complete, up-to-date, and right at hand," she said. The patients have more confidence in our doctors, and have received more face-to-face interaction time during their visits, she said. "We have a high standard of care that we did not want to compromise, and with tablet PCs, wireless laptops, and the Siemens PDAs—we have everything we need to access lab reports, scheduling, and more."

HHOA provides services to 80–100 patients a day—an increase in patient load since installing IMPAC. With 12 busy exam rooms and only 6 physicians, they use IMPAC's online transcription and report management system to quickly and accurately document patient encounters and manage them online. In addition, HHOA uses a structured noting system for patient documentation within the EMR. All incoming lab results also are downloaded into the system via interface, and available from any laptop at the practice, ensuring the patient record is complete, up-to-date, and easily accessible to physicians and staff. "From an administrative and economic perspective, our mobile access to EMRs has meant that we did not need to purchase additional antivirus software and miscellaneous upgrades. We've saved a lot of money, while increasing efficiency, security, and reliability," White said.

For six years, HHOA used pcAnywhere™ in the physicians' homes to access the office. However, they have found remote access to the EMR from IMPAC to be faster, more reliable, and readily accessible from anywhere. There are six physicians on staff at HHOA, all with different technical knowledge, but "they are all comfortable with IMPAC's EMR," White explained. "They can get any reports they need and print right through the system when they are off-site."

---

[5]©2005 IMPAC Medical Systems, Inc. Used with permission.

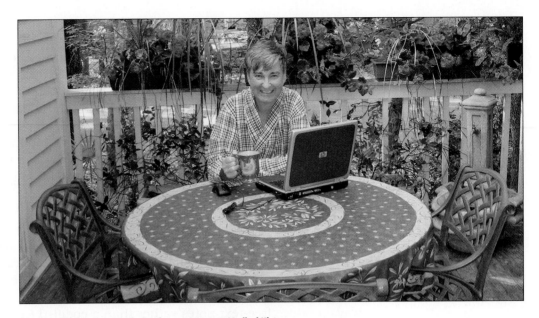

Courtesy of Primetime Medical Software & Instant Medical History.

▶ **Figure 9-19 Dr. Wenner Cleaning Up "Paperwork" from Home.**

home computer. This method prevents unauthorized persons from accessing the system. There are, however, several drawbacks to this method. First, it requires a modem and phone line for every user who needs remote access at the same time as someone else. This is why it is not usually used in clinics with more than a few doctors. The other drawback is that the clinicians can only access the EHR from phone numbers that have been preprogrammed for the modem to dial back.

The other means of getting remote access is by using the Internet. This allows the clinician to access the records from anywhere they can connect to the Internet. Security for direct access to the office computer on the Internet usually requires a VPN, which stands for Virtual Private Network. A VPN encrypts the data going in both directions. This encryption means that the connection can safely be made over a public network such as the Internet, yet the EPHI remains protected. Any computer that intercepted the data from a VPN connection would see only gibberish. A VPN is an ideal for medium to large practices because it is not limited by the number of phone lines the practice has, but running programs over a VPN is usually somewhat slower. A VPN is also complicated to set up and maintain. Your practice will need to have an IT professional manage a VPN.

A third method of remote access is provided by the EHR system itself. Some EHR vendors have created special software within their system that allows the clinician to access and interact with the EHR through the Internet via a secure Web site. The features vary by vendor, but typically the clinician can retrieve patients, review and sign charts, lab results, and look at anything in the patient chart. For most clinicians, this level of remote access is sufficient. This method may be preferred by your IT department because it limits the remote user's access to designated functions of the EHR and, therefore, does not present the level of risk to the computer network as a remote sign-on does. It is also desirable for smaller practices because it does not require a complicated VPN; transmission encryption is handled by the Secure Socket Layer (SSL) of the host Web site.

Speech Recognition

Another useful computer tool for clinicians is speech recognition. Speech recognition software recognizes the patterns in your speech as words and turns them into text. It has been the dream of many doctors that they could create a complete encounter note just by speaking about the patient visit.

Having clinical dictation instantly and automatically transcribed by a computer reduces turn-around time and eliminates the cost of a transcription service, but it does not necessarily produce a codified medical record.

Ray Kurzweil, a scientist and inventor, brought the first commercial large vocabulary speech recognition system to medicine in 1985. By 1990, his system was able to create structured medical records by voice recognition alone. (These were not codified medical records as we have defined them because this was before any national coding standard.) Today, speech recognition systems have advanced considerably and have a low error rate. However, they almost always produce free-text notes rather than a codified EHR.

For specialties such as radiology and pathology, the result of their work is often a report that is primarily text anyway. For them speech recognition is ideal. It can be used with a headset microphone that frees their hands for manipulation of the images or x-rays being read. Modern voice recognition software can send commands to other software on the computer. This allows the clinician to select patients, open orders, save reports, zoom images, or change contrast without using their hands.

Integration of speech recognition with an EHR can ensure the radiologist or pathologist report is automatically tied to the patient chart. In other specialties speech recognition is sometimes used to add free-text comments to findings in the codified medical record. This is especially popular with providers who use a Tablet PC if it does not have a keyboard.

Most people speak at least 160 words per minute but type fewer than 40 words a minute, so speech recognition should be a lot faster. Systems have improved considerably and can achieve up to 99% recognition, but most people seem to average about 95%. This means that a full-length dictation will have one or more errors that must be corrected. The time spent backing up and making corrections slows down the overall rate of efficiency. The good news is that speech recognition systems improve as they are used. Each time the speaker makes a correction, the system learns a little more about the speaker's voice patterns. Recognition is also improved by use of special medical versions, which recognize medical terms that might not be used in a layman's vocabulary. If you would like to know more about speech recognition read the technical explanation, How Speech Recognition Software Works.

> **Note**
>
> ## How Speech Recognition Software Works
>
> The first step in speech recognition is to transform the sound of your voice into a digital file the computer can use. A noise-canceling microphone discards background noise and sends your voice as an analog signal to the PC sound card, which converts it into a digital format. At that point, it is still just a stream of data that must be processed by speech recognition software. Here is what is involved.

You may think of a word you hear as a sound, but most words are really made up of multiple sounds called phonemes. This idea may seem new but you have actually used it for years. Look up any word in the dictionary and you will find its pronunciation represented with symbols for its phonemes (for example: fo' něm). In English, there are about 16 vowel sounds and 24 consonants making about 50 phonemes. Computer scientists measuring electrical patterns of sound waves found that phonemes were represented by differing levels of energy across various frequency bands, over a period of time.

Using mathematical calculations, the speech recognition software identifies the phonemes in the digital data. The phonemes are then compared to the "language model" of the software. Phonemes do not appear in every order; certain sounds would be impossible to articulate. Therefore, only certain sequences of phonemes correspond to words or word syllables. Although English has 10,000 possible syllables, even these will normally appear only in certain combinations and sequence.

In the early days of speech recognition software, the speaker was required to pause between each word. This simplified the analysis because in most cases pattern recognition could find a word with the matching phonemes in the correct order. For example, the phonemes b + el instantly match "bell," whereas t + el match "tell." However, pausing between every word was unnatural and users were dissatisfied. Today, speech recognition software processes "continuous speech" (the way that we speak naturally).

Recognition of continuous speech is not as easy as it sounds. The software must not only match the phonemes, but it also must group them correctly into words. Most people speak about three words a second, and there is an average of six phonemes per word. This means the computer must process about 18 phonemes per second. In addition, many words such as *they're*, *their*, and *there* sound alike. To identify the correct word, the software creates groups of three to four words, called trigrams, and compares them to common speech patterns in the language model to help it decide on the correct word. For example, if you dictated: "There appears to be a blockage . . ." then software would recognize that you didn't mean "their" or "they're" by the word's placement.

Once the correct words are identified, they are displayed on the screen as though you typed them. Usually there is a lag of a few seconds between the words you just spoke and the appearance of the text on your screen. If the software misidentifies a word, you can back up and correct it.

Each time the software misrecognizes a word and you correct it using the software, the computer stores your pronunciation for the corrected word. Then, the next time that you dictate that word, it will identify it correctly.

Speech recognition software also must deal with the diversity of regional accents and the variety of ways that we pronounce words. Most programs start with a simple training session in which you read into the software a document that it already recognizes. It then compares your pronunciation of the words to its existing language model and adjusts accordingly. It continues to build a personal profile of your speech by learning from its mistakes.

Modern speech recognition software typically comes with a vocabulary of about 150,000 words, most of which you do not have to train. However, the software cannot recognize words that it does not have in its vocabulary; the vocabulary usually does not include medical terms. Special versions of the software have language models made for medical dictation. If you are planning on using speech recognition for a health care setting, make certain you purchase a "medical" version.

One of the factors that made advances in speech recognition software possible was the evolution of faster and more powerful computers. As you may have inferred from the technical portions of the previous discussion, there is a lot of computing going on when the software analyzes your words and turns them into text. To get the best results from voice recognition software, use the fastest computer you can buy and add plenty of RAM.

Including Annotated Drawings in the EHR

Another method of entering data about the patient into the EHR involves the use of anatomical drawings of the body and body systems. These are particularly useful on a Tablet PC, but the same or similar result can be achieved on a laptop or workstation computer as well.

Some EHR systems have navigation pages that allow the clinician to quickly locate findings by pointing to a particular body part in a drawing which opens a list of findings relevant to that body system. The clinician then selects the findings appropriate to the visit. In this case, the pictures do not become part of the patient note; they are just a visual tool for navigation (refer back to Figure 9-6 for an example). Think of this as searching with pictures rather than words.

Certain specialists, however, routinely record information about the physical exam in the form of drawings or sketches. Two examples are dermatologists, who sometimes note the location of *nevi* (moles) on an outline of the body, and ophthalmologists, who frequently document observations on a drawing of the eye. These annotated drawings have long been a part of the patient's paper chart and most EHR systems today support a tool to annotate drawings in the computer. The images created using the tools in the EHR become part of the electronic encounter, and are useful for patient education as well.

Annotated images in an EHR are often attached to the note using special findings. These images might be annotated with the size and location of *nevi*, but handwritten notes within the images are not codified data. This means that for the purpose of subsequent analysis of the EHR records, the system will be able to locate patient records with a finding that denotes an attached image, but it would not be able to find patients with "> *20 nevi*" unless the clinician had entered them as findings in the narrative as well.

Hands-On Exercise 49: Annotated Dermatology Exam

This exercise will give you an opportunity to practice the annotation of a drawing using a simplified tool in the Student Edition software. As with previous exercises, the purpose here is to let you experience a function that is often available in commercial EHR systems. The drawing tools you will use here will be similar in principle but not identical to those you might use in your medical office. The method of invoking the annotation tool and the manner in which a drawing is subsequently merged into the patient note will vary by EHR vendor.

In this exercise, the patient has a large number of moles on his back, which the doctor has been monitoring through regular follow-up visits. In addition to the exam notes created at those visits, the clinician finds it useful to save annotated drawings, which show the placement of the moles. In subsequent visits, the doctor will compare the drawings from past encounters to the current state of the patient's skin to quickly identify new moles or changes from a previous visit.

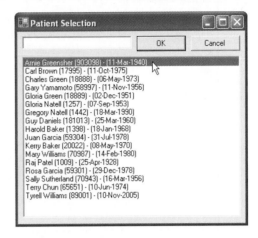

▶ Figure 9-20 Select Patient Arnie Greensher.

Step 1

If you have not already done so, start the Student Edition software.

Click Select on the Menu bar, and then click Patient.

In the Patient Selection window, locate and click on **Arnie Greensher**, as shown in Figure 9-20.

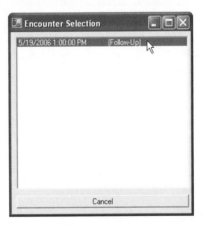

▶ Figure 9-21 Select Existing Encounter for May 19, 2006.

Step 2

Click Select on the Menu bar, and then click **Existing Encounter**.

A small window of previous encounters will be displayed. Compare your screen to the window shown in Figure 9-21.

Select the encounter dated **5/19/2006 1:00 PM (Follow-Up).**

The exam note from that date will be displayed as shown in Figure 9-22.

► Figure 9-22 Patient Exam
Note for May 19, 2006
Encounter.

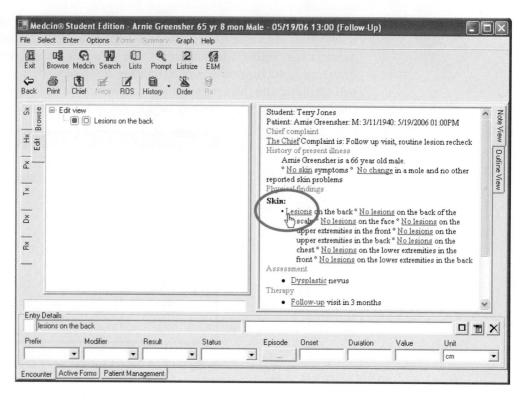

Step 3

In the right pane of your screen, locate and click on the underlined portion of the finding labeled "Lesions on the back" (circled in red). The left pane should change to Edit view, as shown in Figure 9-22.

► Figure 9-23 Click the
Context Button (circled in
red) and Select "Add Object
to Finding."

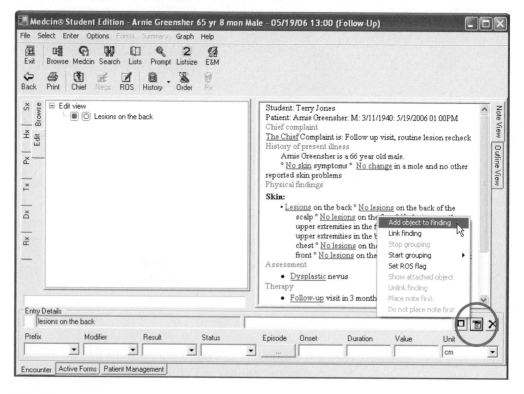

Step 4

Locate the three buttons in the lower right corner of the window. The Context button is the center button (circled in red in Figure 9-23).

Click on the Context button to display a list of advanced actions that can be used with a finding.

► **Figure 9-24 Template Image of Trunk and Back.**

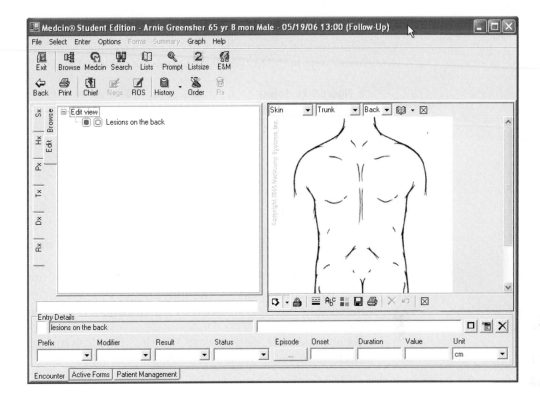

Click the first option in the list labeled "Add object to Finding." This will invoke the annotation tools in the right pane of the window (shown in Figure 9-24).

The software contains various anatomical illustrations, which may be selected for annotation. The right pane displays one of the images.

Above the image is a navigational bar consisting of three fields with drop-down lists. These are used to select images of other body systems and views.

◆ The first field can be used to select the body system to be presented (skin, circulatory, skeletal, etc.).

◆ The center field is used to select the image region within that system (full body, head and neck, lower extremities, etc.).

◆ The third field is used to select the view of the image (front, back, left, etc.).

The gender of the image as well as the age range of the image is automatically determined by the demographics of the current patient. The default body system for the image is automatically determined by the selected finding.

Compare your screen to Figure 9-24; if the image is not of the back of a man's trunk, click the down arrow of the center or right field to change the view. Select Trunk and Back from the respective drop-down lists.

► **Figure 9-25 Draw Toolbar (enlarged to show detail).**

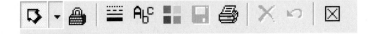

At the bottom of the image is the drawing toolbar, which is shown enlarged in Figure 9-25. We will discuss each of the buttons on the drawing toolbar, from left to right.

Select Tool The first icon on the toolbar shows the currently selected drawing shape or tool. The icon of the button will change according to the current selection. The down arrow next to the button displays a list of choices.

▶ **Figure 9-26 Select the Shape "Circle" from the Drop-Down List.**

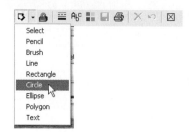

Step 5

Click the down arrow next to the Select button to display the list of tools.

Figure 9-26 shows the drop-down list of shapes of the drawing tool. Most are self-explanatory, except the first one, Select. The Select option is used to select items that have been added to the drawing so they can be deleted or modified.

Locate and click on the word "Circle." The drawing tool button will display a circle in place of the pointer.

Step 6

Lock Button The icon resembles a padlock. This is used to "lock" the selected shape. When it is "locked," the button will appear depressed and the selections you have made for shape or the other drawing tool buttons (discussed later) stay set. When it is not "locked" (does not appear depressed), the drawing toolbar buttons return to their default state after each use.

Locate and click on the "lock" button in the drawing toolbar.

Step 7

Style button icon consists of different horizontal lines. This button invokes the Style Selection window, which sets the pattern and thickness of the tools you will use to annotate the drawings. The style sets not only the line but also the solidity and thickness of other shapes.

▶ **Figure 9-27 Style Selections Window.**

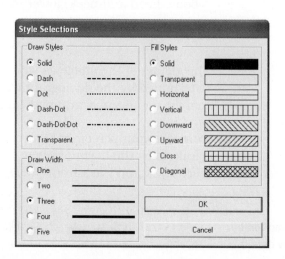

Locate and click on the Style button in the drawing toolbar. A window similar to Figure 9-27 will be invoked.

Click on Draw Width **Three** and click on Fill Style **Solid** as shown in Figure 9-27. Click on the OK button to close the window.

Font button has an icon consisting of the letters a-b-c. It is used to set the font and size of type for the text tool.

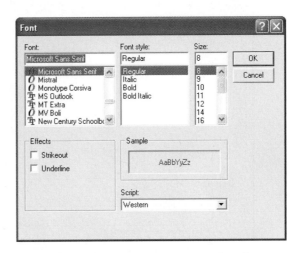

▶ **Figure 9-28 The Font Window Is Used to Change the Font for the Text Tool.**

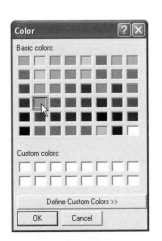

▶ **Figure 9-29 Select Orange in the Color Pallet Window.**

You may, optionally, click on the button to view the window, but do not change any of the settings; alternatively, you may study Figure 9-28 without invoking the window.

Step 8

Color The "Color" button selects the color for the annotations. The button icon consists of four colored squares.

Locate and click on the Color button and select orange by clicking on the orange square, as shown in Figure 9-28. Click the OK button to close the Color selection window.

The next two buttons on the drawing toolbar are:

Save (not used in Student Edition). The icon resembles a floppy disk.

Print (used at the end of the exercise to print a copy of your drawing). The icon resembles a printer. Do not click it until instructed.

Step 9

In this step, you will learn how to draw on the displayed image.

Position the mouse over the patient's left shoulder in the drawing. The cursor should be shaped like a large plus sign. If it is, then hold down the left mouse key while making a slight movement. A circle should appear. The size of the circle is controlled by how far you move the mouse before releasing the mouse button. You are annotating the location of moles. Make a *small* circle.

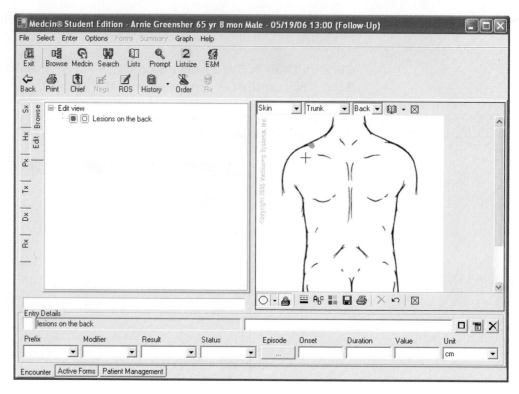

▶ Figure 9-30 Draw a Circle on the Left Shoulder to Represent the Position of a Mole.

Compare your screen to Figure 9-30.

Step 10

The remaining buttons on the drawing toolbar are:

Delete (icon is an X and resembles other Delete buttons in the Student Edition software). It is used to delete a selected portion of the drawing.

Undelete (icon is an arrow curved to the left). Used to restore the last item deleted from the drawing.

Exit (icon resembles an X in a square box). Closes the drawing and restores the exam note narrative view. Do not click it until instructed to do so.

In this step, you will learn how to Delete an item you have added and how to use the Undelete button.

Restore the Drawing tool to the Select pointer by clicking on the down arrow in the drawing toolbar and clicking the first option, "Select."

Locate and click on the padlock to unlock the toolbar.

Position the mouse pointer over the mole created in Step 9; the pointer should change to look like a small hand (as shown in Figure 9-31).

Click on the mole. It will change to an outline of dotted lines when selected.

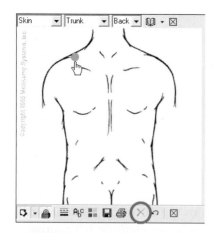

▶ Figure 9-31 Selecting an Object to Delete (Delete button circled in red).

Locate and click on the Delete button in the drawing toolbar (circled in red in Figure 9-31). The mole will be removed from your drawing.

The Undelete button may be used to restore the last deleted item on the drawing. In this case, you deleted a mole.

Locate and click on the Undelete button (the icon resembles a curved arrow). The mole should reappear. Your drawing should once again look like Figure 9-30.

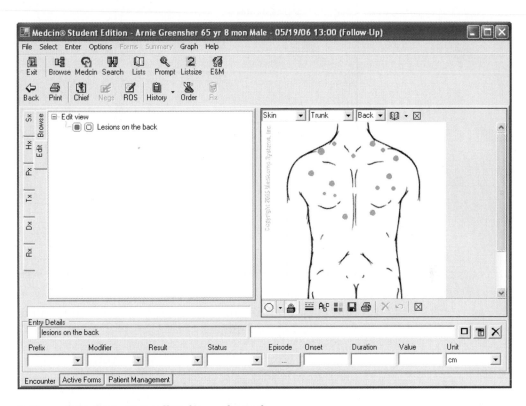

► **Figure 9-32 Draw 15 Small Moles on the Back.**

Step 11

Using what you have learned in step 9, you will now illustrate the location of moles on Mr. Greensher's back using the circle tool.

Click on the down arrow in the toolbar and reselect the circle from the drop-down list as you did in step 5. Locate and click on the padlock to lock the circle shape.

Draw **15** *small* moles on the patient's back, as shown in Figure 9-32. You do not have to place them exactly as they are in the figure; just get reasonably close.

Step 12

Clinicians also can annotate the images by adding text directly on the drawing canvas with the text tool. The clinician also can select a different color for the text. It is wise to do so, as it will help the text stand out from the color and the background of the drawing.

Locate and click on the down arrow next to the Select button. Choose Text from the drop-down list.

Locate and click on the Color button in the drawing toolbar. When the Color pallet window is displayed, select blue, and then click OK.

> **Note**
>
> **If at any time during this step your shape tool reverts to the mouse pointer, just unlock the padlock and reselect the Circle shape, and click on the padlock to relock the shape.**

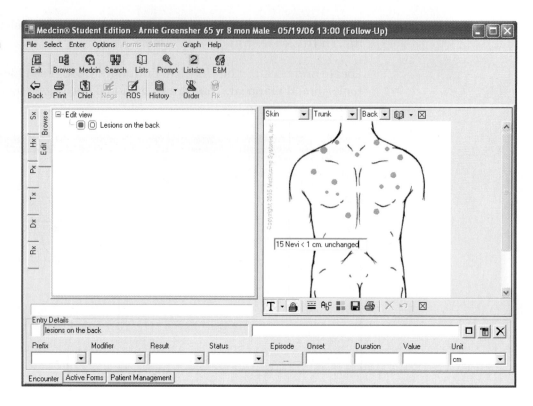

► **Figure 9-33 Type "15 Nevi < 1 cm. Unchanged" in Text box.**

Now click over an empty portion of the drawing and a text box will appear, as shown in Figure 9-33.

If the text box is not positioned where you would like it, click elsewhere. It will move to wherever you click your mouse.

Type the following text in the box: **15 Nevi < 1 cm. unchanged**

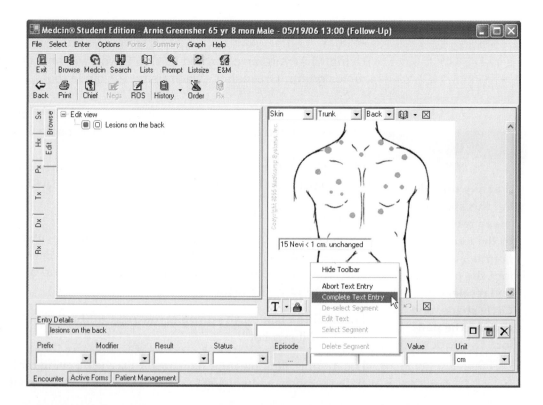

► **Figure 9-34 Right Click Elsewhere in Drawing and Select "Complete Text Entry."**

Step 13

When you have finished typing, merge the text into the drawing by clicking the right mouse button anywhere on the canvas *except* in the text box. A drop-down menu will appear, as shown in Figure 9-34.

Locate and click on the option "Complete Text Entry."

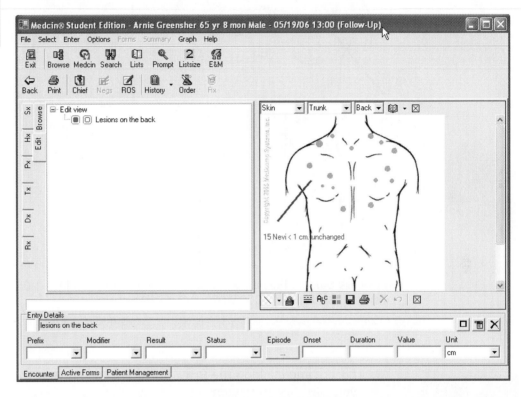

▶ **Figure 9-35 Draw a Blue Line from Text to Region of the Moles.**

Step 14

Another useful drawing tool is the line, which can be used to connect text to the drawing points.

Click on the down arrow in the toolbar and select Line from the drop-down list.

Position your mouse on the canvas just above the text. Hold down the left mouse button as you drag the mouse upward toward the moles on the back. When you release it, the line will end.

Compare your screen to Figure 9-35.

Step 15

In commercial EHR systems, you can merge your finished drawing into the narrative exam notes for the patient visit. In the Student Edition you will only print your drawing, not merge it, because students from other classes share the data.

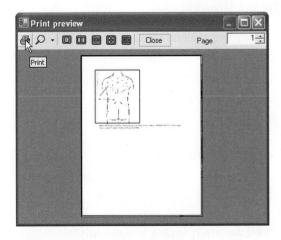

▶ **Figure 9-36 Print Preview Window.**

Select the print button on the *drawing toolbar*, **not** the print button on the main toolbar. A print preview window will be invoked. The Preview window (see Figure 9-36) shows a small copy of the document to be printed.

▶ **Figure 9-37**
Printout of Annotated Drawing for Arnie Greensher.

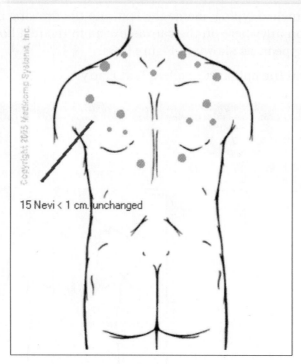

Medcin® Student Edition - Arnie Greensher 65 yr 8 mon Male - 05/19/06 13:00 (Follow-Up)
Terry Jones, Printed: 05/19/06 13:47:47 PM

Locate and click on the Print button in the Preview window to print a copy that you can turn in to your instructor.

Step 16

Compare your printout to Figure 9-37.

When you have a printout of your annotated drawing in hand, close the Preview window. Locate and click on the button labeled "Close" in the top of the Preview window. Save the printed copy to give to your instructor.

Step 17

Return to the Exam Note View by exiting the Drawing tool.

Locate and click on the Exit button in the drawing toolbar (circled in red in Figure 9-38). Use only this button in this step, not any other Exit button in the window.

> **Note**
>
> if you have been using Print To HTML for your exercises, ask your instructor for instructions, as Drawing Images do not have Print To HTML capability.

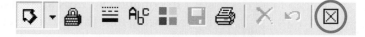

▶ **Figure 9-38 Exit Drawing Tool Using Button Circled in Red.**

> **!** **Alert**
>
> *Do not close or exit the Drawing tool until you have a printed copy in your hand. You could lose your work if you exit before printing has completed.*

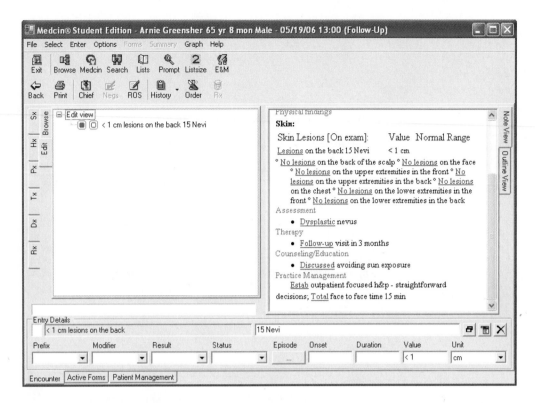

Step 18

Annotated drawings provide an excellent means of recording the location and size of certain observed findings in a physical exam. However, as we have discussed several times, the contents of the image are not codified, searchable records. In this example, the text added to the drawing became part of the image and as such can only be read by a person, not the computer.

Therefore, the clinician also will record the text of the findings in the exam note. This will result in the best of both worlds, codified data for the computer, and a visual record of the location of moles for use in future exams.

With the finding "Lesions on the back" still selected for edit, you will add data to the finding.

Locate the Note field just below the right pane and type: **15 Nevi**

Locate the Value field in the Entry Details section at the bottom of the screen and type: **< 1**

Press the enter key. Compare your screen to Figure 9-39.

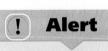

! Alert

*Do not close or
exit the Encounter
until you have a
printed copy in
your hand.* You
will lose your
work if you exit
before printing.

Step 19

Click File on the Menu bar, and then click Print Encounter or Print To HTML (as directed by your instructor).

If you are printing your work, you may alternatively click the Print button on the toolbar at the top of your screen.

Compare your printout or file output to Figure 9-40. If it is correct, hand it in to your instructor *accompanied by the printout of your annotated drawing* (from step 15).

If there are any differences, review step 18 and correct your error.

Student: Terry Jones
Patient: Arnie Greensher: M: 3/11/1940: 5/19/2006 01:00PM
Chief complaint
The Chief Complaint is: Follow up visit, routine lesion recheck.
History of present illness
  Arnie Greensher is a 66 year old male.
  ° No skin symptoms ° No change in a mole and no other reported skin problems
Physical findings
Skin:

	Value	Normal Range
Skin Lesions [On exam]:		
Lesions on the back 15 Nevi	< 1 cm	

° No lesions on the back of the scalp ° No lesions on the face ° No lesions on the upper
  extremities in the front ° No lesions on the upper extremities in the back ° No lesions
  on the chest ° No lesions on the lower extremities in the front ° No lesions on the lower
  extremities in the back
Assessment
    • Dysplastic nevus
Therapy
    • Follow-up visit in 3 months
Counseling/Education

    • Discussed avoiding sun exposure
Practice Management
      Estab outpatient focused h&p - straightforward decisions; Total face to face
      time 15 min

▶ **Figure 9-40 Printed Exam Note for Arnie Greensher.**

The Internet and the EHR

One of the key technologies impacting our society is the Internet. It has
changed the way that people communicate, research, shop, and do business. It
also is influencing changes in health care.

People shop for doctors online, insurance companies provide online participat-
ing provider lists, physician specialty associations, and state and local medical
societies all offer Web sites that help patients locate a provider near them.

Patients also use the Internet for research. Many clinicians are finding their patients are coming to visits armed with printouts about their conditions gathered
from Web sites. Some of these Web sites provide reliable information, some do not.
One of the most trusted sources of consumer information on the Web is WebMD
Health® (webmd.com). On the WebMD Health consumer portal, patients can access health and wellness news, support communities, interactive health management tools, and more. Online communities and special events allow individuals to
participate in real-time discussions with experts and with other people who share
similar health conditions or concerns. By using sites such as WebMD Health, patients can play an active role in managing their own health care.

Another reliable source of health information on the Internet is a Web site set
up by the patient's physician. Many medical practices today have their own
Web sites. Although some of these sites are limited to information about the
medical practice, clinicians, and office hours, others offer online information

about preventative health measures, diseases, and conditions that the practice treats. Patient educational information on your doctor's Web site has the advantage of being consistent with the medical philosophy of the practice.

Doctors, too, can do research online. No longer is it necessary for a physician to make a trip to the medical library or keep a vast library in the office. Large numbers of research papers and nearly every medical journal is available online. Medscape® (shown in Figure 9-41), the leading Web site for providers, is a source of objective, credible, relevant clinical information and educational tools. Medscape provides online continuing medical education (CME) as well as online coverage of medical conferences, access to over 100 medical journals, and specialty-specific daily medical news.

Decision Support

The quantity of information available to clinicians regarding conditions, disease management, protocols, case studies, and treatments far exceeds their available time to read it. Whereas continuing education classes, medical journals, and Web sites such as Medscape are used by a majority of physicians, they are not always at hand in the exam room during the patient visit.

Decision support refers to the ability of EHR systems to store or quickly locate materials relevant to the findings of the current case. Clinics can imbed links in their forms that, when selected, display any type of helpful material. These might include defined protocols, results of case studies, or standard care guidelines prepared by specialists, medical societies, or government organizations.

In current EHR systems, the decision support documents are selected and linked to the system by each individual practice. (The author is not aware of any system that automatically installs standard decision support documents or links.) The selection of decision support items is generally one of the responsibilities of a practice setting up the EHR. Therefore, the support content of EHR systems will differ from office to office.

Provider-to-Patient E-Mail Communication

The HIPAA Security Rule does not expressly prohibit the use of e-mail for sending electronic protected health information (EPHI). The Security Rule allows for EPHI to be sent over an electronic open network as long as it is adequately protected. However, as you learned in Chapter 8, the security standard for transmission security includes addressable specifications for integrity controls and encryption.

The HIPAA Privacy Rule permits the patient to disclose information to anyone they like, but the covered entity may not. This means a patient can e-mail a doctor or medical practice with any information they want about their medical condition, even if the e-mail is not encrypted. However, the clinician has to be very guarded in replying through unencrypted e-mail; that is, neither a copy of the patient's message should be included nor any specific information revealed. Most important, the patient should consider whether they themselves should send private health information using unencrypted e-mail.

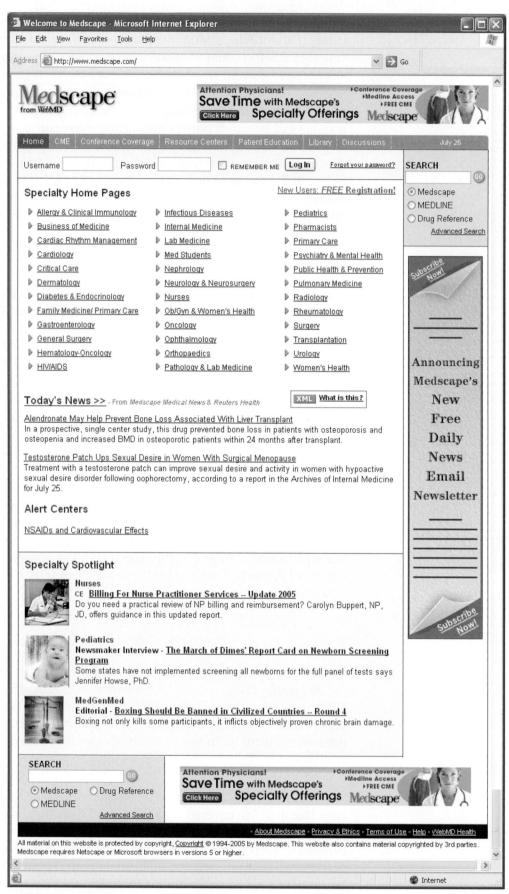

Reprinted with permission from Medscape, http://www.medscape.com © 1994–2005, Medscape.

▶ **Figure 9-41 Medscape Web Site Used by Thousands of Clinicians.**

Although e-mail can be secured by encryption using public/private keys (as discussed in Chapter 8), it becomes difficult to manage on the part of the medical office because keys would have to be kept for thousands of patients, and the appropriate key used for e-mail from each. The preferred alternative is to "e-mail" the clinician using a secure site.

Secure Messaging

Instead of sending an e-mail message from their home or work e-mail system, the patient logs on to the clinician's Web site and types the information in an e-mail screen on the Web page. The Web site handles all the security, protecting the EPHI as required by HIPAA. Even the page the patient is typing in before sending the message is usually a page secured by SSL.

Responses to the patient are handled similarly. The patient checks back to the site for messages, or receives a benign message via their regular e-mail informing them that they have a reply from the medical office waiting. The patient then logs into the secure site to read the message and, if necessary, writes a reply.

Even using secure messages, however, clinicians have concerns about the potential for medical liability, the lack of structure in the messages, and the difficulty of keeping the e-mail exchange as part of the patient's medical record. Also, the doctor doesn't get paid.

E-Visits

Although the banking, brokerage/investing, and travel industries have made Internet-based transactions readily available to consumers, health care as a whole has not. That seems to be changing. One of the developments brought about by the Internet that offers interesting possibilities for enhancing the efficiency of providers and improving the quality of health care for the patients is the e-visit. An e-visit allows the patient to be treated by a clinician for nonurgent health problems without having to come into the office.

An e-visit has all the advantages that e-mail lacks: not only are they secure but also the e-visit gathers symptom and HPI information creating a documented medical exam. When it is integrated with the EHR, the e-visit becomes a part of the patient's chart, just like any other visit.

Equally as important to the clinician, e-visits are reimbursed as a legitimate E&M visit. At the time that this book was published, e-visits (billed using procedure code 0074T) were being paid by Blue Cross/Blue Shield™ plans and other private insurance carriers in 10 states. A study by Price-Waterhouse-Coopers predicted that more than 20% of all office visits could be replaced by an online equivalent by 2010.[6]

---

[6]PricewaterhouseCoopers Report. "HealthCast 2010: Smaller World, Bigger Expectations." November, 1999.

Workflow of an E-Visit

The basic workflow of an e-visit begins with patient entered symptom, history, and history of present illness information, very similar to Instant Medical History, which was discussed in Chapter 6. The following workflow represents a combination of available elements, not necessarily of one particular product currently in use.

The following takes place in a state with a plan that supports e-visits and with a medical office that performs e-visits.

The patient accesses their physician's Web site and signs on. The patient must already be an established patient with the practice, and have medical records on file. E-visits would not be appropriate for a new patient who has never been seen at the practice.

The patient answers a few simple questions and selects the reason for the visit from a list. This allows the software to determine which question sets would be appropriate to ask. The patient also could just enter a free-text complaint, but this is not recommended as free-text messages are not reimbursable by insurance.

The patient answers online interview questions related to their reported complaint, as shown in Figure 9-42. Answers to certain medically significant questions could cause the software to ask different sets of medically related questions automatically. The patient can add free-text clarification at various points in the interview.

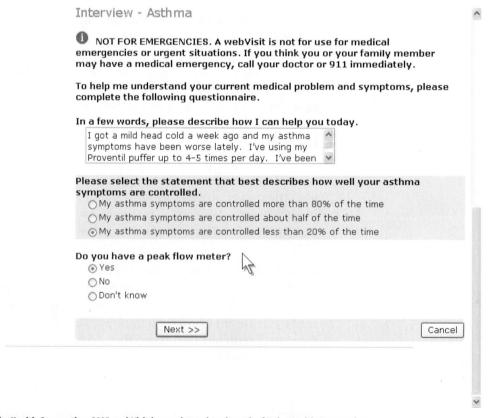

▶ Figure 9-42 Patient Interview Screen for an E-Visit.

E-visits are only used for nonurgent visits. If the condition seems urgent, the patient is advised to seek immediate medical care and the provider is notified. The provider analyzes the patient responses and determines the proper course of action.

If the software determines that the condition is not urgent but that the patient needs to be seen in the office, the patient is given a message to that effect and automatically offered a choice of available appointments.

When the interview is complete, the data entered by the patient is recorded in the EHR and the clinician is notified that an e-visit is ready to review. Even in the event that the patient must come in for the visit, the doctor is better prepared because the symptom and history information is already at hand.

Unlike e-mail, which is directed at a particular individual and therefore not likely to be accessible by another provider, e-visits can be directed to the "doctor on call," allowing practicing partners to share "e-visit" duty, just like they share other on-call services.

The clinician reviews the patient entered data, in a screen similar to Figure 9-43, reviews any relevant patient medical records, and replies to the patient. The system allows the provider and patient to continue to exchange messages, much as a question and answer session in the exam room, except for the factor of time, which is sometimes delayed by one or both parties' responses. A study of e-visits that was done in California found a majority of patients were happy if their provider responded by the next morning. Remember, e-visits are for nonurgent matters.

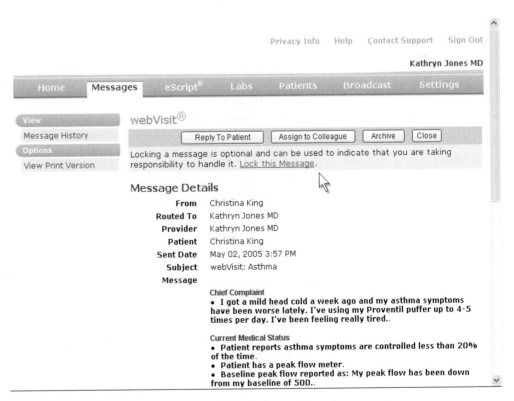

▶ **Figure 9-43 Doctor Reviews Patient-Entered Information for an E-Visit.**

The clinician also can prescribe electronically during the e-visit, just as he or she would during an office visit. When the patient receives the clinician's reply to the e-visit, they are prompted to select their preferred pharmacy from a list (if it is not already known to the EHR) and the prescription is electronically transmitted to the pharmacy by the doctor's system.

The doctor's response also can include patient education material and comments or care instructions from the doctor, all of which are recorded in the care plan. The doctor's practice management system can verify the patient eligibility for the e-visit, and submit the claim electronically.

In an independent study sponsored by Blue Shield of California,[7] most patients and doctors in the study preferred a Web visit to an office visit for nonurgent medical needs. Providers found that the e-visit gathered the important details and eliminated multiple messages back and forth that occur when trying to provide patient care via e-mail. The patients found that the time spent scheduling, driving, parking, and waiting was saved with an e-visit. The reality of on-line medical visits with your doctor is not a question of *if* but *when*.

Patient Access to Electronic Health Records

A small but growing number of medical offices are creating interactive Web sites that actually allow the patient to request an appointment time or a prescription renewal. Web sites for some medical offices even allow patients secure access to information from their medical record. This is usually not the full access the provider has to the chart but, rather, specific portions of the chart, for example, the results of recent lab tests. There also are Web sites for OB practices that use dates from the patient chart to present information relevant to the patient's current month of a pregnancy. In each of these cases, the patient must log in to the Web site using a secure password or pin that authenticates their identity before gaining access to any EPHI.

Online services independent of any one medical group also offer patients the ability to maintain their own EHR online. One of the problems we discussed in Chapter 1 is the fact that, even with growing adoption of EHR in many medical offices, there is seldom any connectivity between those records. Part of the president's 10-year plan for Health Information Technology is to address this, as discussed in Chapter 1.

There is one entity central to the record who can bring records from multiple sources together; that is the patient. An online service allows patients to log on to a secure Web site, and to create and update their records. The patient controls who has rights to access the information and can add or remove permission for clinicians they might visit to view the online record. The clinicians, of course, have their own records, but the medical office record will normally contain only the information gathered at that office. The record maintained online by the patient could contain data from patient visits at multiple practices.

Another advantage of the online EHR is that is available everywhere. Wherever a patient is traveling and needs medical care, the patient can retrieve their own records using the Internet.

---

[7]Relay Health webVisit Study: Final Report; http://www.relayhealth.com ©2002-2003 RelayHealth Corporation.

Optional Exercise 50: Creating Your Own Health Record

The iHealthRecord is a no-cost, secure, and confidential interactive record that allows you to store, update, and share health information with physicians whom you authorize and you have access to it in an emergency situation.

The privacy and security of your iHealth Record are governed by the iHealth Alliance—a not-for-profit organization, chaired by Nancy W. Dickey, M.D., past President of the AMA, President of the Health Science Center, and Vice Chancellor for Health Affairs for Texas A&M University. The Board of Directors is comprised of representatives from a number of the nation's leading medical societies and other organizations whose mission is to protect the privacy and data use of your iHeathRecord.

If you are interested in creating an online EHR record for yourself, and you have Internet access, enter the following address in your Web browser: http://www.ihealthrecord.org.

Enter personal information only if after reading the information on the iHealth site and reviewing their privacy policy you believe that it would be beneficial to you to have an EHR online.

This exercise is completely voluntary. Whether you participate will not affect your grade; no extra credit will be given. Neither the author nor Prentice Hall has any affiliation with the iHealth Web site nor accepts any liability in connection with your decision to use it.

Chapter Nine Summary

In this chapter, we examined how the office environment and the choice of computers, devices, and technology can affect the successful adoption of an EHR. One aspect is the physical layout of your office; how much space is available may determine the type of device you can use. The second aspect is what type of clinician–patient interaction the clinicians hope to achieve. These factors determine how and where you want to use computers to achieve point-of-care EHR.

The third aspect is the mobility of the clinicians:

◆ Does a clinician have a preassigned set of exam rooms used for their patients?

◆ Is the clinician likely to complete the note and all orders while in the exam room?

◆ Where/when will the clinician review lab results, radiology reports, e-mail, and so on:

  ◆ on the move throughout the day

  ◆ at their office desk

  ◆ from home after hours

Each of the devices we discussed had advantages and disadvantages:

◆ Computer workstations are cheap, reliable, dependable, easier for the IT department to manage, and can be upgraded when necessary. But they take up more space and may not fit in the exam rooms.

◆ A laptop computer packages everything in a unit about the size of a notebook. They provide mobility for clinicians who want to take their work from room to room. But they require a wireless network to gain that mobility and they have limited battery life.

◆ The Tablet PC offers the size and portability of a laptop computer and users can move and click the mouse by just touching the screen with a special stylus. However, in tablet mode, it doesn't have a keyboard, so it is less desirable when there is a lot of keyboard input. It works well for EHR systems that primarily involve opening lists and clicking findings with a mouse. Similar to laptops, it requires a wireless network and has a limited battery life.

◆ PDA or Personal Digital Assistants are small, pocket-sized, and convenient for writing prescriptions or reading messages. A PDA that is to be used for an EHR access requires a wireless network and require an EHR "client" software that has been specially written to communicate with their small screen size and limited memory.

"Wi-Fi" is standard on many higher-end laptop computers. Wireless networking has a limited range; therefore, it requires multiple "access points" to be installed throughout the building in close enough proximity that the laptop (or other wireless device) can always find the radio signal.

The style or manner in which the clinicians want to interact with the patient also will determine some of the technology selected. The availability of information from the EHR during the patient visit is an invaluable tool in counseling and patient education. The type of equipment the clinician chooses and how it is arranged enables or discourages the patient's participation in the office visit.

Clinicians may wish to access their EHR by modem or the Internet. Remote access allows them to leave when the last patient is finished, and catch up on messages, review reports, and so on from home. This is usually accomplished through an Internet VPN connection, or a direct dial connection to the office computer using a secure setup.

Although a codified EHR has been discussed many times throughout this book, there are some situations in which text is appropriate. Reports from certain specialties such as radiology and pathology are almost entirely text. Additionally, those clinicians may need their hands for the task at hand. In those cases, speech recognition software may be used. The software recognizes the patterns in your speech as words and turns them into text. When it is integrated with an EHR, the completed text is automatically stored to the correct patient and encounter.

Another method of entering data about the patient into the EHR involves the use of anatomical drawings of the body and body systems. These are particularly useful on a Tablet PC, but the same or similar result can be achieved on a laptop or workstation computer as well. Annotated drawings often are included in the EHR at ophthalmology and dermatology practices.

Some EHR systems have navigation pages that allow the clinician to quickly locate findings by pointing to a particular body part in a drawing, which opens a list of findings relevant to that body system. Think of this as searching with pictures rather than words.

The Internet is one of the key technologies impacting health care. It not only facilitates remote access for the clinician (as described earlier) but provides instant access to medical research and medical libraries. Patients also are researching their conditions and bringing the information to the office visit with them.

Patients also are beginning to e-mail their doctors medical questions about their conditions. Although HIPAA does not expressly prohibit the use of e-mail for sending electronic protected health information, the encryption requirements are too complicated for most practices to handle. Instead, providers are turning to secure Web sites, where information can be exchanged without the use of the more public e-mail systems.

Even using secure messaging, merging the e-mail threads into the patient's EHR or filing an insurance claim for an e-mail consult would be a challenge. An alternative is the e-visit, which allows the patient to be treated by their regular physician for nonurgent health problems without having to come into the office.

The e-visit gathers symptom and HPI information and creates a documented medical exam. It can be integrated into the EHR to become part of the patient's chart, and, equally important to the clinician, e-visits are reimbursed as a legitimate E&M visits in some states.

Patients want to remotely access their medical information just as do providers. A small but growing number of medical offices are creating interactive Web sites that actually allow the patient to request an appointment time or a prescription renewal. Some medical offices even allow patients secure access to information from their medical record.

Testing Your Knowledge of Chapter 9

List the advantages of using each type of computer for an EHR:

1. Workstation

2. Laptop computer

3. Tablet PC

4. PDA

5. Explain how the physical layout of the office impacts the choice of devices.

6. What is used in place of a mouse on a Tablet PC?

7. How does the clinician's mobility affect the choice of EHR devices?

8. List the three styles of the physician–patient relationships.

9. Give an example of a specialty that might use speech recognition to create reports.

10. What types of specialties typically incorporate annotated drawings in an exam note?

11. Discuss the effect of the Internet on health care, and give examples of changes.

12. Describe the differences between provider-to-patient e-mail and e-visits.

13. Discuss patient access to electronic health records.

14. Briefly define and describe Wi-Fi.

15. What CPT code is used to bill for an e-visit?

Comprehensive Evaluation of Chapters 6–9

This comprehensive evaluation will enable you and your instructor to determine your understanding of the material covered in the second half of this book. Complete both the written test and the hands-on exercise provided below. Depending on the time provided, it may be necessary to do this in two separate sessions. Your instructor will advise you. Do not begin the hands-on exercise if there will not be enough class time to complete it.

Part I–Written Exam

1. Where does the data that appears in the patient management tab come from?
2. Why would clinicians use trending of lab results and what type of results can be graphed?
3. Describe the benefits of having patients entering their own symptoms and history.
4. What is triage (as used in this book)?
5. List at least three ways that codified data in the EHR can be used to manage and prevent disease.
6. Describe a problem list and provide at least two reasons why clinicians use a problem list.
7. Describe how to create a flow sheet from a form.
8. What does it mean to cite a finding and how would you do it from a flow sheet?
9. Why are childhood immunizations important?
10. What are "evidence-based" guidelines?
11. Name at least three external sources of data for populating the EHR?
12. What is a growth chart percentile?
13. List the four components of the HIPAA Administrative Simplification Subsection.
14. Compare the difference between Consent and Authorization.
15. Does a provider need the patient's consent to share PHI with an authorized government agency?
16. Name the Covered Entities under HIPAA.
17. Describe how the clinician's style of practice impacts the choice of EHR devices.
18. Give an example of a specialty that might use speech recognition to create reports.
19. Give an example of a specialty that might use annotated drawings in an exam note.
20. How is the Internet changing health care? Give examples of changes.
21. List the three criteria of an Electronic Signature.
22. How does an e-visit differ from provider-to-patient e-mails?

For questions 23–30, select the acronym from the list below that best matches the description, and write it next to the number.

BMI	MMR	PKI
EPHI	OCR	VPN
H&P	PDA	WNL

23. _____ Information protected by the Security Rule

24. _____ Electronic Signature standard

25. _____ Calculation for height/weight ratio

26. _____ Normal findings

27. _____ Three vaccines

28. _____ Enforces HIPAA Privacy Rule

29. _____ Elements of a patient exam

30. _____ Method of Internet Security

Part II–Hands-On Exercise

The following exercise will use features of the software with which you have become familiar. Complete each step in sequential order using the instructions and other information provided.

During the exercise, you will print out two graphs and an annotated drawing; when you have finished the exercise, you will print out the exam note. Hand all four printouts to your instructor. Do not begin the hands-on exercise if there will not be enough class time to complete it. This exercise will use the Student Edition History Program. Make sure that it is running before you begin.

Hands-On Exercise 51: Examination of a Patient with Arterial Disease

Gloria Green is a 54-year-old established patient with a history of hypertension and possible peripheral arterial disease of the legs. During her last visit, she complained of pain in the legs and cold feet following exercise. After performing an ankle-brachial index test in the office, the clinician ordered an angiogram. Gloria is coming today for the results of her test and a follow-up exam.

In this exercise, you use the skills you have acquired to document this exam.

Step 1

If you have not already done so, make sure that the Student Edition History program is running; *then* start the Student Edition software.

Click Select on the Menu bar, and then click Patient.

In the Patient Selection window, locate and click on **Gloria Green**.

Step 2

Click Select on the Menu bar, and then click New Encounter.

Select the date **May 22, 2006**, the time **10:15 AM**, and the reason **Office Visit**.

Make certain that you set the date and reason correctly. Compare your screen to the date, time, and reason printed in bold type before clicking on the OK button.

Step 3

Enter the Chief Complaint by locating the button in the toolbar labeled "Chief" and clicking on it.

In the dialog window that will open, type "**Patient reports leg pain after exercise**."

When you have finished typing, click on the button labeled "Close the Note Dialog."

Step 4

Begin the visit by taking Gloria's Vital Signs and Quick Exam.

Use the form labeled "Hypertension," which you will select from the Forms Manager, invoked on the Active Forms tab (as you have done in previous exercises.)

Enter Gloria's Vital Signs in the corresponding fields on the form as follows:

Temperature:	**98.6**
Respiration:	**28**
Pulse:	**78**
BP:	**130/90**
Weight:	**210**

When you have finished, check your work; if it is correct, proceed to step 5.

Step 5

Remain on the Active Forms tab.

Locate and click on checkbox for hypertension. The small circle will turn red.

- Hypertension   ✓ **Y**

Enter the Quick Exam portion by using the Negs button in the toolbar at the top of your screen. The Quick Exam items should be checked as follows:

Retina	✓ N
Optic Disc	✓ N
Heart Rate And Rhythm	✓ N
Heart Borders	✓ N
Murmurs	✓ N
Heart Sounds S1	✓ N
Heart Sounds S2	✓ N
Heart Sounds S3	✓ N
Heart Sounds S4	✓ N

Step 6

Locate and click on the button labeled "FS Form" in the toolbar at the top of your screen to invoke the Flow Sheet view.

Locate and click on the button labeled "Cite" in the toolbar at the top of your screen.

Move your mouse pointer over the column date "5/17/2006." The pointer should change to include a large question mark. Click on the column date. A window of findings from that encounter will be displayed.

Review the findings and then click the button labeled "Post to Encounter."

Locate and click on the button labeled "Cite" in the toolbar at the top of your screen to turn off the Cite feature. Then locate and click on the button labeled "FS Form" in the toolbar at the top of your screen to return to the Hypertension form.

Step 7

Locate the Section of the Hypertension form labeled "Standard Orders."

Click on the checked boxes to remove the orders for the tests:

☐ **Hematocrit**

☐ **Hemoglobin**

Confirm each deletion by clicking on the OK button in the confirmation dialog box that will appear.

Step 8

Locate and click on the Patient Management tab at the bottom of the screen.

Review the patient's problem list. Locate and click on the problem "Atherosclerosis of the femoral artery."

Locate and click on the button labeled "Flowsheet" in the toolbar at the top of your screen. The Flowsheet view will be invoked for the specific problem.

Locate and click on the button labeled "Cite" in the toolbar at the top of your screen.

Locate the section of the Flowsheet with the label "Tests" (in a teal divider) by scrolling the window.

Cite an individual test result by moving your mouse pointer over the column "**5/18/2006**." The pointer should change to include a large question mark.

Locate the finding, Bilateral Angiography, and click on the column with the abbreviation "POS" (in red). The finding will be recorded in the current encounter.

Cite the findings from the previous exam by moving your mouse pointer over the date "**5/17/2006**" at the top of the column, and click on the date.

A window of findings from that encounter will be displayed.

Review the findings and then click the button labeled "Post to Encounter."

Step 9

Locate and click on the button labeled "Cite" in the toolbar at the top of your screen to turn off the Cite feature. Then locate and click on the button labeled "Flowsheet" in the toolbar at the top of your screen to return to the Patient Management.

Locate and click on the Patient Management tab labeled "Medications." Review the patient's current medications.

When you have reviewed her medications, locate and click on the tab labeled Encounter at the bottom of the window to return to the Exam Note view.

Step 10

Locate and click the assessment "Atherosclerosis of the femoral artery" in the Exam Note. The finding will then be displayed in the left pane on the Edit tab.

Highlight the diagnosis description, then locate and click on the button labeled "Prompt" in the toolbar at the top of your screen.

Locate and click on the Rx tab in the left pane. Locate and click on the following medication:

- (red button) Anticoagulants Warfarin sodium (Coumadin)

This will invoke the prescription writer.

Step 11

Enter the following prescription by selecting the following options as they are presented:

Rx Dosage: **2 mg**

Rx Brand: **Coumadin**

Enter the following data in the prescription fields:

Quantity: **1**

Frequency: **daily**

Days: **30**

Dispense Amount: **30**

Generic: **Y**

Verify that you have entered the information correctly, then click the button labeled Save Rx.

Step 12

Locate and click the button labeled Search in the toolbar at the top of your screen. The search window will be invoked. Type "Low fat diet" and click the Search button.

Locate and select the following findings from the list displayed in the Rx tab:

- (red button) Low Fat Diet
- (red button) Patient Education Dietary Low Fat Cooking
- (red button) Patient Education Dietary Changing Eating Habits

Step 13

In the next steps, you will create some materials to be used for patient education.

Click on the button labeled Search on the toolbar near the top of the screen. The Search String Window will be invoked.

Type the search string "Total cholesterol" and click on the Search button in the window.

The left pane should change to the Tx tab and display several findings with the words "Total Cholesterol" in them.

Locate and highlight the finding "Total plasma cholesterol" (the finding with the red button selected).

Click Graph on the Menu bar, and then click "Current Finding" from the drop-down list. The Graph window will be invoked with a graph of Gloria's recent cholesterol results.

Print a copy of the graph by locating and clicking the print button in the upper left corner of the Graph window. A Print Preview window for graphs will be invoked.

Locate and click on the Print button in the upper left corner *of the Preview window.*

When your graph has printed successfully, click on the button labeled "Close" to close the Print Preview window. Do not close or exit the Preview window until you have your printed copy in hand.

Write your name on your printout and save it to turn in to your instructor.

Step 14

Print a chart of Gloria's weight.

Click Graph on the Menu bar, and then click "Weight" from the drop-down list. The Graph window will be invoked with a graph of Gloria's weight measurements.

Print a copy of the graph by following the print procedures that you used in step 13.

When your graph has printed successfully, click on the button labeled "Close" to close the Print Preview window. Do not close or exit the Preview window until you have your printed copy in hand.

Write your name on your printout and save it to turn in to your instructor.

Step 15

Create an annotated drawing to explain the angiography to the patient.

Scroll the Exam Note in the right pane to locate the imaging study finding "Bilateral Angiography." Click on the word "Bilateral." The left pane should change to the Edit tab.

Locate the context button (the center button of the three buttons in the lower right-hand corner of your window) and click on it. From the drop-down list displayed, choose "Add Object to Finding."

The drawing window will be invoked in the right pane.

If the cardiovascular drawing is not displayed, use the fields at the top of the drawing to select the Cardiovascular, Full Body, Front view from the drop-down lists.

Step 16

Once the correct illustration template is displayed, use the toolbar in the drawing tool to set up the tool.

Locate and click on the down arrow next to the first button; then select "Circle" from the drop-down list.

Locate and click on the Lock button (with the padlock). It should then appear depressed.

Locate and click on the Color pallet button. When the window is displayed, select Blue. Click OK to close the color pallet window.

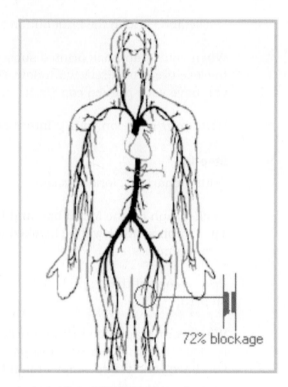

72% blockage

Anatomical Figure © MediComp Systems, Inc.
▶ **Figure 1 Drawing of Annotations to Be
Performed in Exercise 51.**

Step 17

As closely as possible replicate the drawing in Figure 1.

Draw a blue circle over the femoral artery midway between the groin and the knee (as shown in Figure 1).

Change the drawing tool.

Locate and click on the down arrow next to the first button, then select "Line" from the drop-down list.

Draw a horizontal line from the circle to the blank area of the drawing on the right.

Next, change the color to Red by selecting the Color pallet button.

In the blank area of the drawing, draw two vertical, parallel lines to represent an enlarged view of the artery.

Change the drawing tool.

Locate and click on the down arrow next to the first button, then select "Brush" from the drop-down list.

Using the Brush, make a thick line on the interior of each of the parallel lines to represent the blockage in the artery (similar to Figure 9-44).

Annotate the drawing.

Locate and click on the down arrow next to the first button, then select "Text" from the drop-down list.

Click your mouse in the image to the right of the knee and a text field will open. Type "72% blockage."

Right click anywhere on the drawing *except in the text box* to display a list of options; click on "Complete Text" from the list displayed.

Compare your drawing to Figure 1. If you need to correct the line or circle change the tool button to "Select" and click on the object. Use the delete button in the toolbar and then redraw the correct element.

Step 18

When your drawing is satisfactory, select the print button on the *drawing toolbar* (**not** the print button on the main toolbar). A Print Preview window will be invoked.

Locate and click on the Print button in the Preview window to print a copy that you can turn in to your instructor at the end of this exercise.

When your drawing has printed successfully, click on the button labeled "Close" to close the Print Preview window. Do not close or exit the Preview window until you have your printed copy in hand.

Step 19

Locate and click on the Exit button in the drawing toolbar to close the drawing tool and redisplay the exam note.

Locate and click on the button labeled "E&M" in the toolbar at the top of the screen to invoke the E&M Calculator.

Click on the Check box labeled ">50% time spent counseling."

Set Face to face/floor time to 50 minutes.

Click on "Existing Patient."

Click on the button labeled "Calculate E&M code."

The Code field should display "99215: Estab Outpatient Comprehensive H&P—High Complex Decisions."

If this is the code displayed in your window, locate and click on the button labeled "Post To Encounter."

Step 20

Locate and click on the finding "Counseling" in the exam note. The finding should appear on the Edit tab in the left pane.

In the free-text field, type "30 minutes of visit spent on dietary and Coumadin counseling."

Press the Enter key.

Note

If the calculated code is not 99215, verify that you have followed step 19. If it is still not correct, click on the Cancel button, and review steps 4–13 to find your error and correct it.

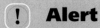

Alert

Do not close or exit the Encounter until you have a printed copy in your hand. You will lose your work if you exit before printing.

Step 21

Click File on the Menu bar, and then click Print Encounter or Print To HTML (as directed by your instructor).

If you are printing your work, you may alternatively click the Print button on the toolbar at the top of your screen.

Hand in the following printouts to your instructor:

1 Graph of Total Cholesterol

2 Graph of Gloria Green's Weight

3 Annotated drawing of femoral artery

4 Printed exam note for May 22, 2006, for Gloria Green.

Appendix A
CMS Documentation Guideline Tables

Examine the two tables provided in this appendix. Figure A-1 is the guideline for a General Multisystem Exam and Figure A-2 is the guideline for a single organ system/body area exam for ENT (Ears, Nose, and Throat).

The contents, or individual elements, of the examination pertaining to that body area or organ system are identified by bullets (•) in the right column.

Compare the tables for the two types of exams. Notice that certain sections of Figure A-2 are outlined with a shaded border. This shaded border will be referred to in Chapter 5 in the table in Figure 5-10.

Notice also that in Figure A-2, five of the body systems are not required and have no bullets at all. However, the sections for constitutional, head and face, ears, nose, mouth, and throat have bullets, are outlined and "shaded."

To count toward the Exam level, a bullet must satisfy any numeric requirements of the element. For example, locate the first body system (Constitutional) in Figure A-1. The element requires "Measurement of any three of the following seven vital signs...." Similarly, elements with multiple components but with no specific numeric requirement require documentation of at least one component. For example, locate Gastrointestinal; the bullet "Examination of liver and spleen" requires examination of at least one of the organs to satisfy the requirement of the bullet.

When you have compared the two tables, return to Chapter 5.

Table of General Multisystem Examination Content and Documentation Requirements		
Level of Exam		**Perform and Document**
1 *Problem Focused*	*	1–5 elements identified by a bullet (•)
2 *Expanded Problem Focused*	*	At least 6 elements identified by a bullet (•)
3 *Detailed*	*	At least 2 elements identified by a bullet (•) from each of 6 systems/body areas **OR** at least 12 elements identified by a bullet (•) in 2 or more systems/body areas
4 *Comprehensive*	*	Perform **all elements** identified by a bullet (•) in at least 9 systems/body areas and document at least 2 elements identified by a bullet (•) from each of 9 systems/body areas
* Note Bullets (•) referred to are shown below		

▶ **Figure A-1 General Multisystem Examination from the 1997 Guidelines**[1]

---

[1]Chart adapted from the 1997 Documentation Guidelines for Evaluation and Management Services, U.S. Department of Health and Human Services, Health Care Finance Administration, 1997.

Elements of General Multisystem Examination	
System/Body Area	**Exam Elements**
Constitutional	• Measurement of any three of the following seven vital signs: (1) sitting or standing blood pressure, (2) supine blood pressure, (3) pulse rate and regularity, (4) respiration, (5) temperature, (6) height, (7) weight (may be measured and recorded by ancillary staff) • General appearance of patient (e.g., development, nutrition, body habitus, deformities, attention to grooming)
Eyes	• Inspection of conjunctivae and lids • Examination of pupils and irises (e.g., reaction to light and accommodation, size and symmetry) • Ophthalmoscopic examination of optic discs (e.g., size, C/D ratio, appearance) and posterior segments (e.g., vessel changes, exudates, hemorrhages)
Ears, Nose, Mouth, and Throat	• External inspection of ears and nose (e.g., overall appearance, scars, lesions, masses) • Otoscopic examination of external auditory canals and tympanic membranes • Assessment of hearing (e.g., whispered voice, finger rub, tuning fork) • Inspection of nasal mucosa, septum, and turbinates • Inspection of lips, teeth, and gums • Examination of oropharynx: oral mucosa, salivary glands, hard and soft palates, tongue, tonsils, and posterior pharynx
Neck	• Examination of neck (e.g., masses, overall appearance, symmetry, tracheal position, crepitus) • Examination of thyroid (e.g., enlargement, tenderness, mass)
Respiratory	• Assessment of respiratory effort (e.g., intercostal retractions, use of accessory muscles, diaphragmatic movement) • Percussion of chest (e.g., dullness, flatness, hyperresonance) • Palpation of chest (e.g., tactile fremitus) • Auscultation of lungs (e.g., breath sounds, adventitious sounds, rubs)
Cardiovascular	• Palpation of heart (e.g., location, size, thrills) • Auscultation of heart with notation of abnormal sounds and murmurs Examination of: • carotid arteries (e.g., pulse amplitude, bruits) • abdominal aorta (e.g., size, bruits) • femoral arteries (e.g., pulse amplitude, bruits) • pedal pulses (e.g., pulse amplitude) • extremities for edema and/or varicosities
Chest (Breasts)	• Inspection of breasts (e.g., symmetry, nipple discharge) • Palpation of breasts and axillae (e.g., masses or lumps, tenderness)
Gastrointestinal (Abdomen)	• Examination of abdomen with notation of presence of masses or tenderness • Examination of liver and spleen • Examination for presence or absence of hernia • Examination (when indicated) of anus, perineum and rectum, including sphincter tone, presence of hemorrhoids, rectal masses • Obtain stool sample for occult blood test when indicated

Elements of General Multisystem Examination	
System/Body Area	**Exam Elements**
Genitourinary	**Female:** **Male:** Pelvic examination (with or without specimen collection for smears and cultures), including: • Examination of external genitalia (e.g., general appearance, hair distribution, lesions) and vagina (e.g., general appearance, estrogen effect, discharge, lesions, pelvic support, cystocele, rectocele) • Examination of urethra (e.g., masses, tenderness, scarring) • Examination of bladder (e.g., fullness, masses, tenderness) • Cervix (e.g., general appearance, lesions, discharge) • Uterus (e.g., size, contour, position, mobility, tenderness, consistency, descent, or support) • Adnexa/parametria (e.g., masses, tenderness, organomegaly, nodularity) Male column: • Examination of the scrotal contents (e.g., hydrocele, spermatocele, tenderness of cord, testicular mass) • Examination of the penis • Digital rectal examination of prostate gland (e.g., size, symmetry, nodularity, tenderness)
Lymphatic	Palpation of lymph nodes in **two or more** areas: • Neck • Axillae • Groin • Other
Musculoskeletal	• Examination of gait and station • Inspection or palpation of digits and nails (e.g., clubbing, cyanosis, inflammatory conditions, petechiae, ischemia, infections, nodes) Examination of joints, bones and muscles of **one or more of the following six areas**: (1) head and neck; (2) spine, ribs and pelvis; (3) right upper extremity; (4) left upper extremity; (5) right lower extremity; and (6) left lower extremity. The examination of a given area includes: • Inspection or palpation with notation of presence of any misalignment, asymmetry, crepitation, defects, tenderness, masses, effusions • Assessment of range of motion with notation of any pain, crepitation, or contracture • Assessment of stability with notation of any dislocation (luxation), subluxation, or laxity • Assessment of muscle strength and tone (e.g., flaccid, cog wheel, spastic) with notation of any atrophy or abnormal movements
Skin	• Inspection of skin and subcutaneous tissue (e.g., rashes, lesions, ulcers) • Palpation of skin and subcutaneous tissue (e.g., induration, subcutaneous nodules, tightening)
Neurologic	• Test cranial nerves with notation of any deficits • Examination of deep tendon reflexes with notation of pathological reflexes (e.g., Babinski) • Examination of sensation (e.g., by touch, pin, vibration, proprioception) • extremities for edema and/or varicosities
Psychiatric	• Description of patient's judgment and insight Brief assessment of mental status including: • orientation to time, place, and person • recent and remote memory • mood and affect (e.g., depression, anxiety, agitation)

Table of Ear, Nose, and Throat Examination Content and Documentation Requirements		
Level of Exam		**Perform and Document**
1	*Problem Focused*	*	1–5 elements identified by a bullet (•)
2	*Expanded Problem Focused*	*	At least 6 elements identified by a bullet (•)
3	*Detailed*	*	At least 12 elements identified by a bullet (•)
4	*Comprehensive*	*	Perform all elements identified by a bullet (•); document every element in each box with a shaded border and at least 1 element in each box with an unshaded border.
* Note Bullets (•) referred to are shown below		

Elements of Ear, Nose, and Throat Examination	
System/Body Area	**Exam Elements**
Constitutional	• Measurement of any three of the following seven vital signs: (1) sitting or standing blood pressure, (2) supine blood pressure, (3) pulse rate and regularity, (4) respiration, of accessory muscles, diaphragmatic movement) (5) temperature, (6) height, (7) weight (may be measured and recorded by ancillary staff) • General appearance of patient (e.g., development, nutrition, body habitus, deformities, attention to grooming) • Assessment of ability to communicate (e.g., use of sign language or other communication aids) and quality of voice
Head and Face	• Inspection of head and face (e.g., overall appearance, scars, lesions, and masses) • Palpation or percussion of face with notation of presence or absence of sinus tenderness • Examination of salivary glands • Assessment of facial strength
Eyes	• Test ocular motility including primary gaze alignment
Ears, Nose, Mouth, and Throat	• Otoscopic examination of external auditory canals and tympanic membranes including pneumo-otoscopy with notation of mobility of membranes • Assessment of hearing with tuning forks and clinical speech reception thresholds (e.g., whispered voice, finger rub) • External inspection of ears and nose (e.g., overall appearance, scars, lesions, and masses)

▶ **Figure A-2 Ear, Nose and Throat Examination from the 1997 Guidelines**[2]

---

[2]Ibid.

Elements of Ear, Nose, and Throat Examination	
System/Body Area	**Exam Elements**
	• Inspection of nasal mucosa, septum, and turbinates
	• Inspection of lips, teeth, and gums
	• Examination of oropharynx: oral mucosa, hard and soft palates, tongue, tonsils, and posterior pharynx (e.g., asymmetry, lesions, hydration of mucosal surfaces)
	• Inspection of pharyngeal walls and pyriform sinuses (e.g., pooling of saliva, asymmetry, lesions)
	• Examination by mirror of larynx including the condition of the epiglottis, false vocal cords, true vocal cords and mobility of larynx (use of mirror not required in children)
	• Examination by mirror of nasopharynx including appearance of the mucosa, adenoids, posterior choanae and eustachian tubes (use of mirror not required in children)
Neck	• Examination of neck (e.g., masses, overall appearance, symmetry, tracheal position, crepitus)
	• Examination of thyroid (e.g., enlargement, tenderness, mass)
Respiratory	• Inspection of chest including symmetry, expansion, or assessment of respiratory effort (e.g., intercostal retractions, use of accessory muscles, diaphragmatic movement)
	• Auscultation of lungs (e.g., breath sounds, adventitious sounds, rubs)
Cardiovascular	• Auscultation of heart with notation of abnormal sounds and murmurs
	• Examination of peripheral vascular system by observation (e.g., swelling, varicosities) and palpation (e.g., pulses, temperature, edema, tenderness)
Chest (Breasts)	
Gastrointestinal (Abdomen)	
Genitourinary	
Lymphatic	• Palpation of lymph nodes in neck, axillae, groin, or other location
Musculoskeletal	
Extremities	
Skin	
Neurological/Psychiatric	• Test cranial nerves with notation of any deficits Brief assessment of mental status including:
	• Orientation to time, place, and person
	• Mood and affect (e.g., depression, anxiety, agitation)

▶ **Figure A-2 (continued)**

Appendix B

Information About the Student Edition History Program

The classroom environment provides a challenge for computer programs because the exercises require multiple students to simultaneously retrieve patient charts and enter findings for the same patient, without disturbing the sample data for the next class.

To accommodate this, a special software program loads previous patient history into the computer's memory just for these exercises. The program must be running during the time you are performing the exercises in Chapter 6, Chapter 7, and the comprehensive evaluation exercise in Chapter 9.

Warnings at key steps in the exercises will explain how to detect if the History Program needs to be restarted before you can continue.

If you reach a point in an exercise when you believe the History Program is not running, and your computer is part of a school network, alert your instructor to the problem. The instructor will restart the History Program. Note to Instructors: go to your network server and follow the steps listed here. Have all students log out of the Student Edition software, and then log back in after the History Program has been started.

If you are working on a computer that is not networked, or if you are working outside the classroom, the History Program needs to be started on your individual workstation before you start the Student Edition software each time that you work on exercises in Chapters 6, 7, or 9. Follow the steps here.

Instructions for Starting History Program Software

Step 1

Exit the Student Edition software on all affected workstations.

Step 2

Click on the Windows Start button.
Locate and click on Programs or All Programs.

From the list of programs displayed, locate and click on the program labeled: "Medcin History Pool Loader." This is the Student Edition History Program.

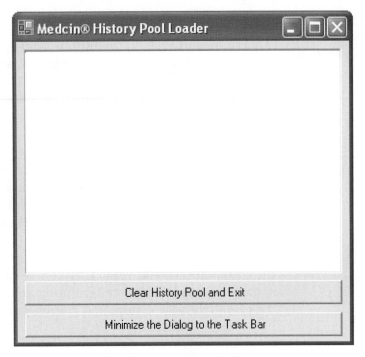

▶ Figure B-1 Medcin History Program Window

Step 3

The Medcin History Pool Loader window shown in Figure B-1 will be displayed; patient names will be displayed as their charts are loaded into memory.

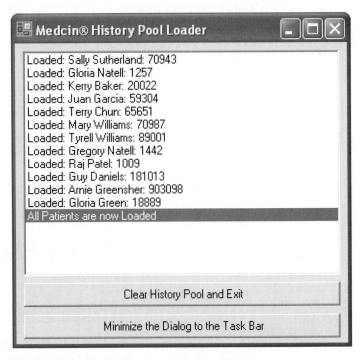

▶ Figure B-2 History Program Showing All Patients Loaded

Step 4

When the program has loaded all the patients, the message "All Patients Are Now Loaded" will be displayed at the end of the list, as shown in Figure B-2.

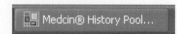

▶ Figure B-3 History Program Running Minimized

Step 5

Locate and click on the button labeled "Minimize the Dialog to the Task Bar" in the History Program window (shown in Figure B-2).

While the History Program is running minimized, it will appear in the Windows Taskbar, as shown in Figure B-3.

Schools sharing a network computer should keep the program running on the network server on which the Medcin server has been installed. Note to instructors: consult with your school IT administrator about adding Medcin History Pool Loader to the list of programs that start automatically whenever the network server is rebooted. This will ensure that the program is running for every class.

Students working on a computer that is not networked, or if working outside of the classroom, should verify they can see an item in their Windows Taskbar as shown in Figure B-3 before beginning any exercise in Chapter 6, Chapter 7, or the Comprehensive Evaluation Exercise in Chapter 9.

Stopping the History Program

Normally the History Program will stop automatically when you shut down the computer. Should you need to close the History Program manually, use the following steps.

Step 1

Make sure there is no one running the Student Edition software on the network.

Step 2

Locate and click on the minimized Medcin History Program in the Windows Taskbar (as shown in Figure B-3).

Step 3

Locate and click on the button in the History Pool Window labeled "Clear History Pool" and Exit (as shown in Figure B-2).

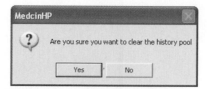

▶ Figure B-4 Confirmation Dialogue to Clear the History Pool

Step 4

When the confirmation dialog shown in Figure B-4 appears, click OK to clear the history pool and exit the History Program. This will stop the History Program.

The table in Figure B-5 provides a list of conditions that will occur during the exercises if the History Program is not running. However, once these occur, the student will have to exit the Student Edition software, start the History Program, and then restart the exercise. In most cases, the student will have completed some portion of the exercise before receiving the error message. Therefore, **it is better to make sure the History Program is running before beginning the exercise.**

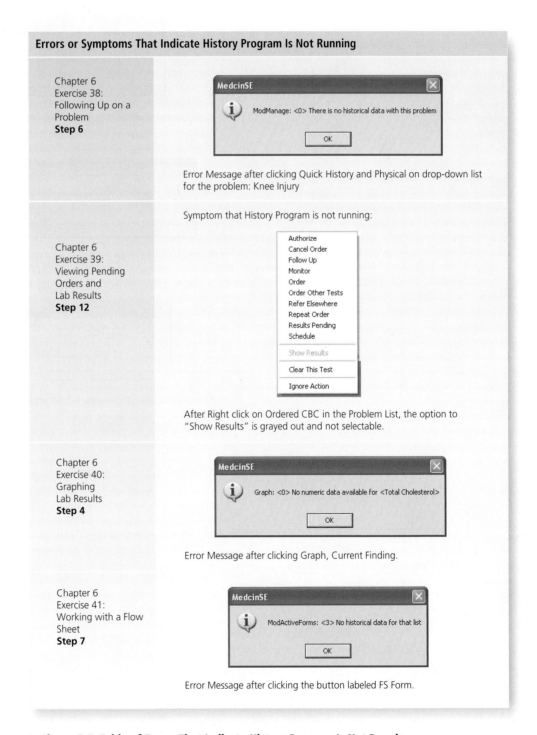

Errors or Symptoms That Indicate History Program Is Not Running

Chapter 6 Exercise 38: Following Up on a Problem **Step 6**	ModManage: <0> There is no historical data with this problem Error Message after clicking Quick History and Physical on drop-down list for the problem: Knee Injury
Chapter 6 Exercise 39: Viewing Pending Orders and Lab Results **Step 12**	Symptom that History Program is not running: Authorize Cancel Order Follow Up Monitor Order Order Other Tests Refer Elsewhere Repeat Order Results Pending Schedule Show Results Clear This Test Ignore Action After Right click on Ordered CBC in the Problem List, the option to "Show Results" is grayed out and not selectable.
Chapter 6 Exercise 40: Graphing Lab Results **Step 4**	Graph: <0> No numeric data available for <Total Cholesterol> Error Message after clicking Graph, Current Finding.
Chapter 6 Exercise 41: Working with a Flow Sheet **Step 7**	ModActiveForms: <3> No historical data for that list Error Message after clicking the button labeled FS Form.

▶ **Figure B-5 Table of Errors That Indicate History Program Is Not Running**

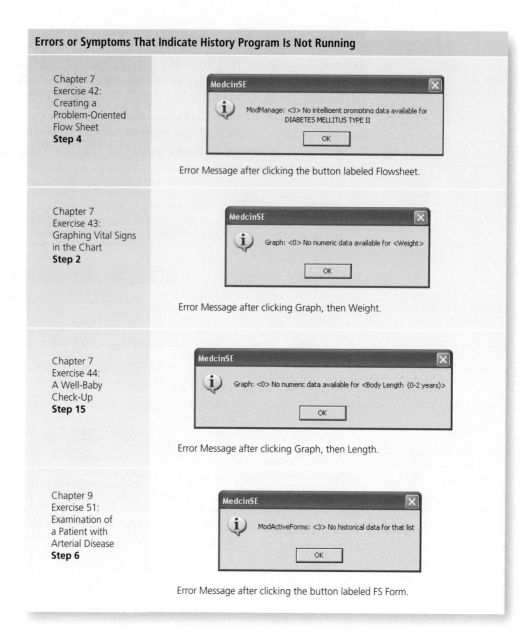

Errors or Symptoms That Indicate History Program Is Not Running

Chapter 7 Exercise 42: Creating a Problem-Oriented Flow Sheet **Step 4**	**MedcinSE** ⓘ ModManage: <3> No intelligent prompting data available for DIABETES MELLITUS TYPE II [OK] Error Message after clicking the button labeled Flowsheet.
Chapter 7 Exercise 43: Graphing Vital Signs in the Chart **Step 2**	**MedcinSE** ⓘ Graph: <0> No numeric data available for <Weight> [OK] Error Message after clicking Graph, then Weight.
Chapter 7 Exercise 44: A Well-Baby Check-Up **Step 15**	**MedcinSE** ⓘ Graph: <0> No numeric data available for <Body Length (0-2 years)> [OK] Error Message after clicking Graph, then Length.
Chapter 9 Exercise 51: Examination of a Patient with Arterial Disease **Step 6**	**MedcinSE** ⓘ ModActiveForms: <3> No historical data for that list [OK] Error Message after clicking the button labeled FS Form.

▶ **Figure B-5   (continued)**

Glossary

ABC An acronym for Alternative Billing Codes, which are used to bill for alternative medicine such as acupuncture, behavioral health, homeopathy, and others.

ABN An acronym for Advance Beneficiary Notice—information presented to the patient in advance that the test or procedure will not be covered by Medicare or insurance. The same acronym is sometimes uses as the abbreviation for Abnormal.

Access Control (HIPAA) Technical policies and procedures to allow access only to those persons or software programs that have been granted rights to access EPHI.

Acetaminophen A medicine used as an alternative to aspirin to relieve pain and fever. The active ingredient in Tylenol.

Active Forms Tab A tab in the EHR software window that uses Forms for data entry and from which form-based flow sheets may be viewed. *See* Forms.

Acute Severe, but of short duration.

Acute Self-Limiting Problems that normally resolve themselves over a short period of time.

Administrative Safeguards (HIPAA) These are the administrative functions that should be implemented to meet the standards of the HIPAA Security Rule. These include assigning security responsibility to an individual and security training requirements.

Administrative Simplification (HIPAA) The Administrative Simplification Subsection of HIPAA covers providers, health plans, and clearinghouses. It has four distinct components: Transactions and Code Sets, Uniform Identifiers, Privacy, and Security.

AHRQ An acronym for Agency for Healthcare Research and Quality, a Public Health Service agency in the Department of Health and Human Services to support research designed to improve the quality, safety, efficiency, and effectiveness of health care for all Americans.

Alert A warning, message, or reminder automatically generated by EHR systems based on logical rules.

Allergy (tab) A feature on the Patient Management tab that provides a list of the patient's allergies, or the fact that the patient has no known allergies. This information is reviewed before writing a prescription.

AMA An acronym for American Medical Association.

Ambulatory Setting Outpatient setting.

Amoxicillin An oral antibiotic; a synthetic penicillin derived from ampicillin.

ANA An acronym for the American Nurses Association.

Angina Pectoris A disease marked by brief, recurrent pain, usually in the chest and left arm, caused by a sudden decrease of the blood supply to the heart muscle.

Angiogram An x-ray (roentgenogram) of the flow of blood after injecting a contrast material.

Angiography *See* Angiogram.

Annotated Drawing Anatomical drawings of the body and body systems on which the clinician has marked observations and text notes. Medcin-based software is capable of linking an annotated drawing to a relevant finding.

ANSI An acronym for American National Standards Institute, a private, nonprofit organization that administers and creates product and communication standards in the United States. ANSI uses a voluntary consensus process to arrive at and maintain standards not only in health care but also in many diverse areas of industry and manufacturing.

Assessment (chart) The diagnosis or determination arrived at by the clinician from the medical examination, subjective and objective findings, and test results.

Asthma A generally chronic disorder often caused by an allergic origin, characterized by wheezing, coughing, labored breathing, and a suffocating feeling.

Auscultation Listening (in this text, listening with a stethoscope).

Authorization (HIPAA) Authorization differs from consent in that it does require the patient's permission to disclose PHI. Under the HIPAA Privacy Rule, authorization is required for most disclosures of PHI other than for treatment of the patient, seeking payment, or operation of the health care facility.

Auto-Negative *See* Negs (button).

Blood Glucose Level The amount of glucose (a type of sugar) in the blood at the time the specimen is taken. A random blood glucose test is done without regard to when the patient last ate. A fasting blood glucose test is done after a patient has not had food or drink (except water) for 12 hours.

BMI An acronym for Body Mass Index, a number that shows body weight adjusted for height.

Bradycardia Abnormally slow heart rate (less than 60 beats per minute.)

Bronchitis A disease marked by inflammation of the bronchial tubes.

Browse (button) Displays the current finding's position in the Medcin nomenclature hierarchy. Also a tab in the software.

Bullets (for E&M) A bullet is a typographic character that looks like this: ● (a solid black circle). Bullets are printed in the E&M guideline tables next to certain individual elements of the examination pertaining to a body area or organ system. The level of the examination component when calculating E&M code is determined by the number of findings in the exam that corresponded to elements in the guideline table with bullet characters printed next to them.

Business Associate Agreement The HIPAA Privacy Rule requires covered entities that use the services of other persons or businesses to obtain a written agreement that the business associate will comply with the protection of PHI under the Privacy Rule.

Button (software) A raised or indented object in the software used to invoke an action or change of state when clicked on with a mouse. Found in most Windows software programs, buttons usually contain a word or icon representing their function.

Bypass Surgery *See* Cardiac Bypass.

Cardiac Bypass A surgical shunt to divert blood supply from one circulatory path to another.

Cardiac Catheterization A test to evaluate the heart and arteries. A thin flexible tube is threaded through a blood vessel into the heart, then a contrast material is injected to trace the movement of blood through the coronary arteries.

Cardiovascular The heart and the system of blood vessels.

Care Plan (tab) A feature on the Patient Management tab that provides a view of the plan from each previous encounter in a problem-oriented view. It is organized by problem and encounter date for which the patient was seen for that problem.

CAT scan Computerized Axial Tomography uses multiple x-rays and a computer to generate images of cross sections of the body.

CBC An acronym for Complete Blood Count, which is a lab test that includes separate counts for both white and red blood cells.

CC *See* Chief complaint.

CCC An acronym for Clinical Care Classification system used by nurses to codify documentation of patient care in any setting. It is an evolution of the HHCC nursing codes.

CDA An acronym for Clinical Document Architecture, an HL7 standard for incorporating clinical text reports or other information in a Claim Attachment.

CDC An acronym for the Centers for Disease Control, an agency of the U.S. Department of Health and Human Services.

CDISC An acronym for Clinical Data Interchange Standards Consortium, an organization that has created standards that enable sponsors, vendors, and clinicians to acquire and exchange data used in clinical drug trials. CDISC has become part of HL7.

CHCS II An acronym for Composite Health Care System II, the U.S. Department of Defense Electronic Health Record System.

Chief Complaint A concise statement describing the symptom, problem, condition, diagnosis, physician recommended return, or other factor that is the reason for the encounter, usually stated in the patient's words.

Chronic Disease or problem that lasts a long time or recurs often.

Cite (software) A feature of the software that allows follow-up visits to be quickly documented by bringing forward findings from previous exams into the current encounter. While doing so, the clinician can update or make any changes to the finding without affecting the previous encounter.

Clearinghouse *See* Healthcare Clearinghouse.

Clinical Terminology An organized list of medical phrases and codes. *See* Nomenclature.

Clinical Vocabulary An organized list of medical phrases and codes. *See* Nomenclature.

CMS An acronym for the Centers for Medicare and Medicaid Services, an agency of the U.S. Department of Health and Human Services (formerly HCFA).

COB Coordination of Benefits; when a patient is covered by more than one health insurance plan, the plans involved determine how much each plan is to pay. A HIPAA transaction permits the plans to do this electronically.

Codified Data (chart) EHR data with each finding assigned a standard code assures uniformity of the medical records, eliminates ambiguities about the clinician's meaning, and facilitates communication between multiple systems.

Comprehensive Metabolic Chem Panel A blood test to determine blood sugar level, electrolytes, fluid balance, kidney function, and liver function. The panel measures (in blood) the sodium, potassium, calcium, chloride, carbon dioxide, glucose, blood urea nitrogen (BUN), creatinine, total protein, albumin, bilirubin, alkaline phosphatase transferase (ALP), aspartate amino transferase (AST), and alamine amino transferase (ALT).

Consent (HIPAA) Under the revised HIPAA Privacy Rule, a patient gives consent to the use of their PHI for purposes of treatment, payment, and operation of the health care practice by acknowledging that they have received a copy of the office's privacy policy. HIPAA privacy consent should not be confused with consent to perform a medical procedure.

Contingency Plan Strategies for recovering access to EPHI should a medical office experience an emergency, such as a power outage or disruption of critical business operations. The goal is to ensure that EPHI is available when it is needed.

Covered Entity (HIPAA) HIPAA refers to health care providers, plans, and clearinghouses as Covered Entities. In the context of this book, think of covered entity as the medical practice and all of its employees.

CPOE An acronym for Computerized Physician Order Entry, also for Computerized Provider Order Entry.

CPRI An acronym for Computer-Based Patient Record Institute, formed to promote the universal and effective use of electronic health care information systems to improve health and the delivery of health care was merged into HIMSS in 2002.

CPT-4 An acronym for Current Procedural Terminology, fourth edition. CPT-4 are standardized codes for reporting medical services, procedures, and treatments performed for patients by the medical staff. CPT-4 is owned by the American Medical Association.

Cross-walk (codes) A reference table for translating a code from one set to a code with the same meaning in another code set. For example, the Medcin and SNOMED-CT nomenclatures each have tables for translating a finding code to an ICD-9CM code.

Cruciate Ligament (of the knee) Two ligaments in the knee joint that cross each other from the femur to the tibia. The anterior one limits extension and rotation.

CT (codes) An acronym for Clinical Terms. *See* Read codes.

CT Scan Computerized Tomography (*see* CAT Scan).

DAW The acronym for Dispensed As Written is used on a prescription as an instruction to dispense the exact brand of medication specified. Do not substitute a generic equivalent drug.

Decision Support *See* Medical Decision Support.

Decryption A method of converting an encrypted message back into regular text using a mathematical algorithm and a string of characters called a "key." *See also* Encryption.

Description (entry detail) The Description field (in entry details) presents the text of the currently selected finding exclusive of any attached free-text. The user can not enter or modify the description in this field.

Diabetes Mellitus A chronic form of diabetes; characterized by an insulin deficiency, an excess of sugar in the blood and urine, and by hunger, thirst, and gradual loss of weight.

Diagnosis A disease or condition; or the process of identifying the diseased condition. Generally codified using ICD-9CM.

DICOM An acronym for Digital Imaging and Communication. It is a standard for communication and file structure for transfer of digital images between equipment and computer systems.

Digital Images (chart) EHR data in image format. This includes diagnostic images, digital x-rays, as well as documents scanned into the EHR (*see also* Scanned Images). Image data usually requires specific software to view the image.

Discrete Data (chart) EHR data in computer format. Discrete data is typically either Fielded or Codified. Fielded data identifies the type of information by its position in the EHR record. Codified data pairs each piece of information with a code that identifies the information in uniform way.

DOQ-IT An acronym for Doctors' Office Quality Information Technology, a demonstration project that aims to provide implementation, education, and quality improvement assistance for small- to medium-sized physician offices migrating from paper charts to an EHR.

Drop-down List A standard feature in most Windows software, which displays a list of items the user may select when a mouse is clicked in the field or on a down-arrow button next to the field.

Drug Formulary Drug formularies are used to look up drugs by names or therapeutic class, provide an updated list of the drugs that are available in the inventory, provide information on costs, indications for use, treatment recommendations, dosage, guidelines, and prescribing information. Health insurance programs use the term *formulary* for plan-specific drug lists.

DTaP An acronym for Diphtheria, Tetanus, acellular Pertussis (whooping cough); a combination vaccine.

DUR An acronym for Drug Utilization Review, which is the process of comparing a prescription drug to a patient's history and recent medications for contraindications, overdosing, underdosing, allergic reactions, drug-to-drug interactions, and drug/food interactions.

Duration (entry detail) The Duration field is used to enter a number and a unit of time related to the duration of the currently selected finding. The time unit can be "second," "minute," "hour," "day," "week," "month," "year," or their plurals. A window with keypad for entering duration can be invoked by double-clicking the mouse in the Duration field.

Dx An abbreviation for Diagnosis (also diagnosis tab in the software).

Dx/Mgt Options An abbreviation used in the E&M Calculator for Diagnosis and/or Management Options. The number of possible diagnoses and management options are factors in the Medical Decision Making component when determining the E&M code.

Dysplasic Polyp Abnormal growth, a tumor.

E&M (codes) An acronym for Evaluation and Management codes, which are a subset of CPT-4 codes used to bill for nearly every kind of patient encounter, such as physician office visits, inpatient hospital exams, nursing home visits, consults, emergency room doctors, and scores of other services. *See also* Key Components.

E&M Calculator A pop-up window in EHR software, which calculates then displays Evaluation and Management codes by analyzing the findings in the current exam note.

ECG An acronym for Electrocardiogram.

EDI An acronym for Electronic Data Interchange. Information exchanged electronically as data in codified transactions.

EHR An acronym for Electronic Health Records—the portions of a patient's medical records that are stored in a computer system as well as the functional benefits derived from having an electronic health record. Also known as Electronic Medical Records, Computerized Patient Records, or Electronic Chart.

Electrolyte Panel A blood test that measures the levels of the minerals sodium, potassium, and chloride in the blood. The test also measures the level of carbon dioxide, which takes the form bicarbonate when dissolved in the blood. Certain medications can create in electrolyte imbalance, which is often the reason an Electrolyte Panel is ordered for patients on those medications.

Electronic Signature A method of marking an electronic record as "signed" having the same legal authority as a written signature. The electronic signature process involves the successful identification and authentication of the signer at the time of the signature, binding of the signature to the document and nonalterability of the document after the signature has been affixed. *See also* How Electronic Signatures Work in Chapter 8.

EMR An acronym for Electronic Medical Record.

Encounter The medical record of an interaction between a patient and a health care provider.

Encryption A method of converting an original message of regular text into encoded text, which is unreadable in its encrypted form. The text is encrypted by means of an algorithm using a private "key." *See also* Decryption.

Endoscopy Examination of the digestive tract using a flexible tube with a light and camera.

ENT An acronym for Ears, Nose, and Throat.

Entry Details The bottom portion of the Student Edition software window contains 10 fields that can be used to enter additional information about, or modify the meaning of, the finding that is selected at that time. (*See* Description, Prefix, Modifier, Results, Status, Episode, Onset, Duration, Value, Units, or Note Textbox.)

EPHI (HIPAA) Protected Health Information in electronic form.

Episode (entry detail) The Episode button is used to display the episode dialog window. This window is used to enter or edit data regarding the frequency or interval of occurrence of the currently selected finding.

ER An abbreviation for Emergency Room.

E-Visit An E-visit is a patient encounter conducted over the Internet, without an office visit. The patient enters symptom, history, and HPI information, which is then reviewed by a clinician who communicates via the Internet to ask additional questions, provides a diagnosis, treatment orders, and patient education. E-visits are used only for nonurgent visits and are reimbursed by a growing number of insurance plans.

Exacerbate To cause a disease or its symptoms to become more severe; to aggravate the condition.

Face-To-Face Time The total time both before and after a patient visit (in the office or other or outpatient setting) such as taking patient history, performing the exam, reviewing lab results, planning for follow-up care, and communicating with other providers about the patient's case.

Family History (tab) A feature on the Patient Management tab that provides a list of the patient's family history items recorded in the EHR during all previous encounters.

FDA An acronym for Food and Drug Administration, an agency of the U.S. Department of Health and Human Services. This federal agency regulates prescription and nonprescription drugs.

FEIN Federal Employer Identification Number—a number assigned by the U.S. Internal Revenue Service, also known as a business tax ID.

FEV$_1$ Forced Expired Volume in one second; the volume of air expired in the first second of maximal exhalation after a full inhalation. This can be used to measure of how quickly full lungs can be emptied.

Finding A precorrelated combination of terms from a nomenclature or clinical terminology into a clinically relevant phrase.

Floor/Unit Time The total time both before and after a patient visit (in the hospital or nursing facility) such as taking patient history, performing the exam, reviewing lab results, planning for follow-up care, and communicating with other providers about the patient's case.

Flow Sheet (software) A feature of the software that presents data from multiple encounters in column format resembling a spreadsheet. Flow sheets allow findings from any previous encounter to be cited into the current note. Flow sheets can be created based on a list, a form, or a problem.

Forms (software) Forms are used to consistently display a desired group of findings in a presentation that allows for quick entry of not only the selected findings but of any entry details as well. Forms are selected from the Forms Manager on the Active Forms Tab. Multiple forms may be used to document an encounter.

Forms Manager A window in the EHR software used to organize and select Forms. *See* Forms.

Formulary *See* Drug Formulary.

Free-text EHR data that is not codified; may be attached to a codified finding as supplemental notes.

FVC An acronym for Forced Vital Capacity.

Gallop An abnormal heartbeat marked by three distinct sounds, like the gallop of a horse.

Gastrointestinal The stomach and the intestines.

Generalized Pallor An unusual paleness, a lack of color especially in the face.

Genitourinary The genital and urinary organs.

GI/GU An acronym for Gastrointestinal/Genitourinary body systems.

Glucose Monitors Home device used by diabetes patients to monitor glucose levels.

GMDN An acronym for Global Medical Device Nomenclature is used to identify the medical devices for ordering, inventory, or regulatory purposes but does not provide for the codification of data from the devices.

Google™ An Internet Web site that provides a free, high-speed index of nearly every piece of information on the World Wide Web. The name is derived from Googol, the mathematical term for the number 1 followed by 100 zeros. Access Google by typing the address http://www.google.com in an Internet browser.

Grid (buttons) A button on the Toolbar in the Patient Management tab toolbar that allows the user to increase the amount of detail that can be viewed in a grid on the left pane of Patient Management by changing the height of the rows of data. The button toggles between two states that "expand" or "collapse" the height of the rows in the grid.

H&P An acronym for History and Physical.

HCFA An acronym for the Health Care Financing Administration, which has since been renamed CMS. *See* CMS.

HCPCS An acronym for Healthcare Common Procedure Coding System. HCPCS is an extended set of billing codes for reporting medical services, procedures, and treatments including codes not listed in CPT-4 codes.

HDL High Density Lipoprotein cholesterol in blood plasma sometimes referred to as good cholesterol because of its tendency to pull LDL cholesterol out of the artery wall.

Health Maintenance EHR system component to provide preventative health recommendations.

Healthcare Clearinghouse A computer system or covered entity that performs the specific function of translating nonstandard EDI transactions into HIPAA-compliant transactions.

HEENT An acronym for Head, Eyes, Ears, Nose, Mouth, Throat (body system).

Hematocrit A blood test to determine the ratio of packed red blood cells to the volume of whole blood; also the result of the test.

Hematologic Blood and blood forming organs (discussed in the text as a component of a physical exam).

Hemoglobin A1c A test that measures the average amount of sugar in the patient's blood over the past 3 months.

Hepatic Function Panel A blood test used to determine liver function and liver disease. The panel measures total protein, albumin, bilirubin, alkaline phosphatase transferase (ALP), aspartate amino transferase (AST), and alamine amino transferase (ALT).

HepB An acronym for Hepatitis B (vaccine).

HHCC An acronym for Home Health Care Classification nursing codes developed to codify documentation by home care nurses, the code set has evolved for use in all clinical settings and is now referred to as CCC.

HHS An acronym for U.S. Department of Health and Human Services.

Hib An acronym for Haemophilus Influenza Type B (vaccine).

HIMSS An acronym for Healthcare Information and Management Systems Society, which is an organization that provides leadership in health care for the management of technology, information, and change through member services, education and networking opportunities, and publications. Members include health care professionals, hospitals, corporate health care systems, clinical practice groups, HIT supplier organizations, health care consulting firms, and government agencies.

HIPAA An acronym for Health Insurance Portability and Accountability Act (of 1996). HIPAA law regulates many things; however, medical offices often use the term HIPAA when they actually mean only the Administrative Simplification Subsection of HIPAA. *See* Administrative Simplification (HIPAA).

History Pool (software) Previous patient history loaded into the computer server memory just for the Student Edition exercises. A special software program called the History Program allows multiple students to simultaneously perform the same exercise on the same patient without disturbing the data used by other classes. The program must be running while performing the exercises in Chapter 6, Chapter 7, and the evaluation exercise in Chapter 9.

HIT An acronym for Health Information Technology, also Healthcare Information Technology.

HIV An acronym for Human Immunodeficiency Virus (disease).

HL7 An acronym for Health Level Seven, the leading messaging standard used to exchange clinical and administrative data between different health care computer systems.

Holter Monitor A device worn by the patient to record the heart rhythm continuously for 24 hours. This provides a record that can be analyzed by a cardiologist to determine any irregular or abnormal activity of the heart. Named for Dr. Norman Holter, its inventor.

HPI An acronym for History of Present Illness, which is a chronological description of the development of the patient's present illness from the first sign or symptom or from the previous encounter to the present.

Hx An abbreviation for History. (Also the history tab in the software.)

Hyperlipidemia High levels of fat in the blood, such as cholesterol and triglycerides.

Hypertension A disease of abnormally high blood pressure.

Hypotension Abnormally low blood pressure.

ICD-9CM An acronym for International Classification of Diseases, Ninth Revision, Clinical Modifications, a system of standardized codes to classify mortality and morbidity. ICD-9CM is currently published in three volumes. The first two volumes provide a listing and an index of diagnosis codes. The third volume, however, lists codes for hospital inpatient procedures.

ICD-10 An acronym for International Classification of Diseases, Tenth Revision, a revision of the ICD-9 codes and used in the United States only for codifying the cause of death on death certificates.

ICD-10-PCS International Classification of Diseases, Tenth Revision, Procedure Coding System (but not derived from the ICD-10 codes). PCS stands for Procedure Coding System, and it is intended to replace inpatient procedure codes in ICD-9CM volume 3. The ICD-10-PCS is not used for billing at this time.

ICNP An acronym for International Classification for Nursing Practice is intended as an organizing structure for mapping other nursing terminologies.

Icon (software) In computer software, a small image usually used on a button to represent the purpose of the button—for example, a picture of a printer on the Print button.

ICU An acronym for Intensive Care Unit, a special section of the hospital with monitoring equipment and staff for seriously ill patients.

IHS An acronym for Indian Health Service, an agency of the U.S. Department of Health and Human Services responsible for providing federal health services to American Indians and Alaska natives.

Immunologic The immune system; discussed as a component of evaluation during a physical exam.

Implementation Specifications An additional detailed instruction for implementing a specific security standard under the HIPAA Security Rule.

Incidental Disclosures (HIPAA) HIPAA Privacy Rule permits incidental uses and disclosures of protected health information when the covered entity has in place reasonable safeguards and minimum necessary policies and procedures to protect an individual's privacy.

Information System Activity Review (HIPAA) A regular review of records such as audit logs, access reports, and security incident tracking reports. The information system activity review helps to determine if any EPHI is used or disclosed in an inappropriate manner.

Inpatient A hospital patient who stays overnight.

IOM An acronym for Institute of Medicine of the National Academies, a nonprofit organization created to provide unbiased, evidence-based, and authoritative information and advice concerning health and science policy.

IPV Inactivated Polio Virus (Salk vaccine).

JCAHO Joint Commission on Accreditation of Healthcare Organizations.

Key Components There are seven components that are evaluated to calculate the CPT-4 code for E&M services. Three of the components, history, examination, and medical decision making, are called the key components because they are used to determine the level of E&M services. *See also* E&M Codes.

Kiosk An unattended computer terminal for use by the patients in the waiting area.

LAN An acronym for Local Area Network, a network of computers that share data and programs located on a central computer called a server.

Laparoscopy Examination of the abdominal cavity through a small incision using a fiber optic instrument.

Laptop Computer A self-contained, battery-operated computer, which typically includes the screen, keyboard, mouse, and speakers, in a package about the size of a standard notebook.

LDL Low Density Lipoprotein cholesterol in blood plasma; sometimes referred to as bad cholesterol it is often associated with clogged arteries.

Leapfrog Group A coalition of 150 of the largest employers who created a strategy that tied purchase of group health insurance benefits to quality care standards, promoted Computerized Physician Order Entry, and the use of an EHR.

Lipids Test Panel A blood test that measures the levels of lipids (fats) in the bloodstream. A lipids profile measures total cholesterol, triglycerides, HDL (high-density lipoprotein), and LDL (low-density lipoprotein).

LIS An acronym for Laboratory Information System, a computer system that connects to and collects data from lab test instruments.

List A subset of findings (typically) used for a particular condition or type of exam making it easier to read and navigate.

List (button) A button on the Student Edition software Toolbar that invokes the List Manager. *See* List Manager.

List Manager A window from which the user may select and load a List.

List Size (button) A feature of the software that controls how many findings are displayed in the nomenclature tree. List Size 1 displays the least number of findings; List Size 3 displays the most.

Login A computer screen requiring the user to enter their name or ID (and password) before gaining access to the programs; or the action of entering a program through such a screen. EHR software typically requires the user to "log in." Note that some systems use the term "log on" for this function.

LOINC An acronym for Logical Observation Identifier Names and Codes. LOINC was created and is maintained by the Regenstrief Institute, affiliated with the Indiana University School of Medicine, and is an important clinical terminology for laboratory test orders and results.

Lymphatic System A network of lymph nodes and small vessels that collects lymph and returns it to the bloodstream.

Macular Degeneration A disease marked by the loss of central vision in both eyes.

Malicious Software Software such as viruses, Trojans, and worms create an unauthorized infiltration to computer networks that can damage or destroy data or cause expensive and time-consuming repairs. Malicious software is frequently brought into an organization through e-mail attachments and programs that are downloaded from the Internet. One requirement of the HIPAA Security Rule is to protect against malicious software.

Mammogram An x-ray of the breast that can be used to detect tumors before they can be seen or felt.

Mammography *See* Mammogram.

MDM An acronym for Medical Decision Making (a key component).

Med/Surg Med/Surg is an abbreviation for Medical/Surgical History on a tab in the Patient Management feature. It provides a list of the patient's past medical or surgical history items recorded in the EHR during all previous encounters.

MEDCIN A medical nomenclature and knowledge base developed by Medicomp Systems, Inc. Recognized as a national standard, it is incorporated in many commercial EHR systems as well as the U.S. Department of Defense CHCS II system.

Medical Decision Making A key component in calculating the level of E&M code; the level of complexity in Medical Decision Making is determined by the number of diagnoses and management options, the amount or complexity of data to be reviewed, and the risk of complications or morbidity or mortality.

Medical Decision Support Computer- or Internet-based systems used to improve the process and outcome of medical decisions by delivering evidence-based information to the clinician who is determining the diagnosis or treatment orders.

Medication List (tab) A feature on the Patient Management tab that provides a list of the medications that the patient currently is taking. The Medication list is always reviewed before writing new prescriptions.

Menu Bar The Menu Bar consists of a row of words across the top of the Student Edition software screen: File, Select, Enter, Options, Forms, Summary, Graph, and Help. Clicking the mouse on any of the words on the Menu Bar will display list of related software functions. Clicking the mouse on an item in the list will invoke that function.

Metformin An oral medication used along with a diet and exercise program to control high blood sugar in diabetic patients.

Microscopy Studies or images of studies performed using a microscope.

Minimum Necessary Standard (HIPAA) A standard in the HIPAA Privacy Rule intended to limit unnecessary or inappropriate access to and disclosure of PHI beyond what is necessary. The minimum necessary standard does not apply to disclosures to or requests for information used by a health care provider for treatment of the patient.

MMR An acronym for a combination of vaccines to immunize against Measles, Mumps, Rubella (German measles).

MODEM An acronym for modulate-demodulate. It is a device that converts computer data into signals that can be sent over a standard telephone connection. A second modem on the receiving end converts the signals back to data for the receiving computer.

Modifier (entry detail) The Modifier field (in entry details) is used to modify a selected finding. For example, the finding "Pain" may be qualified as mild, severe, and such.

Morbidity A diseased state or symptom.

MOU An acronym for Memorandum of Understanding (between government entities). It can be used between government agencies to meet the HIPAA Security rule requirement in lieu of Business Associate agreements.

Mouse (computer) A computer device for moving the pointer or cursor on the screen, selecting items, and invoking actions in Windows software.

Mouse Button A button on the mouse that when pressed causes a Windows software program to invoke some action. The Student Edition software requires a mouse that has at least two buttons (left and right click). The left button is most frequently used to highlight items (single-click) or select items. Some programs require a double-click of the left mouse button to invoke an action. (Double-click is to press the left button twice in quick succession.) The right button generally invokes a small drop-down list or menu of options related to a particular item or area of the Window program. In most software, the right click option is only available for selected areas of the program.

Mouse Pointer Typically an arrow shape that moves over the Window program in relationship to the movements of the mouse by the user. It also is sometimes referred to as a "cursor." When using flow sheets or forms, the Student Edition software may change the shape of the mouse pointer to a large question mark or the shape of a hand, indicating a different mode of functionality is temporarily in effect.

MRI An acronym for Magnetic Resonance Imaging, which uses magnetic fields and pulses of energy to create images of organs and structures inside the body that cannot be seen by x-ray or CAT scan.

Musculoskeletal Components of the physical exam involving both the musculature and the skeleton.

MVV An acronym for Maximal Voluntary Ventilation that is a measurement of the total volume of air that a person can breath in and out of the lungs in 1 minute.

NANDA An acronym for the North American Nursing Diagnosis Association, which has developed the Taxonomy II Nursing Diagnosis code set. It can be used to identify and code a patient's responses to health problems and life processes.

NASA An acronym for National Aeronautics and Space Administration.

Nasal Turbinate Spongy, spiral-shaped bones in the nose passages.

NCVHS An acronym for National Committee on Vital and Health Statistics, an advisory panel within the U.S. Department of Health and Human Services, which selects national standards for HIPAA and recommends standards for the federal government initiatives on Electronic Health Records.

NDC An acronym for National Drug Code. The NDC is the standard identifier for human drugs. It is assigned and used by the pharmaceutical industry.

NDF-RT A nonproprietary terminology being developed by the Veterans Administration that classifies drugs by mechanism of action and physiologic effect.

NEC An acronym for Not Elsewhere Classified (diagnosis codes.)

Negs (button) Auto-Negative; a button that will automatically set all the findings (that are not already set) to "normal." The Negs button is operative only on Symptom or Physical Exam findings.

Neurological Disorders Disorders of the nervous system.

Nevi Moles on the skin; plural of nevus.

NHII An acronym for National Health Information Infrastructure, a plan to make EHR records available wherever the patient is treated.

NHS An acronym for National Health Service, the national medical system in the United Kingdom.

NIC An acronym for Nursing Interventions Classification, which is a code set designed for codifying nursing interventions in any clinical setting.

NLM An acronym for the United States National Library of Medicine; a unit of the National Institute of Health, it is the world's largest medical library.

NMDS An acronym for Nursing Minimum Data Set, which defines the minimum set of basic data elements for nursing in a computerized patient record.

NOC An acronym for Nursing Outcomes Classification, which is a code set used in conjunction with NIC for codifying the outcome of nursing interventions.

Nomenclature A system of names created by a recognized group or authority and used in a field of science. An EHR nomenclature is an organized list of medical phrases and codes that helps to standardize the way clinicians record information. These are also referred to as clinical vocabularies or clinical terminologies.

NOS An acronym for Not Otherwise Specified (diagnosis codes).

Note Textbox (entry detail) The Note textbox (in entry details) is used to enter or view a free-text note attached to the currently selected finding. Free-text also may be added through a Note window, allowing easier entry of a longer note. The note dialog window can be invoked by clicking the note button to the right of the note textbox. (*See also* Free-Text.)

NPI An acronym for National Provider Identifier for doctors, nurses, and other health care providers. Established under HIPAA Uniform Identifier Standards, the NPI was not in use at the time this book was published.

OB Obstetrics is the field of specialty concerned with pregnancy, childbirth, and the period following.

Objective (chart) The clinician's observations and findings from the physical exam.

OCR (computer) An acronym for Optical Character Recognition, which is software that can analyze scanned document images, identify typed characters, and convert them into computer text.

OCR (HIPAA) An acronym for Office for Civil Rights, an agency of the Department of Health and Human Services that enforces the HIPAA Privacy Rule, in addition to other federal laws.

OIG An acronym for Office of Inspector General (Department of Health and Human Services).

Omaha System (codes) The Omaha System is the oldest standardized terminology for nursing documentation.

Onset (entry detail) The Onset field (in entry details) is used to enter a number and a unit of time related to the onset of the currently selected finding. The time unit can be "second," "minute," "hour," "day" "week," "month," "year," or their plurals. A window with keypad for entering onset can be invoked by double-clicking the mouse in the onset field. Alternatively, a calendar in the window can be used to record a specific date of onset.

Order (button) Prefaces the highlighted finding with the prefix "Ordered" and records the finding in the Plan section. The button is enabled only when a finding is "orderable" but not a medication.

Otitus Media Inflammation of the middle ear, often accompanied by pain, fever, dizziness, or hearing abnormalities.

Otolaryngeal Ears, Nose, and Throat.

Outpatient A patient who is examined or treated at a health care facility but is not hospitalized overnight. In this textbook, outpatient applies to all medical offices and clinics without overnight accommodation.

Pane (software) Two smaller windows within the Student Edition software, each capable of displaying and updating information. The left pane generally displays the nomenclature, or patient management tabs. The right pane generally displays the exam note, outline view, or drawing tools; however, when using forms or flow sheets, the nomenclature tree may temporarily appear on the right to avoid covering a portion of the form or flow sheet.

PC An acronym for Personal Computer, any computer capable of running applications without requiring connection to a server.

PCDS An acronym for Patient Care Data Set, which is a comprehensive set of nursing codes gathered from use in nine hospitals.

PDA An acronym for Personal Digital Assistant, a small handheld computer of a size that will fit in the palm of your hand.

PE An abbreviation for Physical Exam. (*See also* Px.)

PEFR An acronym for Peak Expiratory Flow Rate of air exhaled from the lungs.

Pending Order A lab test or diagnostic procedure that has been ordered but for which no results have been received.

Personal Representative (HIPAA) The HIPAA Privacy Rule allows a patient to appoint a personal representative and requires covered entities to treat an individual's personal representative as the individual with respect to uses and disclosures of the individual's protected health information and the individual's rights under the Privacy Rule.

Pertussis Whooping cough (vaccine).

PET Positron Emission Tomography combines CT (Computer Tomography) and nuclear scanning using a radioactive substance called a tracer, which is injected into a vein. A computer records the tracer as it collects in certain organs then converts the data into a three-dimensional images of the organ, which can be used to detect or evaluate cancer.

PFSH An acronym for Past History, Family History, and Social History, obtained from patient or other family member.

Pharynx The muscular and membranous cavity leading from the mouth and nasal passages to the larynx and esophagus.

PHI (HIPAA) An acronym for Protected Health Information; a patient's personally identifiable health information (in any form) is protected by the HIPAA Privacy Rule.

Phlebotomist A medical technician who draws blood specimens.

Physical Safeguards (HIPAA) The HIPAA Security Rule requirements to implement physical mechanisms to protect electronic systems, equipment and EPHI from threats, environmental hazards, and unauthorized intrusion. They include restricting access to EPHI and retaining off-site computer backups.

PIN An acronym for Personal Identification Number, a secret number used like a password.

PKI An acronym for Public Key Infrastructure, which is used to secure messages or electronically sign documents.

Plan of Treatment Prescribed therapy, medication, orders, and patient instructions for treatment or management of the diagnosed condition.

PMRI An acronym for Patient Medical Record Information.

PNDS An acronym for Perioperative Nursing Data Set nursing codes.

Polydipsia Excessive, abnormal thirst.

Prefix (entry detail) The Prefix field (in entry details) is used to qualify a selected finding. The prefix will sometimes change the section of the note to which the finding is assigned. For example, penicillin normally appears under Medications. When the prefix "Ordered" is used, it will appear under Plan. If the prefix "Allergy to" is used, it will appear under Allergies.

Privacy Official (HIPAA) One individual designated by the medical practice as having overall responsibility for the HIPAA Privacy Rule.

Privacy Policy Covered entities are required to adopt a privacy policy, which meets the requirements of the HIPAA Privacy Rule, and to provide a copy of it to patients.

Privacy Rule (HIPAA) Federal privacy protections for individually identifiable health information.

Problem List Acute conditions for which the patient was recently seen as well as chronic conditions such as high blood pressure, diabetes, and so on, which are monitored at nearly every visit, and can affect decisions about medications and treatments for even unrelated illness.

Problem Oriented Chart A method of documenting or viewing a patient's chart by listing each problem or condition with the correlating symptoms, observations, and treatments related to that assessment.

Proctosigmoidoscopy *See* Sigmoidoscopy.

Prompt (button) Prompt stands for "prompt with current finding." Prompt is a software feature that generates a list of findings that are clinically related to the finding currently highlighted when the prompt button is clicked.

Protocol Standard plans of therapy used to treat a disease or condition.

PSA An acronym for Prostate-Specific Antigen, a test used to detect possible cancer of the prostate gland in men.

Psittacosis An infection acquired from raising birds.

Pulmonary Embolism Obstruction of the pulmonary artery or one of its branches by an abnormal particle such as a blood clot.

Purulent Discharge Pus or puslike discharge.

PVC An acronym for Pneumococcal Conjugate (vaccine).

Px An acronym for Physical Exam (same as PE). Also the Physical Exam tab in the software.

Radiologists Specialists who interpret x-Rays, CAT scans, and other diagnostic tests.

RAM An acronym for Random Access Memory, a measure of the quantity of computer memory.

Read Codes A nomenclature developed by Dr. James Read, later renamed Clinical Terms and merged into SNOMED CT.

RELMA A free software program provided by Regenstrief Institute to assist with LOINC coding. *See also* LOINC.

Remote Access The ability to access the EHR from outside the medical facility network by using a direct-dial connection or a secure connection through the Internet.

Resectable Surgically removable.

Result (entry detail) The Result field (in entry details) is used to enter a result qualifier associated with the current finding. Examples include normal, abnormal, high, or low.

Review of Systems An inventory of body systems starting from the head down, often referred to as ROS. The body systems in a standard ROS are Constitutional symptoms, HEENT (Head, Eyes, Ears, Nose, Mouth, Throat), Cardiovascular, Respiratory, Gastrointestinal, Genitourinary, Musculoskeletal, Integumentary (skin and/or breast), Neurological, Psychiatric, Endocrine, Hematologic/Lymphatic, and Allergic/Immunologic.

Rhinitis Inflammation of the mucus membrane of the nose.

Rhonchi Rattling or snoring sounds heard in the chest when there is a partial bronchial obstruction.

Risk Analysis (HIPAA) Identify potential security risks, and determine the probability of occurrence and magnitude of risks.

Risk Management (HIPAA) Making decisions about how to address security risks and vulnerabilities.

ROS An acronym for Review of Systems. *See* Review of Systems.

ROS (button) A button that toggles On and Off with each click of the mouse. When On, the button appears depressed and history findings are recorded in the Review of Systems section; when Off, history findings are recorded in the History of Present Illness section.

Rx An abbreviation for Therapy (including prescriptions). Also the therapy tab in the software.

Rx (button) Invokes the prescription writer. The button is enabled only if the highlighted finding is a medication.

Rx Norm A nonproprietary vocabulary being developed by the NLM to codify drugs at the level of granularity needed in clinical practice.

Sanction Policy (HIPAA) An office policy to deter noncompliance so that workforce members understand the consequences of failing to comply with security policies and procedures.

Scanned Data (chart) Exam Notes, Letters, Reports, and other documents that have been converted to an image by use of a scanner, then stored in the EHR. The data is accessible by a person viewing the chart, but the image contents cannot be used as data by the system for trend analysis, health maintenance, or similar purposes.

Scroll bar (software) A scroll bar is a feature of most Windows software that automatically appears on the right of a list or text that is too long to fit in the window. The scroll bar has a button that can be moved by pressing the mouse button when dragging the mouse. The information in the window (or window pane) scrolls respective to the movement of the mouse.

Search (button) A word search used to quickly locate all findings in the nomenclature containing either matching words or synonyms of the search word.

Secure Messaging A recommended alternative to sending PHI in e-mail messages; secure messaging uses a secure Web page to read and write messages. The only message sent as e-mail is an alert to the receiving party that the actual message is waiting on the secure site. The contents of secure messages are stored in a secure server not in an e-mail system.

Security Official (HIPAA) One individual designated by the medical practice as having overall responsibility for the HIPAA Security Rule; however, specific security responsibilities may be assigned to other individuals.

Security Reminders (HIPAA) One of the implementation requirements in the HIPAA Security Rule, includes notices, agenda items, and specific discussion topics at monthly meetings, as well as formal retraining about office security policies and procedures.

Security Rule (HIPAA) HIPAA security standards requiring implementation of appropriate security safeguards to protect health information stored in electronic form.

Sig Instructions for labeling a prescription (from Latin *signa*).

Sigmoidoscopy Examination of the rectum, colon, and sigmoid flexure using an illuminated, tubular instrument.

Sinusitis Inflammation of the sinus of the skull.

SNOMED An acronym for Systemized Nomenclature of Medicine had its origins in1965 as Systemized Nomenclature of Pathology.

SNOMED CT A medical nomenclature developed by the College of American Pathologists and United Kingdom's National Health Service. It is a merger of two previous coding systems, SNOMED and the Read codes, and has been recommended to become the core terminology for codified EHR in the United States.

SNOMED RT RT stands for a Reference Terminology, developed in conjunction with Kaiser Permanente to make SNOMED more useable in medical clinics.

SOAP A defined structure for documenting a patient encounter by organizing the information into four sections. The acronym SOAP represents the first letter of each of the section titles: subjective, objective, assessment, and plan.

Social History (tab) A feature on the Patient Management tab that provides a list of the patient's social and behavioral history items recorded in the EHR during all previous encounters.

Speech Recognition (software) Software that recognizes the patterns in human speech as words and turns them into computer text. (See How Speech Recognition Software Works in Chapter 9 for a detailed explanation.)

Spirometer An instrument that measures how much and how quickly air can enter and leave the lungs. Measurements may include VC (Vital Capacity). FVC (Forced Vital Capacity), PEFR (Peak Expiratory Flow Rate), MVV (Maximal Voluntary Ventilation), and FEV (Forced Expired Volume).

Spirometry An objective measurement useful in the diagnosis and management of asthma and other lung conditions. (*See* Spirometer.)

SSL An acronym for Secure Socket Layer that transparently encrypts and decrypts Web pages over the Internet.

Status (entry detail) The Status field (in entry details) is used to add the status of the currently selected finding. Examples include worsening, improving, resolved, and similar designations.

Stress Test An electrocardiogram performed before, during, and after strenuous exercise, to measure heart function.

Subjective (chart) The patient describes in their own words what the problem is, what the symptoms are, and what they are experiencing.

Sx An abbreviation for Symptoms—subjective evidence of disease or physical disturbance. Also the symptom tab in the software.

Tablet PC A self-contained battery-operated computer similar to a laptop computer but utilizing a special stylus and screen to replace the mouse, thus allowing the computer to be used as though the user was writing on a tablet.

Td An abbreviation for Tetanus and Diphtheria toxoids vaccine.

Technical Safeguards (HIPAA) Primarily automated processes used to protect EPHI data and control access to data. They include using authentication controls to verify that the person signing onto a computer is authorized to access that EPHI, or encrypting and decrypting data as it is being stored or transmitted.

Text Data (chart) Information stored in the EHR as word processing, blocks of text, or text reports. The data is searchable but neither codified nor standardized and is generally not indexed.

Toolbar A "Toolbar" is row of icon buttons, the purpose of which is to allow quick access to commonly used functions. The Student Edition software has dynamic toolbars that change the selection of icons depending on the tab the user has selected, as well as special toolbars for functions such as annotated drawings and printing graphs.

Total Cholesterol A blood test that measures the total of all cholesterol in the blood, including both HDL (high-density lipoprotein) and LDL (low-density lipoprotein).

Transactions and Code Sets (HIPAA) HIPAA regulations requiring all covered entities to use standard EDI transaction formats and standard codes within those transactions for claims, remittance advice and payments, claim status, eligibility, referrals, enrollment, premium payments, claim attachments, report of injury, and retail drug claims.

Tree (software) A standard Windows software method of displaying hierarchical lists using small plus and minus symbols to indicate where additional hierarchical levels are hidden from view. The tree structure is used in the Student Edition nomenclature pane. Clicking the mouse on the plus sign next to a finding will "expand the tree" to display additional related findings in an indented list. Clicking on the minus sign next to a finding will "collapse the tree," hiding all findings in the indented list below the selected finding. The purpose of the tree structure is to allow the user to quickly navigate extremely long lists by viewing only the level of hierarchy necessary.

Trend Analysis Comparing data from different dates, tests, or events to correlate the changes in the results with changes in the patient's health.

Triage The screening of patients for allocation of treatment based on the urgency of their need for care. ER triage is often a simplified, organ-specific review of systems conducted by the triage nurse, based on the presenting complaint.

Tx An abbreviation for Tests (performed). Also a tab in the software.

U.S. Preventive Services Task Force An independent panel of experts in primary care and prevention sponsored by AHRQ that systematically reviews the evidence of effectiveness and develops recommendations for clinical preventive services based on the patient's age, sex, and risk factors for disease. These recommendations are published by the AHRQ and also are incorporated in EHR systems from several vendors.

UMDNS An acronym for Universal Medical Device Nomenclature System is used to identify the medical devices for ordering, inventory, or regulatory purposes but does not provide for the codification of data from the devices.

UMLS An acronym for Unified Medical Language System from the National Library of Medicine. UMLS is not itself a medical terminology but, rather, a resource of software tools and data created from many medical nomenclatures to facilitate the development of EHR.

Uniform Identifiers (HIPAA) HIPAA regulations require all covered entities to adopt and use standard identification numbers for plans, providers, and employers in all HIPAA EDI transactions.

Unit (entry detail) The Unit field (in entry details) shows the currently selected unit for the currently selected finding, provided a standard unit exists. If more than one unit is available for selection, the selection will be shown in blue; otherwise, the selection will be shown in black.

URI An acronym for Upper Respiratory Infection. An infection affecting the nose, nasal passages, or upper part of the pharynx.

VA A common abbreviation for U.S. Department of Veteran Affairs.

Vaccine (tab) A feature on the Patient Management tab that provides a list of the patient's immunizations that have been administered at the clinic.

Value (entry detail) The Value field (in entry details) is used to enter a numerical value for those findings that have a numeric value. (For example: BP, weight, test results, and similar designations.) A window with keypad for entering numeric values can be invoked by double-clicking the mouse in the Value field.

Varicella Chicken pox (vaccine).

Vasoconstrictor An agent or drug that initiates or induces narrowing of the lumen (cavity) of blood vessels.

VC An acronym for Vital Capacity, a measure of the amount of air that can be forcibly exhaled after a full inhalation. An indicator of the breathing capacity of the lungs.

Vital Signs Functional measurements recorded at nearly every visit, temperature, respiration rate, pulse rate, and blood pressure; most clinics measure height and weight as well.

Vital Statistics Statistics of birth, death, disease, and health of a population.

VPN An acronym for virtual private network. Data sent over a public network is encrypted and decrypted without user intervention to attain a level of security similar to a private network.

Wellness Conditions Findings that are not disease-related but, rather, used in health maintenance and preventative screening programs to keep healthy patients healthy. Wellness conditions are based on the age, sex, and history of the patient. Examples of preventative recommendations based on wellness conditions include a mammogram for a healthy woman over 35; immunization vaccines at certain ages in children; and a colonoscopy for a healthy person with a family history of colorectal cancer.

WEP An acronym for Wired Equivalent Privacy, a protocol for securing the content of signals sent over a wireless network.

WHO An acronym for World Health Organization.

Wi-Fi An abbreviation for Wireless Fidelity, a type of fast wireless computer networking. *See also* Wireless Network.

Wireless Network A local area computer network using radio signals in place of wired network cables. (See a detailed explanation in Chapter 9.)

WNL (chart) An acronym for Within Normal Limits in medical charts.

Workstation A personal computer, usually connected to a main computer (server) via a network.

X-Ray Traditionally an image made by the passage of short wave radiation through the body onto photographic film. Digital receptors are now able to replace film, allowing the image to be captured and stored in a computer form without photo processing.

Index

consent form, 375
EHR, 176, 184
FS, 322
hypertension, 319, 455
intake, 176
laboratory requisition, 24
multipage, 174
pediatric, 341
short intake, 178
vitals, 226
Forms manager, 110, 120, 161, 243
window, 110, 137, 178
Formulary compliance checking, 32
Free text
adding, 98
additional, 348
field, 99, 119
FS flow off button, 327
FS flow on button, 327
FS form, 322
FS form button, 321, 333
Full exam note, 323

G

GE Healthcare, 36
General multi-system examination, 207, 225, 463. *See also* illustration A-1
elements of, 464
Generic allowed fields, 171
Government
agencies, 379
influence on coding standards, 47
Granular code sets, 49
Graphing
lab results, 300
vital signs, 337
Graph numeric findings, 337
Grid button, 271
Group field, 162, 244
Growth chart, 340, 351
Growth rate of babies, 350

H

Handwriting recognition, 416
HCPCS II codes, 64
Head-related symptoms, 83, 95, 117

Health
and safety, 9
information and data, 3
insurance coverage, 372
maintenance, 6, 46
maintenance systems, 46
maintenance screen, 361
plans, 372, 384
surveillance, 4, 14
system, 58
Health and Human Services department (HHS), 380. *See also* HHS
Health care, 9
clearinghouse functions, 393
decisions, 382
industry, 48, 67
providers, 372, 384
system, 48
Health Care Common Procedure Coding System (HCPCS), 64
Health Care Financing Administration (HCFA), 48
Health information
privacy of, 374
Health Information Technology (HIT), 10, 448
Health Insurance Portability and Accountability Act (HIPAA), 5, 372
Health Insurance Portability and Accountability Act (HIPAA) Administrative Simplification Rules, 380
Health Level Seven, 34. *See also* HL7
HEENT (Head, Eyes, Ears, Nose, Mouth, Throat), 163, 179
Height and weight measurements, 351
Hepatitis B vaccine (HepB), 356
HHS. *See also* Health and Human Services
department, 380
guidance documents, 378
Office of Civil Rights, 383
U.S. department of, 10, 48
High-density lipoprotein, 362
Higher-end laptop computers, 415
High-resolution screens, 415